Harry and Sarah Sneider's **OLYMPIC TRAINER**

Harry and Sarah Sneider's **OLYMPIC TRAINER**

Athletic Excellence through Resistive Rebounding

Published by

THE NATIONAL INSTITUTE OF REBOUNDOLOGY & HEALTH, INC.

Edmonds, WA 98020 • USA

Cover Photo by Gerald Trafficanda
Cover Design by Richard Marin
Inside Photos by Scott Smith

Published by The National Institute of Reboundology and Health, Inc.
7416 - 212th S.W., Edmonds, WA 98020 • USA
(206) 776-6403 or (800) 426-1333
Printed in U.S.A.

Library of Congress Catalog Card No.: 81-84311
ISBN 0-938302-25-6

Dedicated . . .

to our wonderful parents who taught us the rules of success, to our friends at Ambassador College, to Jack LaLanne who is a continual inspiration to us all, to you, our friends in health, who desire to be fit.

YOUR MIRACULOUS BODY

By Albert E. Carter, President,
National Institute of Reboundology & Health, Inc.

Careful study of the muscle cells of the human body will reveal that muscle movement, or contraction, is a cellular function. The muscle is a community of cells banded together to perform a work that an individual cell cannot perform by itself, namely, move a part of the skeletal system. The body is made up of more than 620 of these highly organized communities of individual cells which are able to communicate with each other through a sophisticated, intricate system of neurons, or nerve cells, without which the muscle cells are unable to move.

Coordination is the combination of the exact neural message delivered to precisely the right muscle cells at exactly the right moment to perform an extremely complicated neuromuscular activity. For example, the seemingly simple activity of pitching a baseball is a highly complicated movement involving every part of the muscle-skeletal system all the way from the large bones and muscles in the legs through the large and small muscles, bones and joints of the back including the muscles, joints, and bones through the shoulders, arms, wrists, and hands, and finally to the fingertip, which fine tunes the direction of the projection of the baseball.

The baseball pitcher thinks nothing of the internal activity of his miraculous body as he winds up to pitch. His thoughts are on the man on first, the batter, and the message he receives from the catcher. He doesn't have to think of the internal activities of his body because this miraculous machine performs its millions of miracles automatically once they are learned.

The teachers for the talents that have been developed by the world's greatest athletes are the very same instructors for our newborn infants who are just beginning to learn the art of grasping mother's little finger. They are the very same teachers who taught our space scientists how to calculate the trajectory of an inbound space capsule bearing the very valuable human cargo of our astronauts. Those teachers are none other than the ever present, never changing downward pull of gravity, and the two forces of movement — acceleration and deceleration. Every movement of man or beast is a combination of one or more of these three interacting forces. Our athletes are those who have been able to learn from these three masters.

Rebound exercise uniquely combines these three potent forces. Only with rebound exercise are the forces of gravity, acceleration, and deceleration established in the vertical plane or direction. The phenomenal neuromuscular stimulation of this unique experience can be found nowhere else in this world. Although it is unique, it has never been investigated by the serious athlete except for gymnasts and divers until now. The neural muscular stimulation of rebound exercise is close to phenomenal.

Harry Sneider has combined the universally accepted age old exercise concept of resistance with the revolutionary new cellular exercise concept of rebounding that not only assists in building muscle, bulk, and strength, but also teaches the body the necessary neural talents of balance, coordination, rhythm, timing, dexterity, and kinesthetic awareness. Rebound exercise also provides a refreshing aerobic activity void of the joint jarring shock of hitting a hard surface. I feel this imaginative system of exercises will revolutionize the exercise methods of our world class athletes. It is a system that Harry has already proven successful with some of our best athletes, but it can and should be used by everyone from the weakest to the strongest, from the clumsiest to the most fleet of foot.

Do not be fooled by its simplicity. Prove it with yourself for yourself.

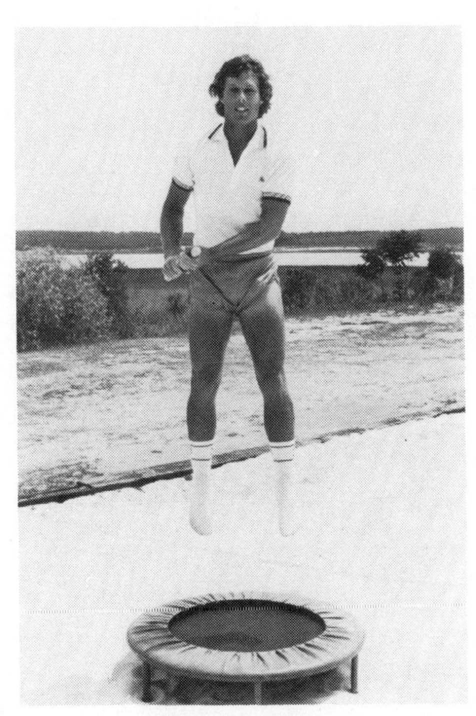

Wayne Grimditch,
water ski champion

Contents

Preface

I've been involved in athletics and fitness all my life and have been a coach and trainer of professional and world class athletes, movie stars, men and women young and not so young for the past twenty years.

Combining many recent athletic training developments to basic fundamentals and my own research, a distinctive training style has evolved which is so effective, it's revolutionary. I believe it could change the entire future trend in professional physical training.

The basic force at work in nearly every exercise form today is **resistance.**

Two years ago, I was introduced to the use of a rebound device for exercise and was struck immediately by numerous benefits previously unavailable in athletic training programs. The simple addition of this exercise medium, commonly called rebounding, to exercise sequences I was using proved its usefulness.

I studied the work done by Albert E. Carter, president of the National Institute of Reboundology and Health, Inc. and sensed an even greater awareness that I was on the verge of a scientific breakthrough in fitness and athletic training.

I now began studying the effect of certain resistive routines I was working with, on and off a rebound unit. The improvement in fitness was astonishing, especially when both resistance and rebounding were involved. We worked with various sequences and measured improvements in all age groups, male and female, from the least to the most developed in skill, in virtually every skill required for every sport.

The systematic application of resistive disciplines applied to the universal regenerative forces in rebounding, produced a breakthrough in what we all strive for in exercise. The alternating weightlessness and increased G-forces combined with a sequence of exercises which extended each muscle group through its full range and produced a balance and harmony resulting in total body fitness and tone. Every single cell, organ and muscle was exercised.

Two physical elements must be present to produce the full effect: (1) a rebound unit; and (2) small calibrated weights suitable for carrying in the hands. We found that relatively light, malleable graduated weights (like sandbags) provided the desired safety in use, the proper stress or resistance and the flexibility to adapt well to all exercise groups as well as to all trainees regardless of skill or state of development.

The procedures and sequences described in this book are proven and produce phenomenal results. You'll see improvement in virtually every sport or physical objective you select.

For additional reading, I recommend *The Miracles of Rebound Exercise,* by Albert E. Carter, president of the National Institute of Reboundology and Health, Inc. The "Institute" is the focal point in the gathering of research verifying and identifying the scientific principles at work in exercise involving rebounding.

Mr. Carter has told me that my work as depicted in this book "represents a major breakthrough in exercise." I believe it does, too. The scientific principles involved begin with Newton and go on from there. Not all of them have been identified yet, but I have proved in case after case that they work on behalf of general health and fitness, better than any other system I've ever tried.

Good reading, and good health!

Harry and Sarah Sneider

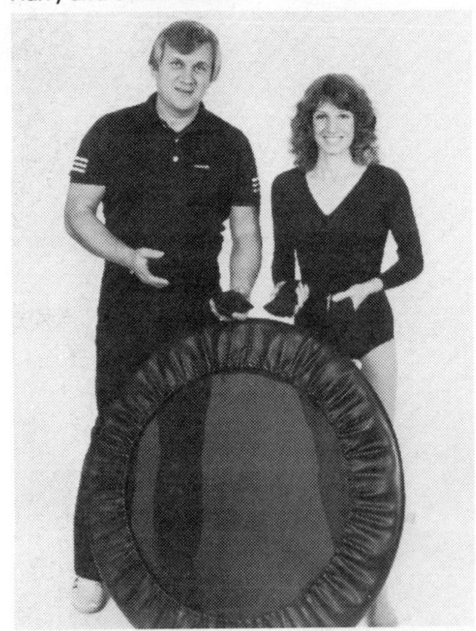

Foreword

The "Harry Sneider Story" is a triumph of spirit over disability. Harry was born in Latvia. His father, a skilled interior decorator, was an athlete, excelling in track; his mother, a person of robust health, never saw the inside of a hospital except to bear children.

Forced to flee Latvia with his family at the age of 2½, due to the chaos of World War II, Harry contracted osteomyelitis as a consequence of poor nutrition and general hardships, losing the ball and socket joint of his right hip after an injury.

Convalescence gave Harry time to nourish dreams of overcoming his handicap. When his family immigrated to the United States and settled in Minnesota, Harry set about rebuilding his crippled body. In school, liking games of all sorts, he learned to throw a football over seventy yards and a baseball 350 feet.

Cheated of a life as a professional athlete, Harry turned to weight training. In a year, he was pressing 225 pounds, weighing only 150. Eventually, he was to "squat" 490 pounds on one leg (using the other for a brace), shattering the world record of 480 pounds (on two legs). World-famous fitness expert, Jack La-Lanne called Harry's lift "one of the most spectacular achievements in all sports."

Sneider began coaching and teaching athletes as a student at the University of Minnesota, his first pupil being his 13-year-old brother, Karl, who later played professional football for the San Diego Chargers and Edmonton Eskimos. Karl once performed a record deadlift of 600 pounds. Sneider's older brother, John, was an Olympic-caliber bike rider, star miler and a powerful weight lifter. Sneider's sister, Ilze, is a student of health and hopes to become a veterinarian. At Minnesota, Sneider studied athletic training in depth, performing research in psychology, philosophy, kinesiology, physical training, coaching, and human relations. His basement became a major community training center which produced a host of high school and college stars. His slogan: "If you don't want to become a champion, don't train here."

Becoming a manager for a health club near Minneapolis, Sneider began developing the training routines that form the foundation of this book. In 1967, his scope of operations enlarged enormously when he became a faculty member and coach at Pasadena's Ambassador College. Today his professional activities include teaching physical fitness to grade school, high school and college students; general fitness training, training of athletes for Olympic Games, television "Superstars" episodes and important amateur and professional competition; preparation of actors and actresses for movie and television roles; and carrying out athletic research with leading medical and health care centers.

Among Sneider's more famous "pupils": Dwight Stones, 10-

time world high jump champion; "Golden Girl" Susan Anton (body building routines); James Butts, Olympic triple jump silver medalist; and Wayne Grimditch, "Superstars" winner. Sneider appears frequently on talk shows and at seminars and clinics. He is advisor and coach to Olympic teams from Canada, Taiwan, Germany and other nations.

Sneider recently has completed research with the National Athletic Health Institute, headed by Dr. Robert Kerlan, head physician for the Los Angeles Rams, Lakers, Dodgers, Kings and other teams. He's also done research in collaboration with Dr. Leroy Perry, Olympic doctor for several nations; and Dr. David Martin, exercise physiologist, Georgia State University, on the subjects of injury prevention, athletic performance and development in the high jump.

From this lifetime of involvement with training techniques and theories has come the raw material for Harry Sneider's development of resistive rebound training which is what this book is all about.

A full-time contributing partner to Sneider's training programs and to this book has been his wife, Sarah. A college graduate who has studied nutrition and human development, Sarah teaches exercise, dance and does fitness testing in the fitness centers.

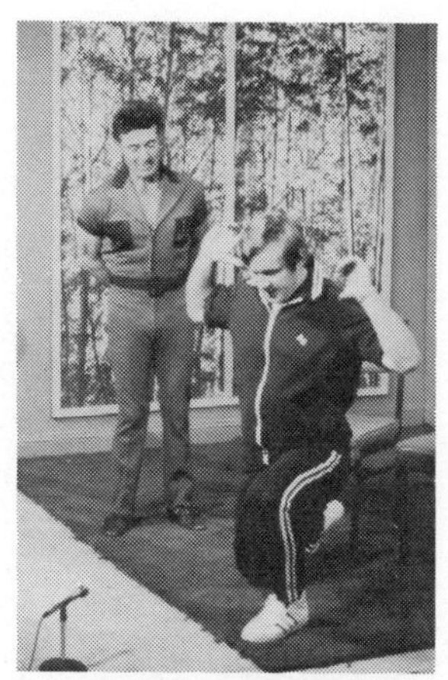

Author demonstrates 490-lb. "squat" lift on national TV as host, Jack LaLanne, watches.

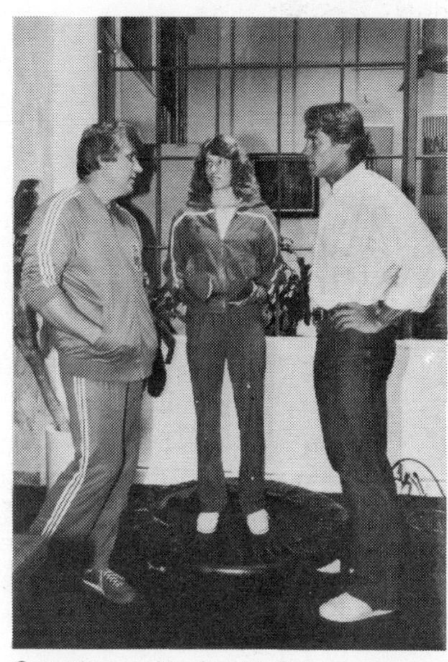

Co-authors with Arnold Schwarzenegger, "Mr. Olympia" and six times "Mr. Universe", body builder and actor.

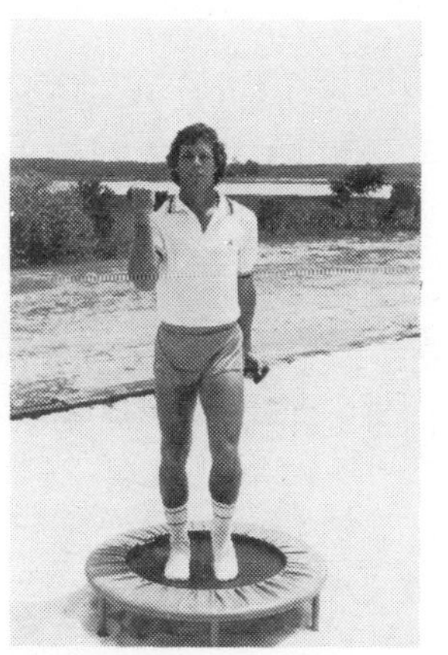

Wayne Grimditch, world's top water skier, "Superstars" competitor and holder of world's water ski distance record.

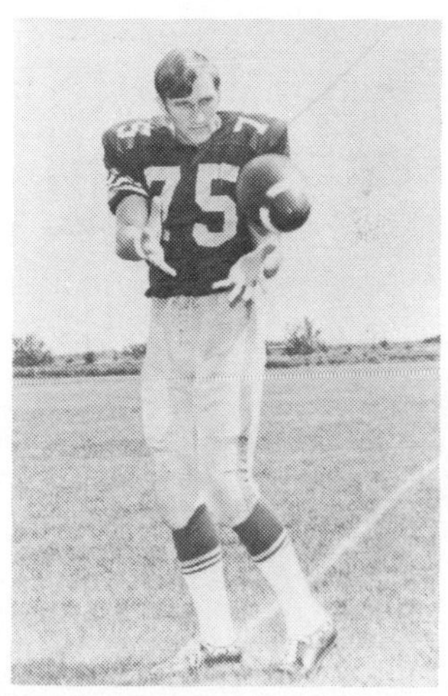

Karl Sneider, trained under Harry, played both college and professional football.

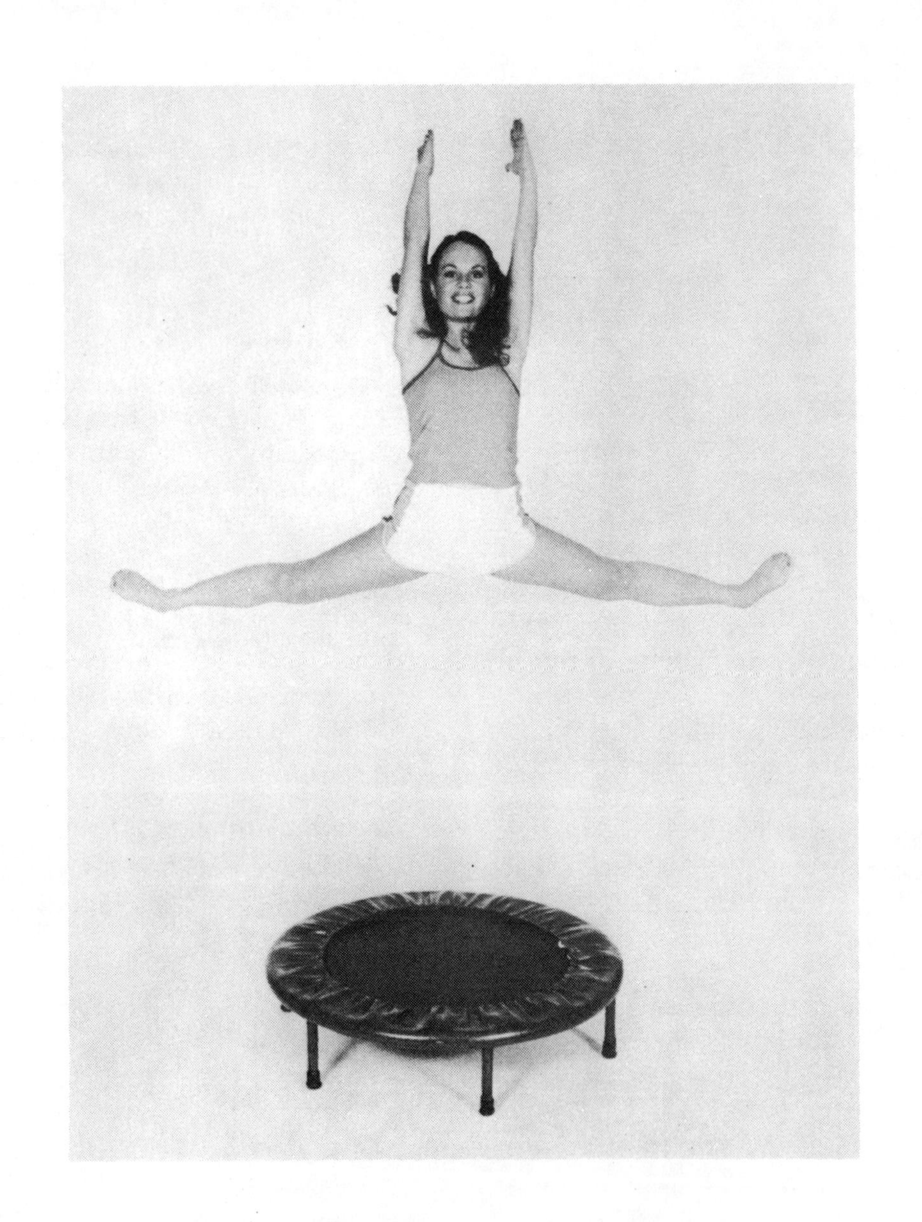

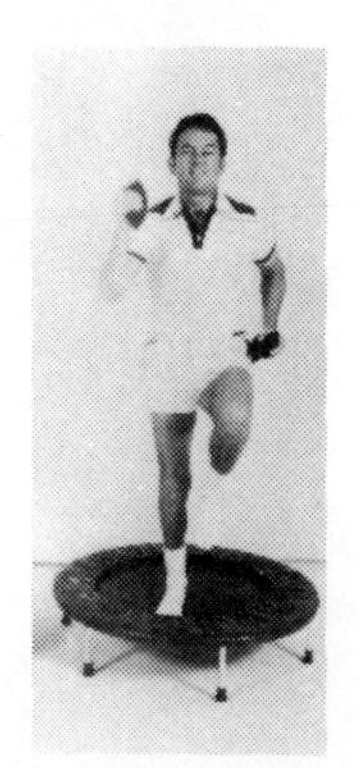

Introduction

Welcome to a world of physical fitness, fun and achievement. You are about to take a giant step toward the realization of your dream of becoming that individual that God created you to be. An individual who is fit, fulfilled, enjoys life to the hilt and who lives up to full potential.

Fitness should not be something that you **have to do.** Fitness should be fun and, at the same time, provide a real benefit to your total health. This book is intended to provide you with both fun and total health.

We are living in the most incredible time in the history of mankind. We have seen man fly to the moon, the heart transplanted, the 3:48.4 mile run in track, and the average American living to 70 years and more. You are witnessing a literal explosion of scientific discovery and enlightenment in all areas of academic inquiry. There has been another explosion of interest in physical exercise. Thanks to science and advances in training techniques and methods, you are living in an age of exercise that will help you live 10, 20 or 30 years longer.

We are just now discovering the fantastic benefits of rebound exercise, which is said by many of its advocates to be the world's most perfect form of exercise. As you read this book and take up your own program of resistive rebounding (rebounding with calibrated weights), you can share in the benefits, which are immediate, many in number and longlasting.

Total fitness includes cardiovascular fitness, correct body alignment, disease prevention, improved strength and stamina and much more. You can achieve this state of all-around fitness if you set aside just a few minutes each day and do these simple exercises. Olympic athletes, executives, housewives, children, senior citizens and people from all walks of life will receive great bonuses of health and well being with these simple daily exercises.

We encourage you to take a little time each day to become a total human being. You can decide what you want — health or disease. The decision is in your hands. Please, may we encourage you to choose health, happiness and the abundant life this program can give you.

Harry and Sarah Sneider
Arcadia, California
March 19, 1981

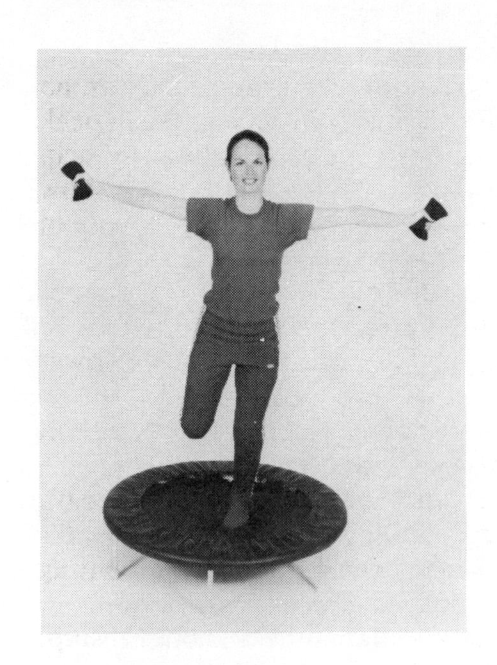

Chapter 1

Resistive Rebounding

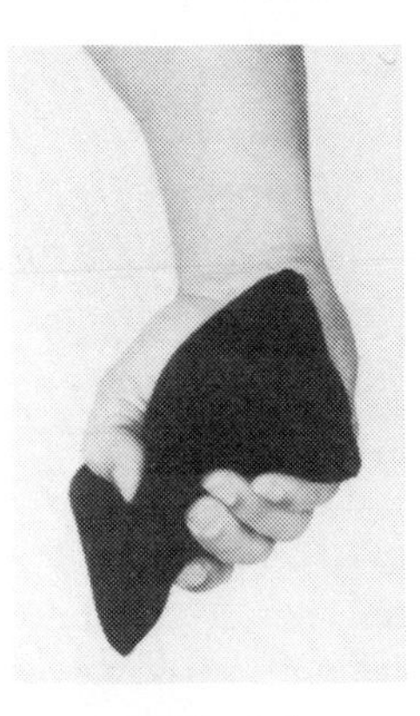

Rebounding and sandbagging — they go together!

The muscular and cardiovascular systems require continuous maintenance in order for you to remain healthy. **Whatever you don't use, you will lose.** The body only improves with use.

Maintaining bodily fitness through use, or exercise, is universally accepted. How to accomplish this most efficiently, quickly and pleasantly is the question. My answer is: rebounding with resistance.

It all begins with your portable rebound unit, this book and the calibrated soft weights or sandbags that come with it.

Each time you jog, bounce or run on your rebound unit, while holding or manipulating the calibrated weights, you are working against gravity. Stated another way: gravity is working for you; gravity and the weights act as **resistance to shape your body** and keep you fit and looking good. Using gravity as an ally with your resistive rebounding program, you possess, for extremely modest cost, the **best home training program in existence today.** You have available infinite exercise variations: standard body-building drills, dance routines, stretching exercise, body-building disciplines and routines for coordination improvement — all of which can be easily performed with light resistance on your rebound unit.

The routines pictured and described in later chapters are very simple, exciting, brand new and, best of all, lots of fun. Compared to the drudgery of heavy weight lifting, the complications of dance routines and the expense of club memberships, this system is, in my opinion, far superior in all respects.

Whether you are an athlete seeking to reach and maintain an Olympic caliber of performance or a citizen wishing to reach peak condition for a robust, active life, resistive rebounding can help you reach your goals in as little as 15 to 20 minutes a day. I know this is possible because I have seen it happen in case after case in my own training programs.

A total fitness program should consist of seven distinct components, all of which can be yours with resistive rebounding:

1. **Flexibility** — Development of fluid movement of the lower neck, hips, knees, ankles, upper back and neck.
2. **Cardiovascular Fitness** — Improvement of circulation, strengthening of the heart and lungs.
3. **Strength** — Development of ability to excel in explosive activities such as sprinting, jumping, lifting.
4. **Lymphatic System** — Cleansing the system, preventing illness.
5. **Coordination** — Improvement of hand/eye relationship, movement, balance, sports techniques.
6. **Body Balance** — Muscular development to support joints to improve posture, body alignment.
7. **Low Cost Fun** — A program you can afford for daily use over a whole lifetime of physical fitness.

Now you've purchased your rebound unit and your resistive rebound kit. Let's have a word about the weights.

The graduated weights come in pairs of .45, .91, and 1.36 kilos each, or 1, 2 and 3 pounds, respectively. One for each hand, naturally, in all three weight classes. They have purposely been made soft and malleable (flexible). Why? Because they are easier on the hands, can be used by any person of any age and because you can do more things with them.

From now on, I'm going to call them "Sanbags," a word I have copyrighted, or "weights" in order to simplify the formal term of "graduated malleable weights."

Sanbags© are excellent for developing the grip in all sports. They increase circulation to the forearm, wrists and hands. They distribute resistance evenly in your hands and they are great for quick movement.

Sanbags© are particularly useful for sculpturing your body in a controllable, individualized way. By squeezing the pliable bags, you can reach those hard-to-develop regions of your body that machines, which work only general areas, cannot. Sanbags© reach these inaccessible muscle groups because with them, movement is unconstrained.

Rapid skill development in all sports is possible with Sanbags©. With them you can emulate sports movements needed for throwing, stroking, gripping, running, or jumping. Sanbags© aid motor learning, hand/eye coordination and are easily adaptable. Thus, they can be used by all, from the wee toddler to the giant football linebacker.

In your Olympic Trainer Kit, you will find six Sanbags© two each in three different weights. Since all Sanbags© weights will be referred to in kilograms (kilos) for the balance of this book, the following table will enable you to convert the metric weight to pounds:

	Kilos, each	Lbs., each
Weight Set One	.45	1.0
Weight Set Two	.91	2.0
Weight Set Three	1.36	3.0

"Big Three" of Fitness

Of the seven components of fitness mentioned earlier, the most important are (1) Cardiovascular Fitness, (2) Flexibility Fitness and (3) Strength Fitness.

The most important element of overall fitness is the cardiovascular system (heart, lungs, arteries). Books have been written on this subject and I don't intend to dwell on it here, except to add my two cents worth to the universal agreement that the health of the cardiovascular system is the key to the health of the whole person.

Rebound exercise is excellent for the cardiovascular system, as well as being a form of exercise that aligns the body and absorbs the shock of gravity, a feature that is of particular importance for overweight, out-of-condition people.

An activity that simply doubles the resting pulse rate is all that is necessary to achieve cardiovascular fitness. How to take your resting and active pulse rates is dealt with in my next chapter. You will see how to achieve this doubling effect in the first chapter on simple resistive rebounding exercises.

A word of caution: Before you start this or any other exercise program, check first with your doctor.

Flexibility is markedly improved with resistive rebounding. It lengthens individual cells, elongates muscles and conditions joints — while easing impact on joints that have been injured or overworked from playing on hard surfaces such as tennis, racquetball or basketball courts or jogging paths. A program for stretching to improve flexibility will be described in a later chapter.

Strength is essential to most daily activities, from lifting the groceries from the trunk of the car to thrusting one's body over a seven-foot high jump bar. A sound program of weight training exercises will strengthen the body. Unfortunately, I've seen far too many programs which concentrate on development of the large muscles to the exclusion of other muscle groups and completely ignoring the other essential components of fitness. You will not be making this mistake if you follow the routines set forth in this book.

Chapter 2

Before You Begin

The Vital, Necessary Preliminaries

There are a few important preliminaries one must attend to before undertaking any regular program of physical conditioning. Most accomplished amateur and professional athletes and quite a few adherents of fitness for fitness' sake **already** are acquainted with them and have done something about them. It may not be necessary for those to read this chapter, although a review of these procedures certainly won't do any harm. I feel that this chapter is a **must** for all others.

Let's take a look at them:

Physical Examination

A physical examination is strongly recommended before beginning any exercise program. Consult your family physician or any qualified sports medical practitioner for an examination to determine your readiness for exercise and advice as to how strenuous a program you can undertake at first.

Taking Your Resting Pulse Rate

Your "resting" pulse rate is an indicator of your cardiovascular fitness. A person in good cardiovascular condition usually has a lower resting pulse (heart) rate than that of a person in poor condition.

The average resting pulse rate for men is 72-80 heart beats per minute, for women, 72-86. You are likely to find that as you become involved in resistive rebounding over a period of weeks, your resting pulse rate will decrease significantly, indicating that your heart has become stronger.

You can take your own resting pulse rate. Just follow the simple procedure indicated in the pictures below:

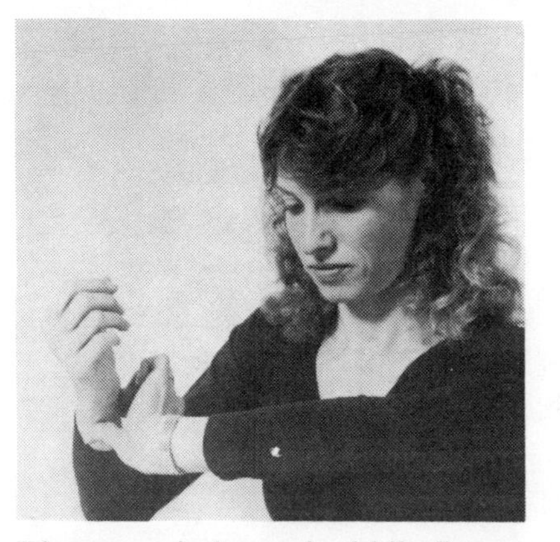

Place your index and middle fingers on the thumb side of your inner wrist, or . . .

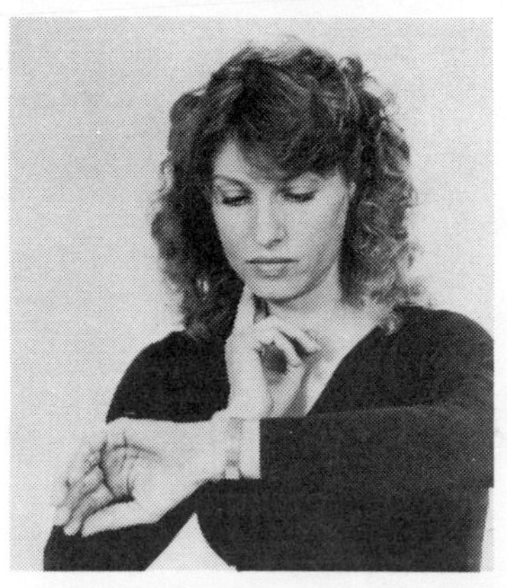

Place your fingers gently at the carotid artery located on either side of the neck.

The ideal time to take your resting pulse rate is before you get out of bed in the morning. Count your pulse with a sweeping second hand for 30 seconds and multiply by two to get your **resting** pulse rate. Once again, if there is any question about this procedure, check with your family physician.

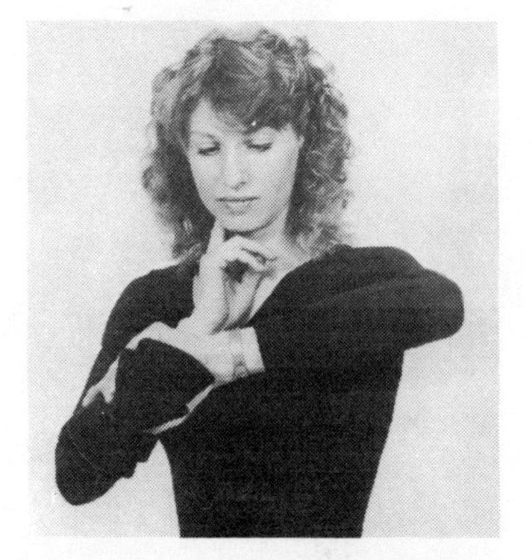

Monitoring Your Working Heart Rate

To achieve cardiovascular fitness, it is necessary to increase the resting pulse rate. Doubling the rate will produce excellent cardiovascular fitness. For example: If your resting pulse rate is 70 beats per minute, multiply by two (70 × 2 = 140). For the beginner, then, 140 beats per minute becomes his or her "working heart rate."

The following chart obtained from the National Institute of Reboundology and Health, Inc. indicates recommended heart rates during exercise (working heart rate):

Target Zones and Maximal Attainable Heart Rates*

Age in Years	Target Zone Beats/Minute	Maximal Attainable Beat/Minute
25	140 to 170	200
30	136 to 165	194
35	132 to 160	188
40	128 to 155	182
45	124 to 150	176
50	119 to 145	171
55	115 to 140	165
60	111 to 135	159
65	107 to 130	153

*From Lenore R. Gzohman, *Beyond Diet . . . Exercise Your Way to Fitness and Heart Health* (Englewood Cliffs, NJ: CPC International, Inc., 1974), p. 15.

— Chart from *Rebounding Aerobics*
by Morton Walker, D.P.M. and Frank Angelo

Start out gradually jogging on your rebound unit with the Sanbags© (begin with the .45 kilo Sanbags©, one in each hand) and monitor your heart rate by stopping after a minute or two and taking your pulse. Using a watch with a sweep second hand, count the heart beats for six seconds. Multiply by ten to get the beats per minute. You now have your working pulse rate.

A good time to take your six-second reading is as you change phonograph records or wait for a new song on the radio.

Monitoring your working heart is extremely important to make sure it doesn't get too high for you (see chart above).

Recovery Heart Rate

The "recovery heart rate" is measured in terms of the time it takes for the working heart to return to its resting rate after cessation of activity. This measurement is taken five to seven minutes after stopping exercise, as follows:

Stop exercise. Find your pulse and count it for six seconds while standing in place. Multiply by ten to get your rate per minute.

If the count is more than 120 beats per minute after five to seven minutes, you are overextending yourself. It's a sign you should cut back on your exercise program a little. After 10 to 12 minutes, take your pulse again. If your pulse rate now is below 100, you are exercising at the proper level.

Resistive rebounding usually improves your recovery heart rate. After several weeks, you should find your heart returning to normal faster than when you began the program.

Exercise to Music

I suggest you exercise to music, preferably to music with a definite beat to keep you moving at a smooth, fairly fast pace. Music makes exercise more fun, too. As you learn the exercises, you can vary them to the flow of the music.

Resistive rebounding, however, is so versatile you can get the benefits of it with or without music. On occasion, you may prefer to exercise while watching a favorite television show, listening to a stimulating radio talk show or while conversing with friends.

What To Wear

Your clothing should be comfortable and allow you to move without restriction. Women should wear a supportive bra while bouncing.

Your Ideal Weight

Before embarking on your resistive rebounding program, it's a good idea to weigh yourself. Then compare this figure with the chart below which gives the ideal weight for a given height and age.

Ideal Weight Chart

WEIGHT	HEIGHT		WEIGHT
Women	Feet	Inches	Men
85-100	5	0	95-110
90-105	5	1	100-115
95-110	5	2	105-121
100-115	5	3	110-126
105-120	5	4	115-132
110-125	5	5	120-137
115-130	5	6	125-143
120-135	5	7	130-148
125-140	5	8	135-154
130-145	5	9	140-159
135-150	5	10	145-165
140-155	5	11	150-170
145-160	6	0	155-176
150-165	6	1	160-181
155-170	6	2	165-187

— Chart Courtesy of The National Institute of Reboundology and Health, Inc.

It is suggested that those who are overweight at first (by 10 to 100 pounds), who are out of condition or who have difficulty maintaining balance on the rebound unit stay with the BIG FOUR series of exercises (see next chapter) for a week or two to help gain balance and confidence before attempting the complete DAILY DOZEN program that follows it.

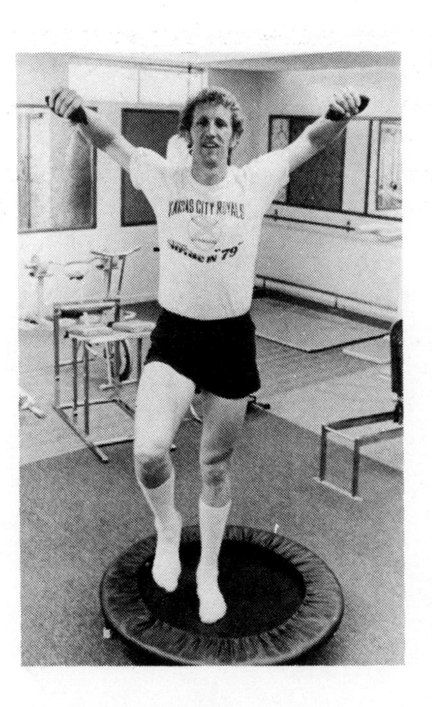

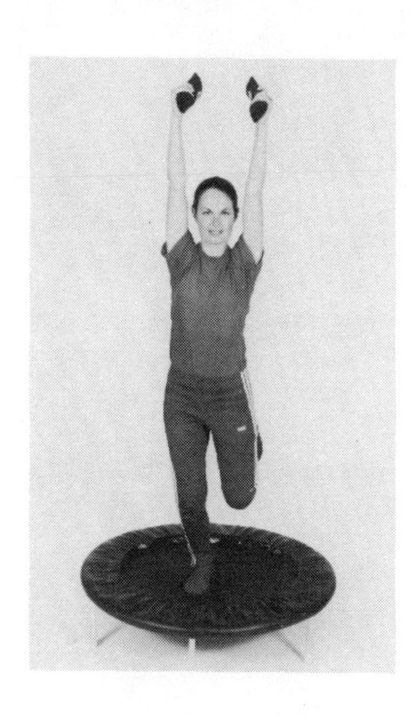

PART ONE

The complete conditioning program for all men, women and children.

ATHLETES: For championship conditioning in your sport, see PART TWO (Page 65)

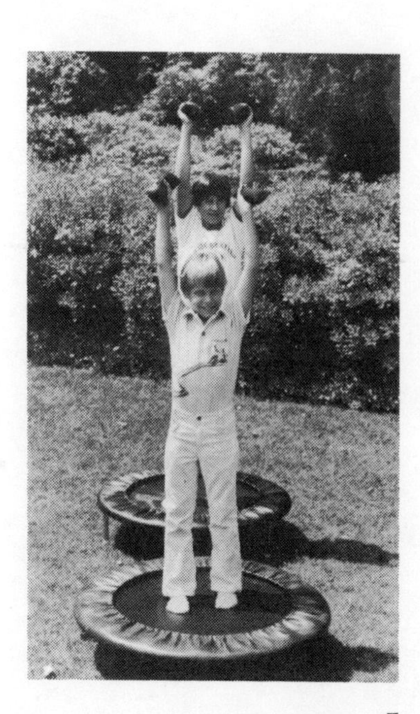

Chapter 3

The 'Big 4'

From beginning to warmup

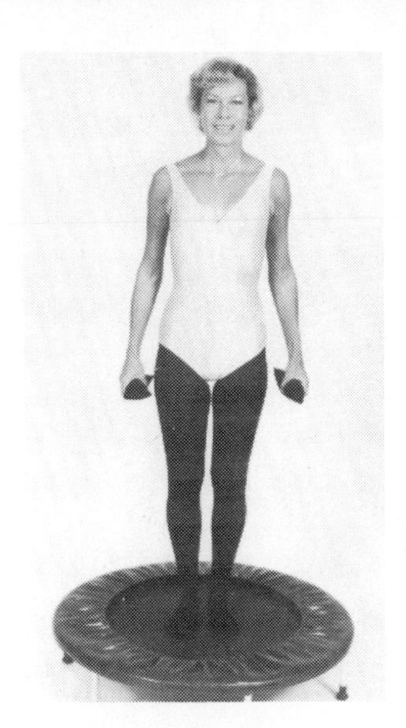

The "Big 4" sequence of resistive exercises represents a complete program for male and female beginners, those who are out of condition or those who are overweight.

As your body condition improves with this program, you should increase the length of time devoted to each one, according to my recommendations. When you feel comfortable with these exercises at the advanced level of time recommended then the "Big 4" becomes your basic warm-up for all other exercise routines that follow.

CAUTION: A physical examination is recommended before beginning any exercise program.

The rate at which you exercise is determined by your physical condition. To help you determine your exercise rate for the "Big 4" and all exercise routines that follow, I have selected three categories. Pick the category that most nearly reflects your present condition.

BEGINNER: Individuals who are overweight by 10 to 100 pounds, out of condition, or who have used a rebound unit one month or less.

INTERMEDIATE: Those who have used a rebound unit for at least one month and whose resting heart rate is 60-80 beats per minute.

ADVANCED: Individuals who have jogged at least one mile per day, whose resting pulse is 40-65 beats per minute, or who have used their rebound unit for three months or more.

Now that you have determined what category you belong in, here are the "Big 4." Be sure and refer to the pictures which illustrate exactly how they are performed:

1. LYMPHATIC BOUNCE **(page 10)**
2. SHUFFLE **(page 10)**
3. JOG **(page 11)**
4. BOUNCE **(page 11)**

Instructions on how to perform each exercise, plus the recommended duration for beginners, intermediates or advanced participants are printed below each picture.

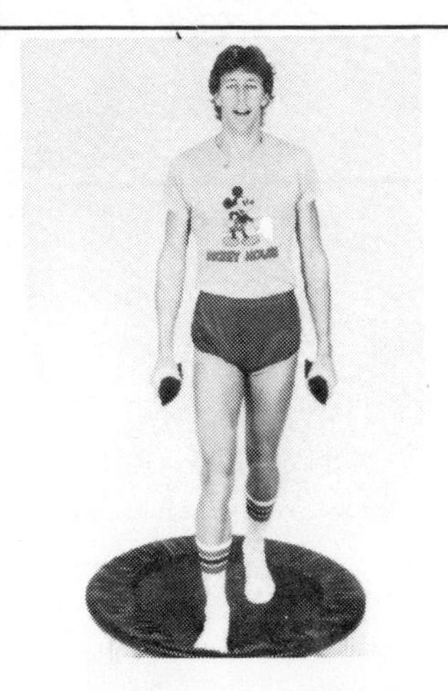

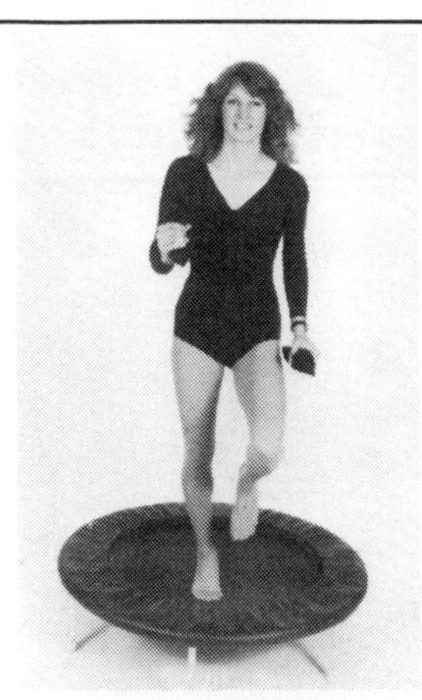

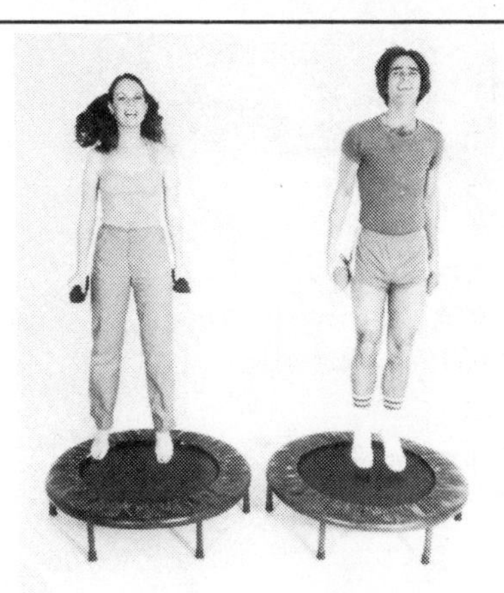

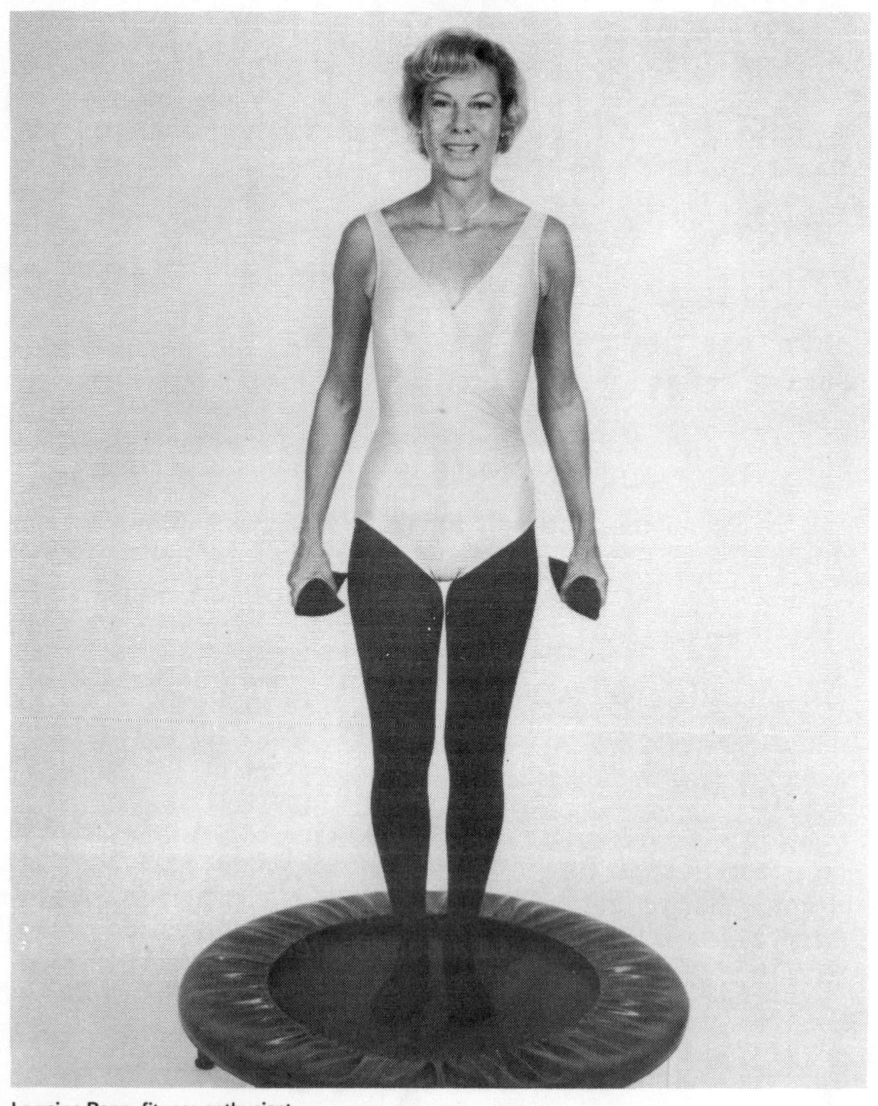

Lorraine Rapp, fitness enthusiast.

1. LYMPHATIC BOUNCE

Bounce in the middle of the mat without feet leaving the mat. Hands are at sides holding .45 kilo weights. Maintain erect posture.

Beginner: Start 10 seconds a day, add 5 seconds every three days.
Intermediate: 30 seconds a day, add 5 seconds every three days.
Advanced: 45 seconds to 1 minute a day, add 5 seconds every three days.

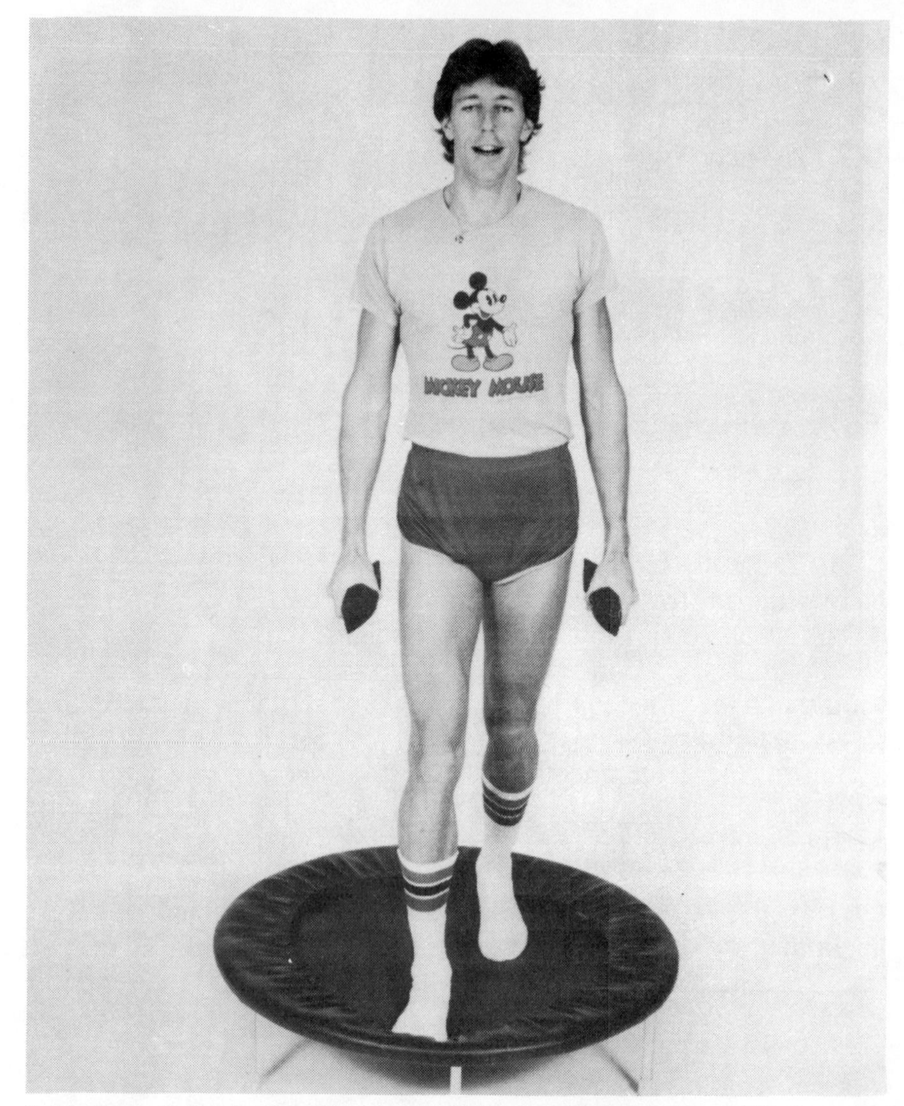

Dwight Stones, holder of ten world high jump records, present American record (7'7 ¼"), two-time Olympic bronze medal winner.

2. SHUFFLE

Move feet across mat with a rhythmic shuffle while bouncing, holding .45 kilo weights in hands.

Program: Same as Lymphatic Bounce.

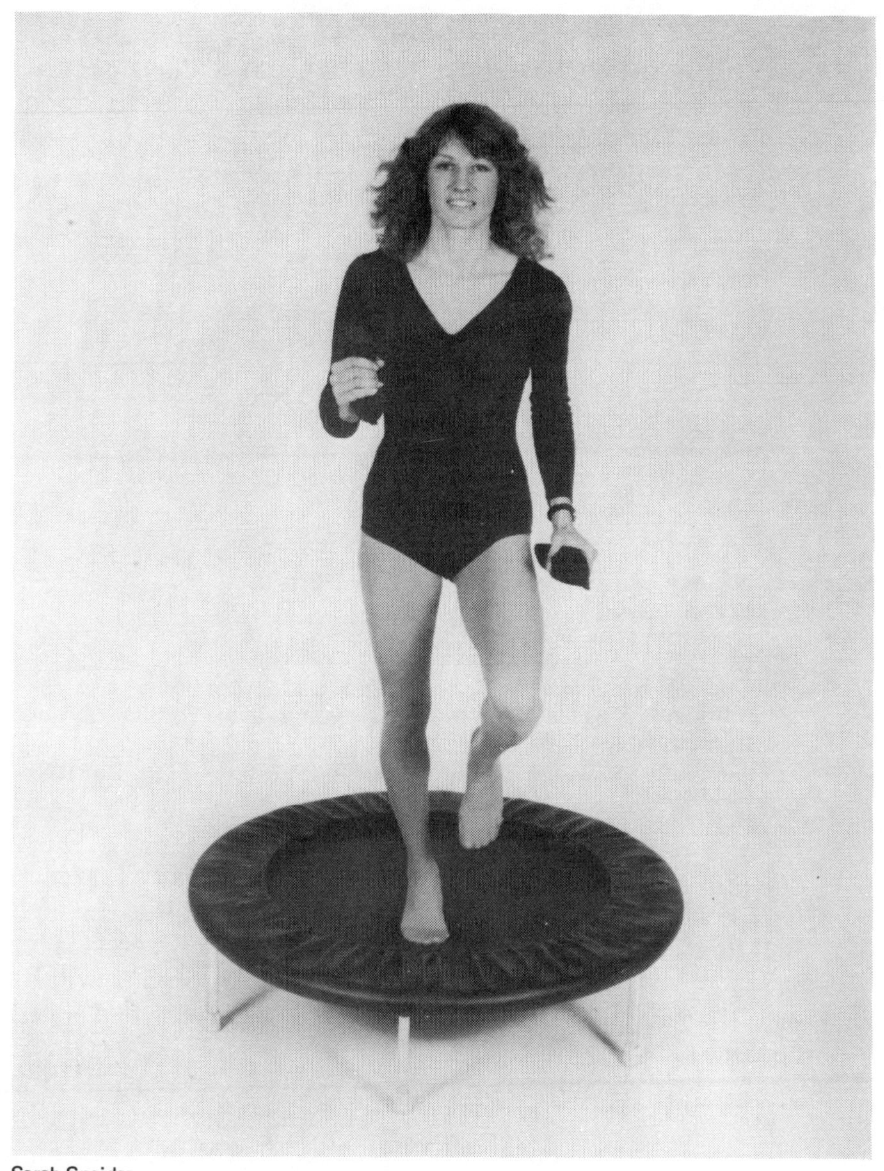

Sarah Sneider

3. JOG

Hold .45 kilo weights in hands. Knees are higher than a walk. Swing arms, keeping elbows high. An easy, rhythmic jog.

Program: Same as Lymphatic Bounce.

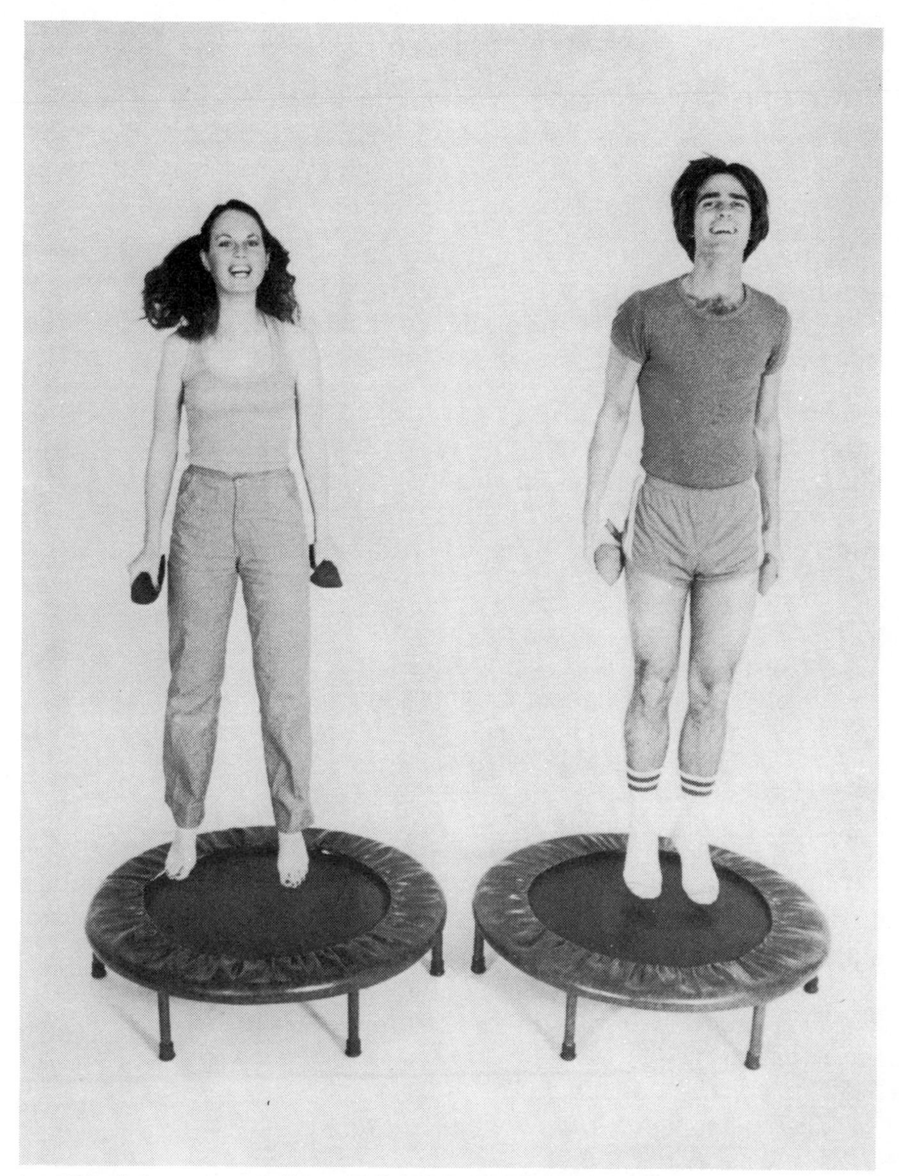

Lynn Grimditch, actress and athlete, with T.J. McCavitt, also actor and athlete.

4. BOUNCE

Holding .45 kilo weights in hands, bounce 2-6 inches off mat.

Program: Same as Lymphatic Bounce.

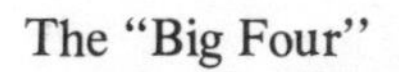

'Big 4' a MUST for everyone!

The "Big 4" will help you maintain a better level of health. This program is a must for all who have a rebound unit. You may use this as an exercise program and achieve excellent results as you reach 15-20 minutes a day.

Remember, beginners should start easy with the recommended progression. You will really improve if you are consistent. Try the "Big 4" every day first thing in the morning. You will love the rest of your day!

The "Big 4" is for any age group. With your weights in hand, your progress will accelerate. Add more resistance every month. Start with the small .45 kilo weights. After 30 days, switch to the .91 kilo weights. In three months' time, you will be up to 15-20 minutes each day in the "Big 4" with 1.36 kilo weights.

Caution: Those who are overweight by 10 to 100 pounds, please stay with the lighter weights until the overweight problem has been corrected. The surplus body poundage coupled with heavier weights could be hard on the joints. TRAIN, DON'T STRAIN.

I have personally used this system with hundreds of my pupils in the health club and Athletic Fitness Center and have received many glowing comments:

"This is easier on my joints than jogging, and I have not lost my wind!"
"I'm not tired as much."
"This is more fun than weight training."
"My clothes are looser."
"I don't have to see my chiropractor as often."
"I haven't missed work due to a cold for months."
"It's so much fun."

The "Big 4" with your graduated weights truly will help you, too.

IMPORTANT NOTE

In order for you really to benefit from all subsequent resistive rebounding routines, it will be important for you to do all exercises **in order,** unless otherwise prescribed. To facilitate this for you, each section of new exercises will contain a table which will look like this:

Exercise	Wt.	Reps.			Sets	Goals
		B	I	A		
1.						
2.						
3.						
4.						
5. etc.						

Explanation of Terms

Exercise: Name of exercise, such as "Curl and Press."
Wt.: Weights used, by kilogram (.45, .91, 1.36 kilo)
Reps: Repetitions, meaning the number of times you perform a particular exercise.
Set: One completion of all designated exercises in any particular routine. To add another set, start with 1. and continue through final exercise.
Goals: The number of sets you have set out to achieve at your selected fitness level.
B-I-A: Beginner, Intermediate, and Advanced, respectively.

For instance, in the following chapter on the "Daily Dozen," you will start from Exercise No. 1 "Curl" and continue through the remaining 11 in numerical order until you reach Exercise No. 12 "Jog Easy." That will constitute Set No. 1. Set No. 2 will be identical. Repeat until you reach your goal as prescribed in **all training routines.**

Resist the temptation to do all your sets of curls, all your sprints and other like exercises in a row. Such an approach will make the program harder and will not be as profitable to you. There are good physiological and psychological reasons for these exercises being in the order they are in, variety being the spice of life, as well as the core of conditioning. You should start from top to bottom, then keep adding repetitions and sets as prescribed in all programs, whether they are for physical conditioning, dance proficiency or athletic achievement.

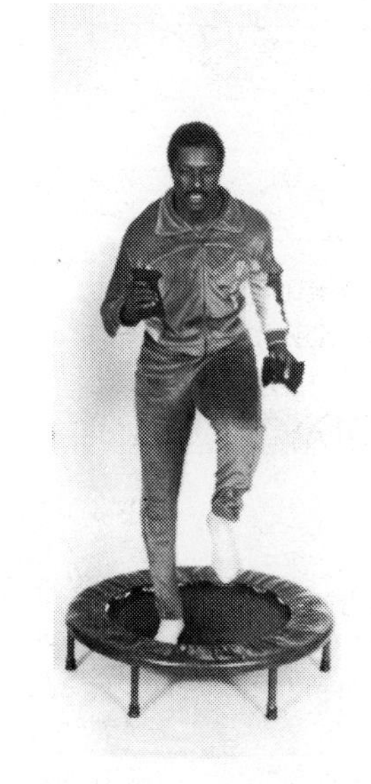

THE DAILY DOZEN CHART

(A Program For All Ages)

Suggested Warm-Up: The "BIG FOUR"

Exercise	Muscles Worked	Reps.			Sets	Goals
		B*	I	A		
1. Curl	Bicep, fore-arms, hands	10	12	15	1	3 sets of 25
2. Press	Shoulders, upper back	10	12	15	1	3 sets of 25
3. Upright Row	Chest, shoulders, arms	10	12	15	1	3 sets of 25
4. Tricep Press	Back of arms, chest	10	12	15	1	3 sets of 25
5. Squeeze	Grip of hand, forearms	10	12	15	1	3 sets of 25
6. Curl & Press	Arms, shoulders, upper back	10	12	15	1	3 sets of 25
7. Side Raise	Shoulders, chest, forearm	10	12	15	1	3 sets of 25
8. Crossovers	Chest, upper back	10	12	15	1	3 sets of 25
9. Sprint High Knee	Legs, entire body, arms	15	20	30 sec.	1	3 sets of 2 min.
10. Press Up & Out	Upper back, arms, chest	10	12	15	1	3 sets of 15
11. Pullover	Chest, arms, stomach	10	12	15	1	3 sets of 25
12. Jog Easy	Legs, entire body, arms	30	45	1 min.	1	3 sets of 4 min.

*B — Beginner, I — Intermediate, A — Advanced

These exercises are done either to bouncing, jogging, or shuffling on your rebound unit.

Chapter 4

The 'Daily Dozen'

Key to excellent fitness and the body and skills you want

A rebound unit and your weights is all you need for a super body building and fitness program. After warming up with the "Big Four," follow the "Daily Dozen Chart" (left), doing the exercises in the order they are given while bouncing, jogging, or shuffling on your rebound unit.

Some of these exercises will require some flexibility in the upper back and arms (such as the pullover and tricep press) and may take time before your body reaches this desired flexibility. Be patient.

All exercises are illustrated on subsequent pages in this chapter.

The Importance of Sequence

The "Daily Dozen" exercises were designed for both men and women to work the muscular system symmetrically, developing body balance, body alignment and fitness improvement. Therefore, it is strongly suggested that they be done in order for maximum benefit.

However, if the participant desires to work one group of muscles more than another, then it is acceptable to do in a row those exercises that will work the same muscle group (curl, curl and press, press, tricep press). This variation will be harder than doing the "Daily Dozen" in order and makes the program similar to those of circuit weight machines, barbells or dumbbells invoking the "Overload Principle."

Resistance Speeds Conditioning

Since you will be using weights as resistance, it will take less time to feel your body being worked. Remember, you are now working your muscular and cardiovascular systems at the same time. This means additional stress over all, so it won't take you as long to reach your pulse rate level for your age as jogging or bouncing without resistance would.

As mentioned earlier, it is recommended that the "Daily Dozen" be done in the order they are listed for greater benefit, but you can mix them for variety. Just remember to warm-up and warm-down with an easy jog or easy curl and jog. You can bounce, jog, or shuffle while doing the "Daily Dozen." Variety can be the greatest asset to your program.

The exercises in the "Daily Dozen" can also be done slowly or quickly. The slower rate will work the muscular system more. Quicken the pace and the cardiovascular system will be trained. Either way you will benefit both systems.

The "Big Four" and the "Daily Dozen" can be used together in a program of exercise. The "Big Four" is used as a warmup and the "Daily Dozen" is a total body building and fitness program. Combine both groups of exercises and receive even more benefit.

CAUTION: Some of these exercises, such as side raise, press up and out, and crossover, may be difficult to do for more than 25 repetitions. Don't become discouraged. It will take you some time to work up to 3 sets of 25 repetitions with .91 or 1.36 kilo weights. DON'T STRAIN, BUT TRAIN. Particularly those of you who are overweight and out of shape. YOU CAN DO IT, but easy does it at first.

Remember, a consistent daily workout will help you reach those goals a little sooner. This program can be done more than once a day, especially if you are advanced in your conditioning program. Don't miss your daily resistive rebounding session. Each day will bring that renewed vigor and a wonderful appearance. My hope is that you will enjoy this program as have the many hundreds in my fitness centers.

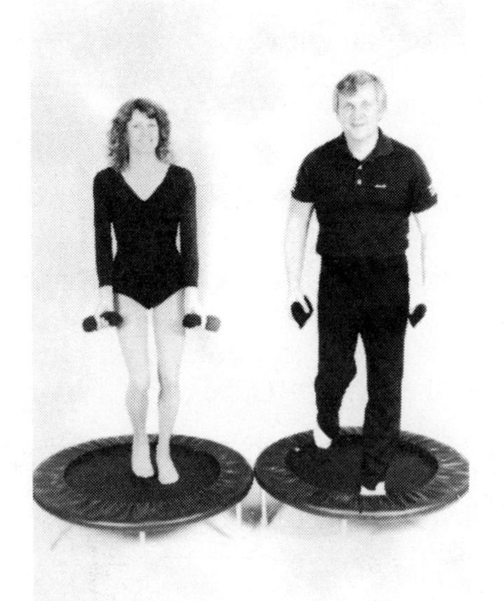
Curl, starting position.

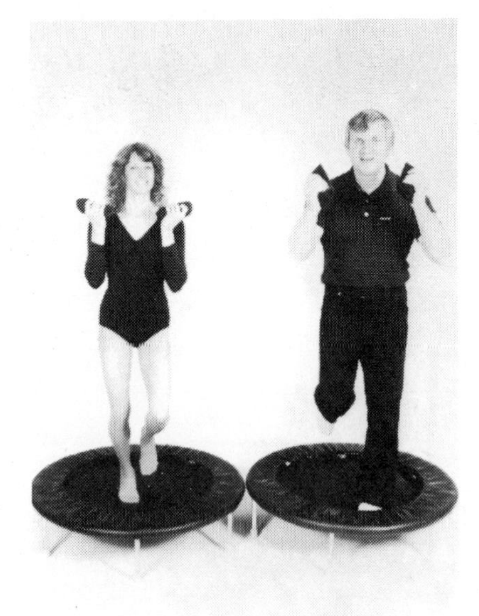
Completion.

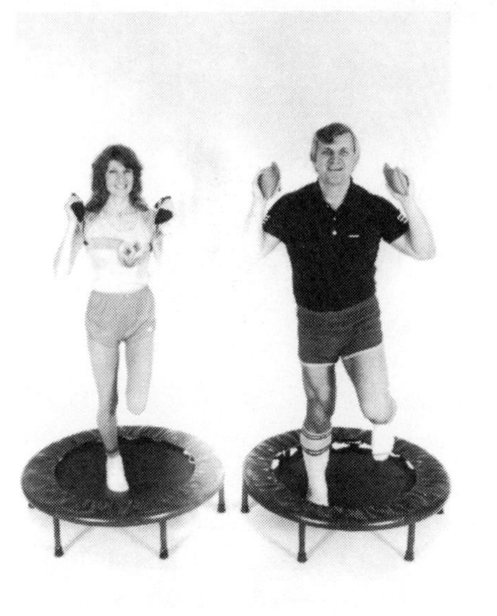
Press, starting position.

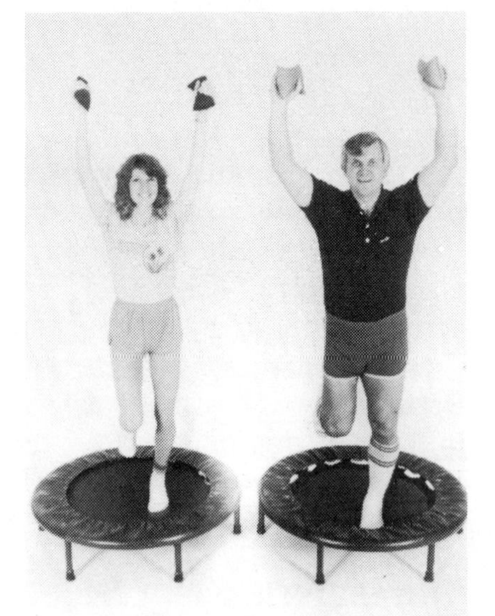
Completion.

1. CURL

Purpose: Great exercise that firms upper arms, forearms and grip. Works entire cardiovascular system.

Beginner:	10 reps
Indermediate:	12 reps
Advanced:	15 reps

Firmly grip your .45 kilo weights in hands. Jog or shuffle in the center of the mat, with your palms up and your elbows close to your side. Raise both weights together to your shoulders, then bring weights back to original position.

2. PRESS

Purpose: Wonderful exercise for upper back, shoulders, arms, grip and excellent overall toning for the arms. Works entire cardiovascular system.

Beginner:	10 reps
Intermediate:	12 reps
Advanced:	15 reps

Firmly grip your .45 kilo weights in hands. Jog or shuffle in the center of the mat. Bring weights to your shoulders, push both arms together overhead, bring back to shoulders after each repetition.

T.J. McCavitt

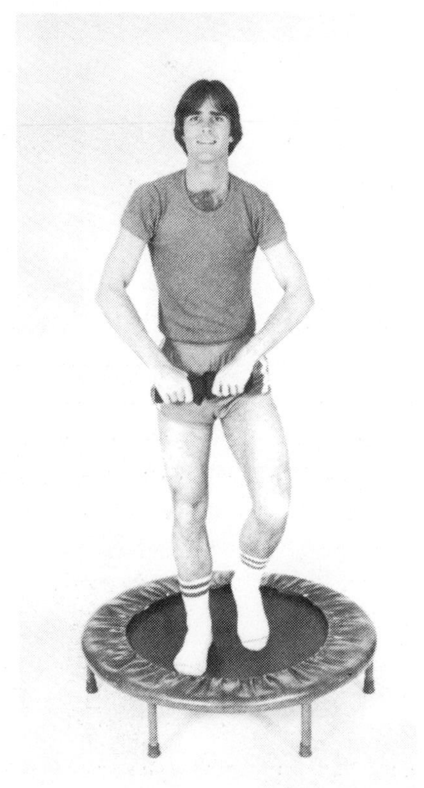

Upright row, beginning.

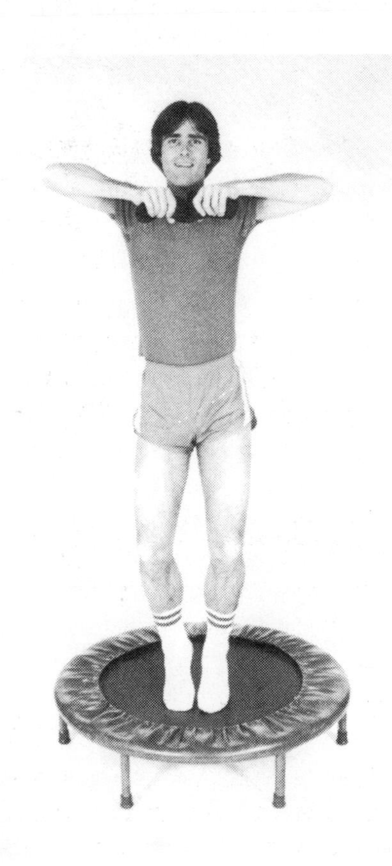

Completion.

Sarah Sneider and T.J. McCavitt

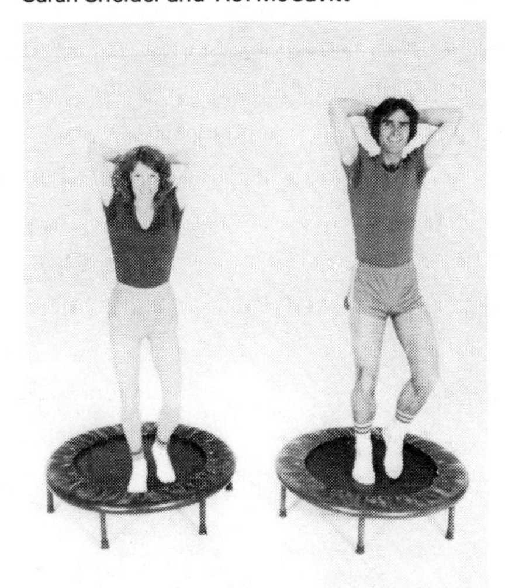

Tricep press, starting position.

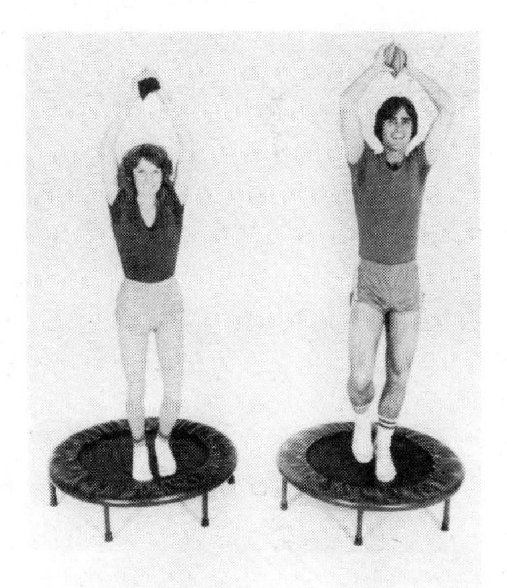

Completion.

3. UPRIGHT ROW

Purpose: Excellent for posture, upper back, shoulders, chest and forearms. Works entire cardiovascular system.

Beginner: 10 reps
Intermediate: 12 reps
Advanced: 15 reps

Firmly grip your .45 kilo weights in hands. Jog, shuffle or bounce in the center of the mat. Pull your hands to your chin (both together) with high elbows, lower to original position after each repetition.

4. TRICEP PRESS

Purpose: A very specific exercise for back of upper arms, shoulders and grip. Works entire cardiovascular system.

Beginner: 10 reps
Intermediate: 12 reps
Advanced: 15 reps

Firmly grip your .45 kilo weights in hands. Jog, shuffle or bounce in the center of the mat. Place hands behind head, extend forearms (together) and then bring back down to original position.

Lynn Grimditch

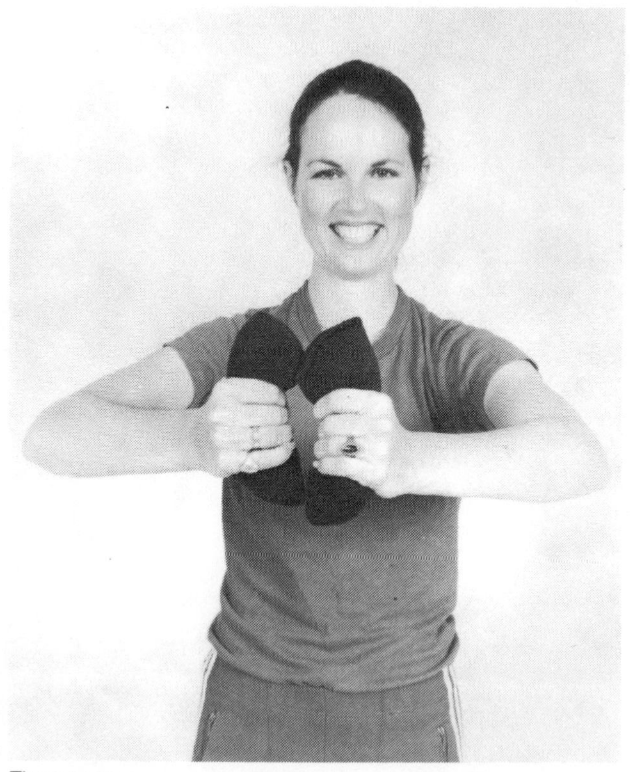
The squeeze.

5. SQUEEZE

Purpose: A wonderful exercise for grip and forearms. Works entire cardiovascular system.

Beginner:	10 reps
Intermediate:	12 reps
Advanced:	15 reps

Firmly squeeze .45 kilo weights in front of your body while you jog, shuffle or bounce in the center of the mat. Squeeze firmly and release.

Sarah and Harry Sneider

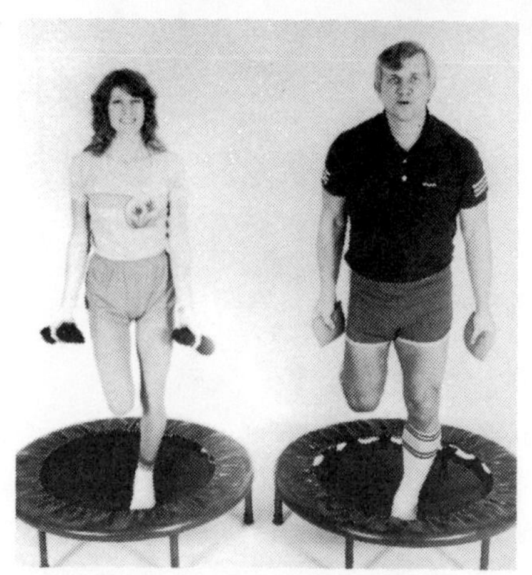
Curl and press, starting position.

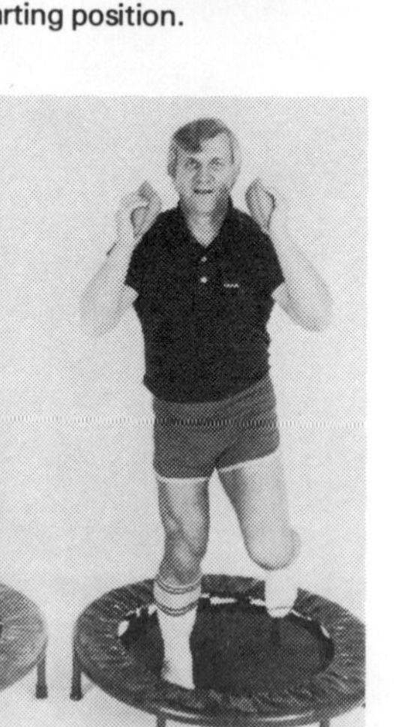
Completion of curl, beginning of press.

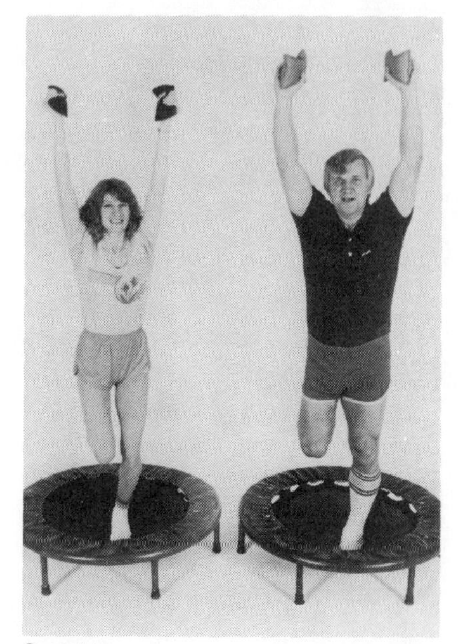
Completion.

6. CURL & PRESS

Purpose: Excellent for shaping the arms both in front and back, upper chest and forearms. Works entire cardiovascular system.

Beginner:	10 reps
Intermediate:	12 reps
Advanced:	15 reps

Firmly grip your .45 kilo weight in hands. Jog, shuffle or bounce in the center of the mat. With palms up, elbows to side, pull weights to shoulders. From the shoulder position, push both weights overhead, bring Sanbags back to shoulders and then down each time.

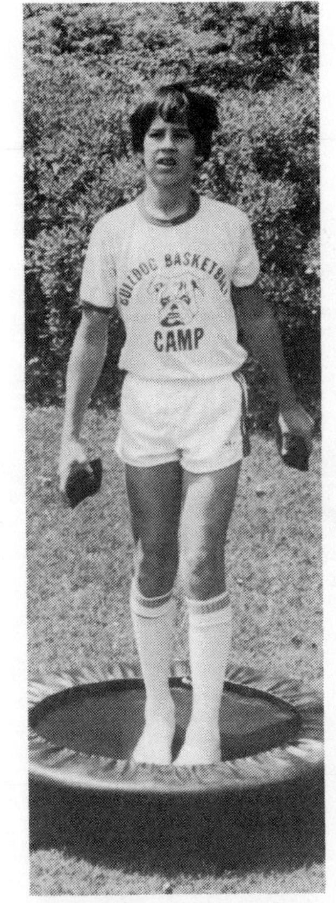

Todd Grinolds, all-around athlete, demonstrates starting routine of side raise.

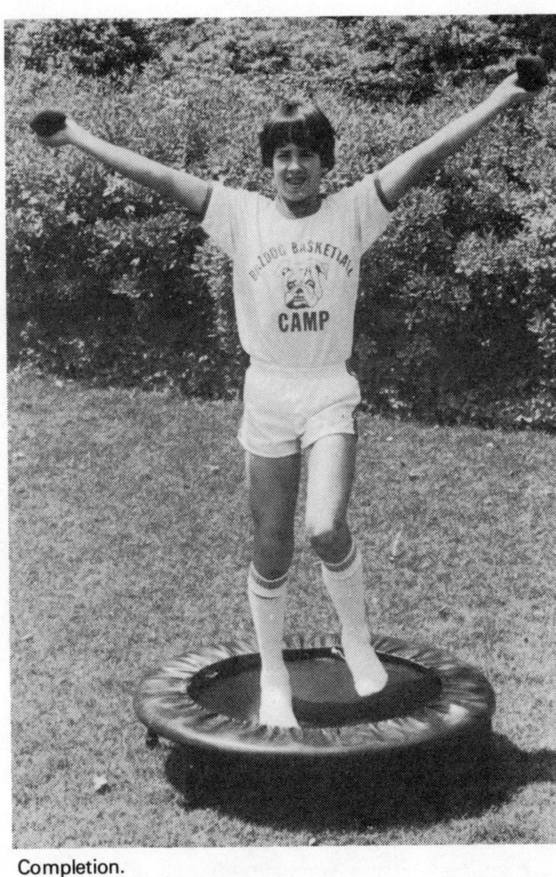

Completion.

7. SIDE RAISE

Purpose: A very specific exercise for shoulders, arms and upper back. Works entire cardiovascular system.

Beginner:	10 reps
Intermediate:	12 reps
Advanced:	15 reps

Firmly grip your .45 kilo weights in hands. Jog, shuffle or bounce in the center of the mat. Raise the weights with straight arms to at least shoulder level, without bending your elbows, and then let them back down to your sides again.

Kenneth L. Sutton, speed roller skater, winner of two gold, one silver in 1978 Pan American Games.

Starting point of crossover.

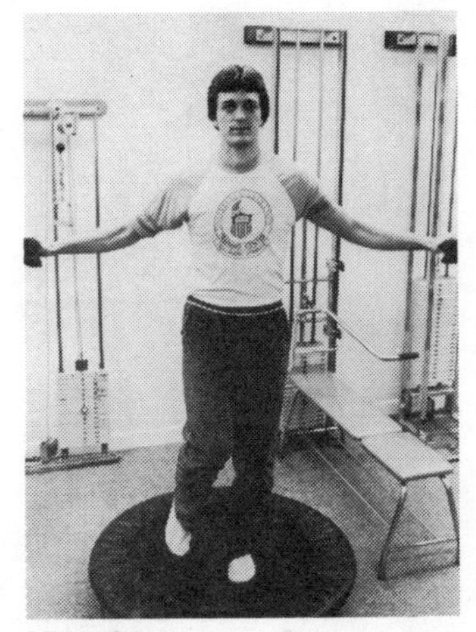

Mid-point.

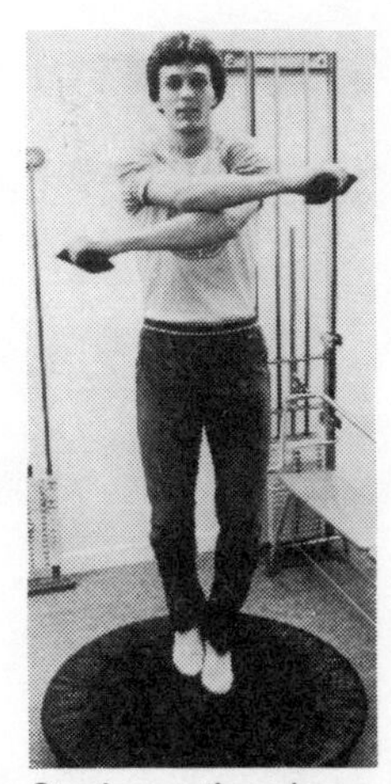

Starting routine, alternating arms.

8. CROSSOVERS

Purpose: This exercise firms upper chest, shapes arms and shoulders and strengthens upper back. Works entire cardiovascular system.

Beginner:	10 reps
Intermediate:	12 reps
Advanced:	15 reps

Firmly grip your .45 kilo weights in hands. Jog, shuffle or bounce in the center of the mat. Raise weights to eye level, bend elbows slightly in front of face. Hug yourself with weights one repetition over your eyes, the next under. The elbows must be bent for effectiveness here.

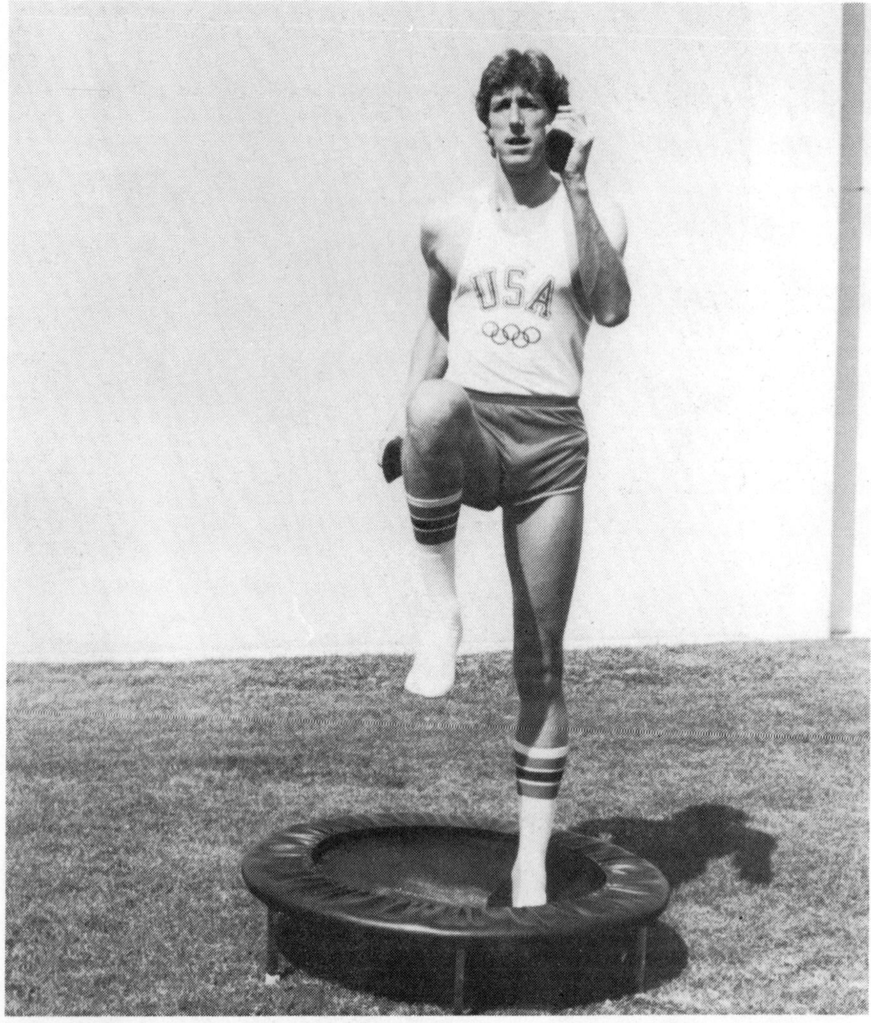

Dwight Stones demonstrates sprint high knee routine.

9. SPRINT KNEE HIGH

Purpose: A wonderful conditioner for all muscles, specifically waist, hips, thighs, calves and upper body, too. Works entire cardiovascular system.

Beginner:	15 seconds
Intermediate:	20 seconds
Advanced:	30 seconds

Firmly grip your .45 kilo weights in hands, begin running with high knee drive and rhythmic arm carry, elbows and knees moving in unison.

Denise and Richard Guthy, fitness directors.

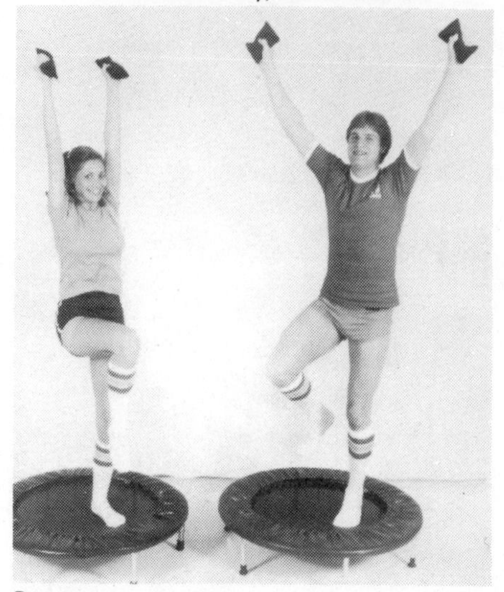

Press up.

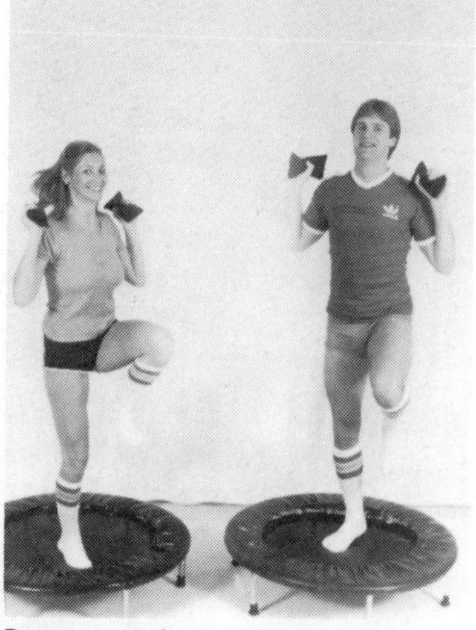

Return to starting position.

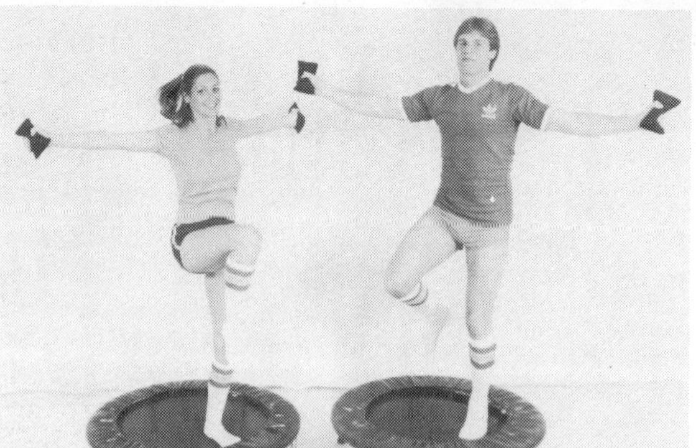

Press out.

10. PRESS UP & OUT

Purpose: Firms upper back, shoulders, arms and chest. Works entire cardiovascular system.

Beginner:	10 reps (Pressing up and out count as 1 repetition)
Intermediate:	12 reps
Advanced:	15 reps

Firmly grip your .45 kilo weights in hands. Jog, shuffle or bounce in the center of the mat. Pull weights to shoulders, push overhead together, bring back to shoulders. Now push weights out to side, then bring back to shoulders. Alternate by pressing overhead and pressing to the side.

Sarah and Harry Sneider

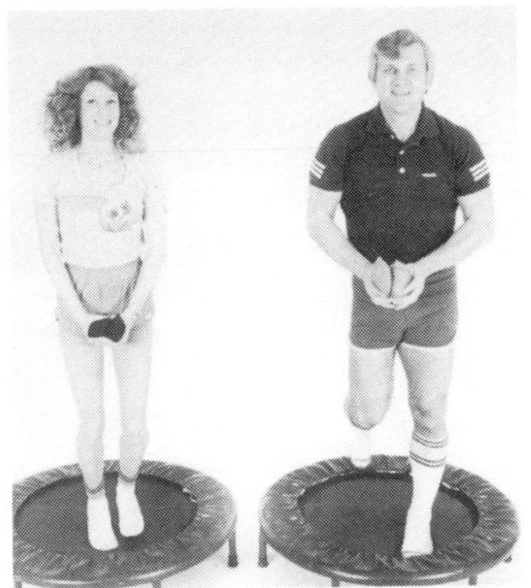
Beginning of pullover.

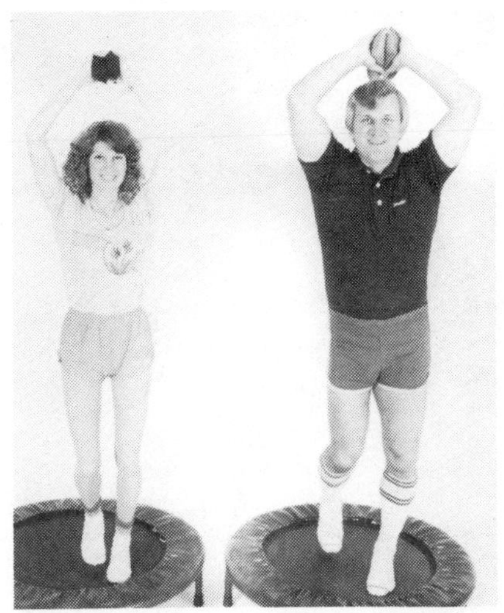
Mid-point.

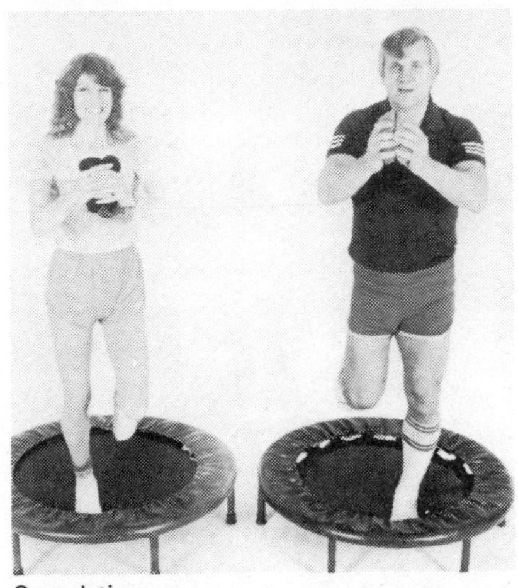
Completion.

11. PULLOVER

Purpose: Excellent shaping exercise for chest, shoulders and arms. It will work waist, too. Works entire cardiovascular system.

Beginner:	10 reps
Intermediate:	12 reps
Advanced:	15 reps

Firmly grip your .45 kilo weights in hands. Jog, shuffle or bounce in the center of the mat. Push both Sanbags together in front of body, pull them overhead touching back of head, bring back to original position. The arms are curled, not straight, when pulled over head.

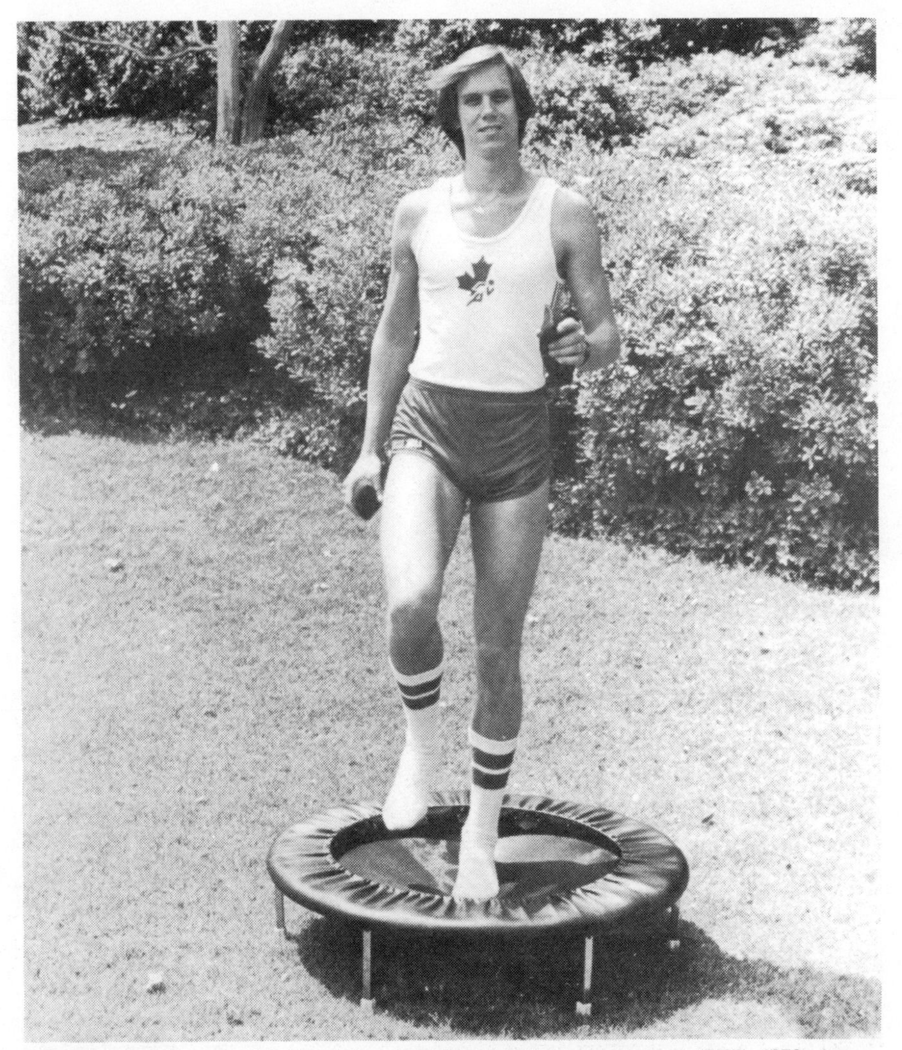
Greg Joy, 1976 Olympic high jump silver medalist, world record high jump (7'7"), 1978, demonstrates easy jog.

12. JOG EASY

Purpose: Overall good body conditioner.

Beginner:	30 seconds
Intermediate:	45 seconds
Advanced:	1 minute

Firmly grip your .45 kilo weights in hands. Jog easy in the center of the mat, elbows and knees moving together in easy cadence.

Julie Nelson, 2, daughter of Sandy Nelson, jogs with stuffed animals.

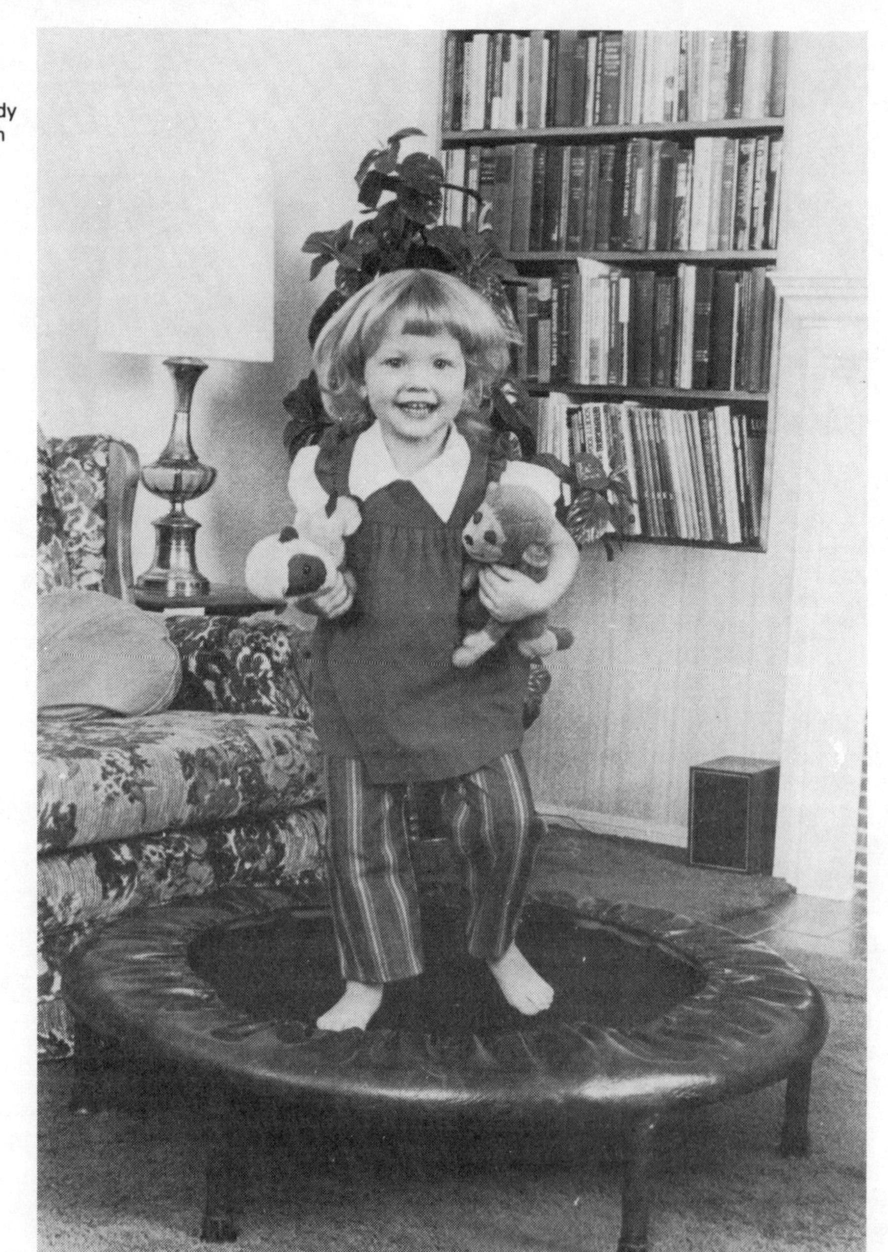

Program for Children

(Children from 1½ to 10 years old)

Bounce, Bounce, Bounce, 1, 2, 3!!

Many of our top pediatricians, psychologists, and educators are telling us that the first six years of life are the most important in developing skills like motor learning, coordination, posture, body alignment, etc. Why not start your child today developing these skills with "Sanbagging."

Take the "Fun Four" and use the light .45 kilo Sanbags, and watch the child's posture improve, fitness develop and his or her academic learning improve. The "Fun Four" could be used up to three times a day. Start with 30 seconds in the Bounce & Jog Easy and work up to two minutes each. Start with 3 sets of 10 reps in the Curl & Press and Squeeze, work up to as many as your child enjoys, such as 3 sets of 25.

In each activity, keep the Sanbags light, not forcing growth, but encouraging your child to develop slowly. This is the age where your child has almost a plastic body. Children's bones are forming, muscles are developing, and tremendous spurts of growth are taking place. With these exercises, you are developing your child to greater fitness and health in the years ahead.

Bouncing through and to the end of a song on a 45 rpm. record, or using a 3-minute timer can be helpful as a motivation. Children also love rewards, a cookie, etc., means a lot to them after a good performance!

Encourage your younger children by counting out loud: 1, 2, 3, etc., as they do each exercise. Or you may count backwards: 10, 9, 8. . . . An enjoyable way to teach the alphabet is to say A, B, C . . . as they do their exercise. You'll be amazed how quickly your younger children learn their letters and numbers.

THE FUN FOUR

(For 1½ to 6 year olds)

Especially good for Small Toddlers
Suggested program as follows using light (.45 kilo) Sanbags

Exercise	Time Reps	Goals
1. Bounce	30 seconds	add 10 seconds every week
2. Curl & Press	10 reps	add 2 reps every week
3. Jog Easy	30 seconds	add 10 seconds every week
4. Jog & Squeeze	10 reps	add 2 reps every week

WORK UP TO 3-5 minutes TOTAL PROGRAM

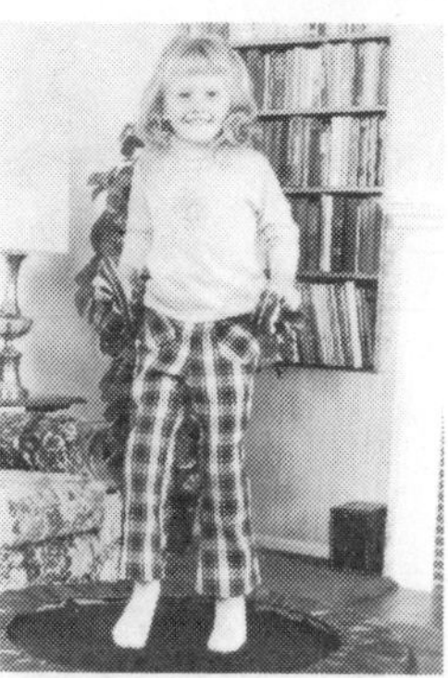

Becky Nelson, 5, bounces with shoes in hand.

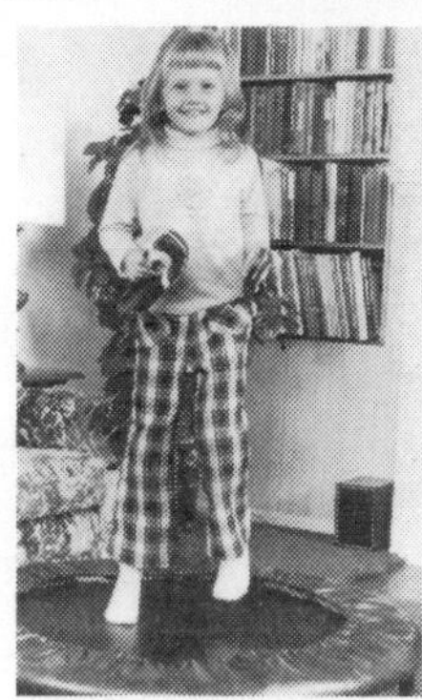

Starting position, curl.

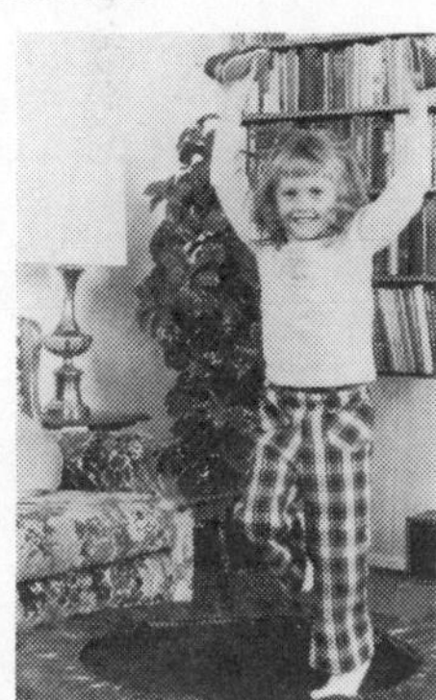

Completion, press.

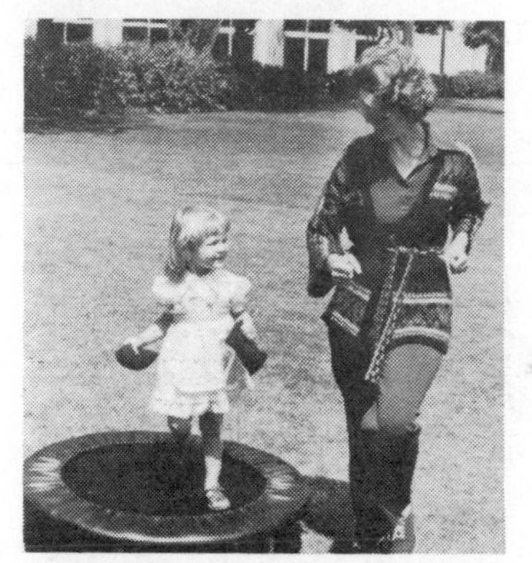

Sandy Nelson helps daughter, Julie, 2, with easy jog.

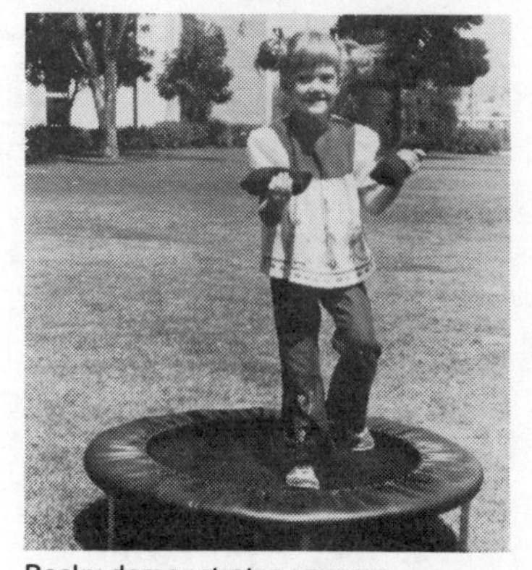

Becky demonstrates squeeze.

CAUTION: The parent should be close to the rebound unit so the child does not fall and hurt himself. The child will improve very quickly if you make a game of the activity. Try to encourage a FUN environment rather than an **arduous must atmosphere.**

You may find the .45 kilo Sanbags are too heavy for your child. You can do all the exercises, including the "Daily Dozen" without the Sanbags — just with open hands. Or, they may use their tennis shoes, a couple of tennis balls, two small stuffed animals, etc., as resistance.

THE TERRIFIC SIX

(For 3½ to 10 year olds)

Here is a moderate program for the child who would enjoy a shorter workout or cannot do the "Daily Dozen" yet. These exercises are especially excellent for the child who has a slower motor learning rate or is overweight.

Suggested program using .45 kilo Sanbags.

Exercise	Reps or Time	Sets	Goals
1. Curl	10 reps	1	HAVE FUN FIRST!
2. Squeeze	10 reps	1	3 sets of 10
3. Curl & Press	10 reps	1	3 sets of 10
4. Sprint High Knee	15 sec.	1	Work up to 1 min.
5. Jog Easy	45 sec.	1	Work up to 4 min.
6. Bounce	30 sec.	1	Work up to 1 min.

Add 1 set every week till you reach 3 sets of 10. Add weight only if you feel the weight is too light. Be cautious not to push. Add 15 sec. on the Sprint High Knee and Bounce every week. (You may include a 5 sec. bounce on the left leg, then 5 sec. bounce on the right leg.) Add approximately 30 sec. per week on the Jog Easy every week. This program should be done **every day,** if possible. Approximate time after 5 weeks or more: 8 minutes. Remember to try to make it a FUN session!!

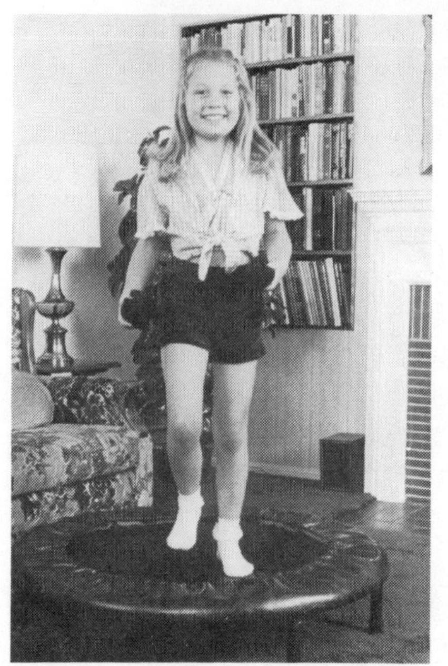

Amy Nelson demonstrates starting position of curl.

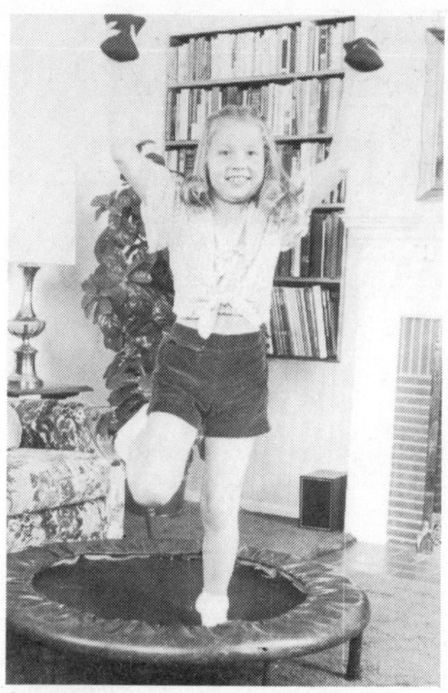

Completion, curl and press.

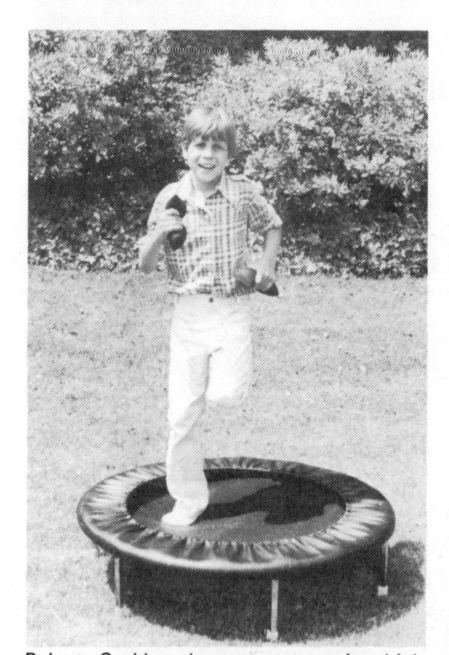

Robert Sneider demonstrates sprint high knee.

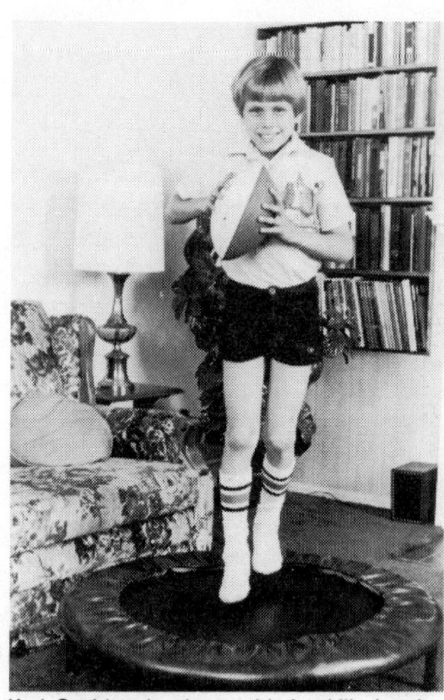

Karl Sneider develops athletic skills jogging with football in hand.

The Daily Dozen

(For 3 to 6 year olds)

The "Daily Dozen" is a very useful body building tool. You will shape not only the muscles, but the bones, too. This program was designed for muscular symmetry and fitness. Your child will surprise you how quickly he or she will respond to this program.

They will be developing their muscular and cellular system, hand-eye coordination, stamina, etc. with this program. You as a parent can start your child on a road to tremendous confidence in all aspects of life. Don't buy your children expensive toys that will be thrown away in a few weeks. Instead, invest in their future with the Sanbagging program. Do your child a big favor and start this program **today.**

THE DAILY DOZEN

(3 to 6 year olds)

An Advanced Program

Suggested program using light (.45 kilo) Sanbags.
Suggested Warm-Up: The "Fun Four"

Exercise	Reps or Time	Sets	Goals
1. Curl	10	1	HAVE FUN FIRST!
2. Press	10	1	5 sets of 10
3. Upright Row	10	1	If child can do more than 10 repetitions, let him do as much as he can benefit from.
4. Tricep Press	10	1	
5. Squeeze	10	1	
6. Curl & Press	10	1	
7. Side Raise	10	1	
8. Crossover	10	1	
9. Sprint High Knee	30 sec.	1	Add 10 sec. per week till you reach 2½ min.
10. Press Up & Out	10	1	
11. Pullover	10	1	5 sets of 10
12. Jog Easy	45 sec.	1	Add 15 sec. per week till you reach 5 min.

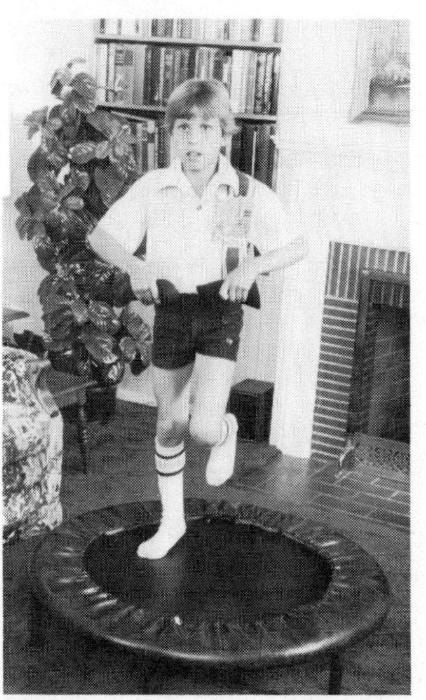

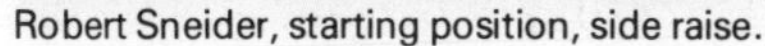

Robert Sneider, starting position, side raise.

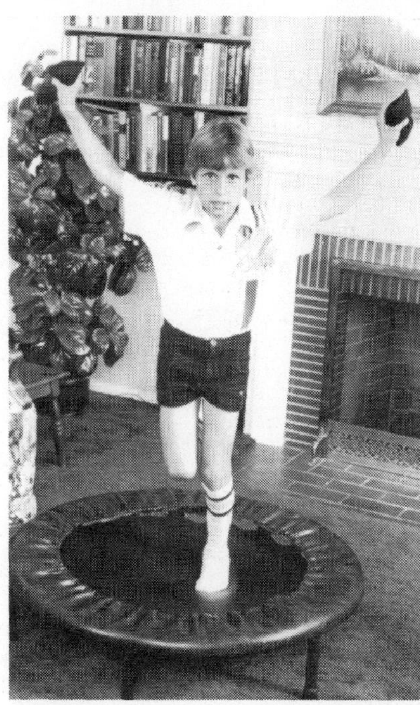

Completion.

1. HAVE FUN FIRST!! Try not to push your child. These exercises can be hard to do, so be patient. If your child has problems doing the "Daily Dozen," refer to the "Terrific Six."
2. If a child can do more than 10 repetitions in each exercise, move them up another set. Don't push it. Just ask if they are ready.
3. A good time limit on one exercise period should be 3-5 minutes (depends on ages).
4. You, as a parent, should do your program of the "Daily Dozen." Remember, example speaks louder than words.
5. Have some music with a tempo and beat. Children will enjoy the fun more than a big push. And the rhythmical work with music is most helpful.
6. Watch them grow before your eyes!!

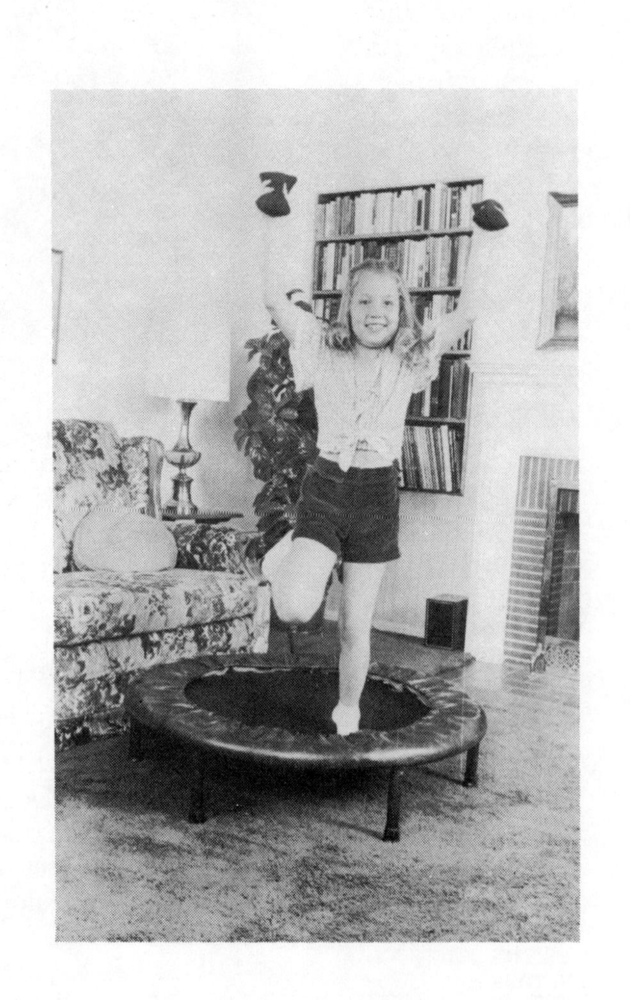

Chapter 6

From 7 Years to Late Teens

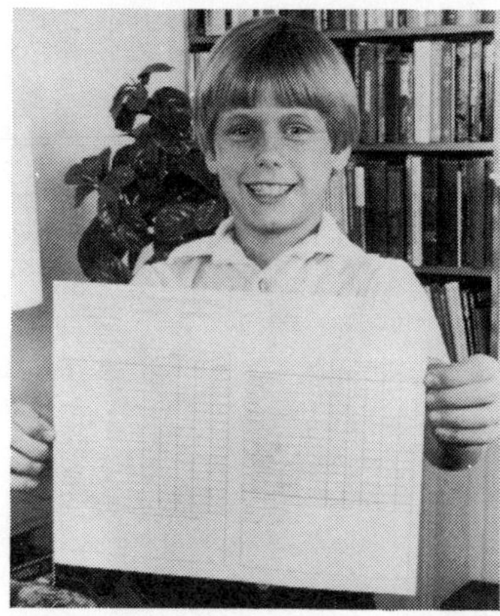

Karl Sneider with improved report card, thanks to rebound exercise.

These wonderful formative years leading into puberty and beyond are your opportunity to develop total fitness with Sanbagging. Having three children in this age group, Debbie 11, Karl 9, and Robert 7, I can attest to the fact that Sanbagging on a rebound unit made a difference in their school work, posture, athletic skills and more.

Many children want to improve their coordination, strength, stamina, and appearance. There may be the pressure of making the soccer team, cheerleading, losing weight, or whatever. The Sanbagging program will help all these areas.

Start your child off with the "Big Four" holding the pliable Sanbags in their hands.

THE BIG FOUR

Exercise	Time
1. Lymphatic Bounce	1. Start 30 seconds in each exercise
2. Shuffle	2. Add 10 seconds per week till you reach 10-15 minutes in all 4 exercises combined.
3. Jog	
4. Bounce	

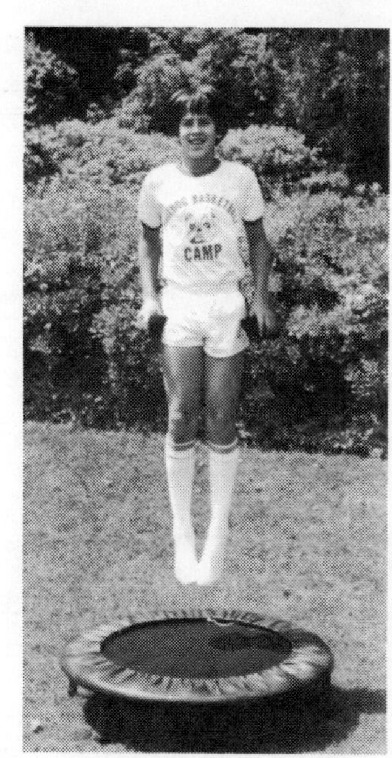

Todd Grinolds demonstrates high bounce.

To make this activity more challenging for those in their teens, add one pound (.45 kilo) to the Sanbag program every month till you are using 3 pound (1.36 kilo) Sanbags.

If your child finds this program too difficult, cut back to a shorter, modified version of 15 seconds in each exercise and work up to a goal of one minute in each exercise of 8 minutes total.

Try to encourage a DAILY program. Consistency in workouts will develop that body just a little more than a haphazard program. You will need to set some goals for your children. Tell them about how they are going to develop their baseball skills, improve posture for gymnastics, slim their bodies, build muscles or improve their grades.

Reward them when they achieve by words of encouragement, new clothes, a bike, or just a loving hug.

The "Daily Dozen" is an excellent fitness and body building program for your child. "Sanbagging" is easier on the joints than most popular machines used in expensive health clubs or studios, and certainly much safer. The price of a health club membership can run into the hundreds of dollars per year. You can have your own health club right in your own living room or gymnasium for a fraction of the cost, and you can be there personally to encourage your children. The principles that are used on very expensive gym equipment can be used in your "Daily Dozen" program. Here is how to really improve:

THE DAILY DOZEN

(For 7 year olds to late teens)

Suggested program using .45 kilo Sanbags.
Suggested Warm-up: The "Big Four."

Exercise	Weight	Reps or Time	Sets	Goals
1. Curl	.45 kilo	10	1	5 sets of 10 with 1.36 kilo "Sanbags"
2. Press	.45 kilo	10	1	
3. Upright Row	.45 kilo	10	1	
4. Tricep Press	.45 kilo	10	1	
5. Squeeze	.45 kilo	10	1	
6. Curl & Press	.45 kilo	10	1	
7. Side Raise	.45 kilo	10	1	
8. Crossover	.45 kilo	10	1	
9. Sprint High Knee	.45 kilo	30 sec.	1	Add 10 sec. per week till reaching 6 min.
10. Press Up & Out	.45 kilo	10	1	5 sets of 10 with 1.36 kilo "Sanbags"
11. Pullover	.45 kilo	10	1	
12. Jog Easy	.45 kilo	45 sec.	1	Add 30 sec. per week till reaching 6 min.

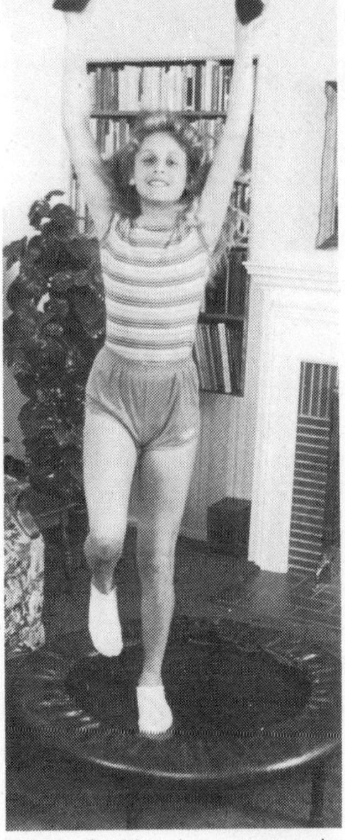

Debbie Sneider demonstrates the press up.

Add one set of each exercise each week till your child can do 5 sets of 10 repetitions in each exercise. Add 15 seconds per week on Sprint High Knee till your child can do this exercise for 2 minutes. On the Jog Easy, add 30 seconds per week till your child can jog over 3 minutes. Add Sanbag weight every month ONLY if the child can handle it.

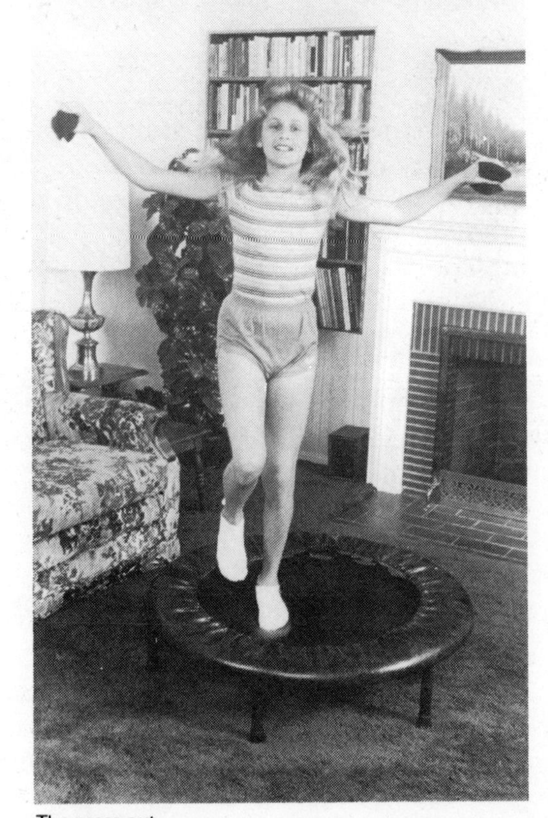

The press out.

For the advanced child in a high physical fitness category who is an athlete, refer to later chapters of this book. These programs are not intended to make muscle men or wonder women out of your child. They are designed to maintain good health, improve coordination, develop balanced muscular structure, develop good self image, etc. The more we are studying the field of rebound exercise with Sanbagging, the more we are amazed at the benefits this program has for growing children. Help your child right now with this program.

If you have more than one child, encourage friendly competition by having the child work up to a set of 25 to 35 repetitions in each exercise using the .45 kilo Sanbags. Do this only if you can see that the child can handle the program easily.

1. One set, start with 10 reps, work up to one set of 35, by adding 1 rep. per day.
2. In the Sprint High Knee and Jog Easy, add 10 seconds per day till your child is up to 8 minutes in Jog Easy and 3 minutes in Sprint High Knee.
3. Remember, the idea is not to strain, but to train. Try not to push your child too fast. Take time with smaller children to build up to these recommended levels.
4. This program is strongly recommended for those who are overweight or underweight, as "Sanbagging" can either help lose inches, or help you gain muscular bodyweight. More activity will reduce bodyweight, especially if the child is dieting along with it.
5. When a child can do more than 1 set of 35 in each exercise, including 1 set of 8 minutes in Jog Easy and 3 minutes in the Sprint High Knee, then have your child do this program twice a day.

There is quite a variation of abilities in what children can do in this age group. Be patient, learn to adapt the program so the child is comfortable. Then as children see it is no longer hard, challenge them. These programs will encourage excellent skills development in other areas, too. Enjoy this program. It is fun to watch children have fun while working hard.

You as parent, teacher, or coach can see that these programs are very **simple.** I wanted to keep it easy on you so at least you would try these exercises. There are **countless hundreds** of exercises you can do with your Sanbag program. Variety is great, I recommend it, but more important is that you are consistent in these basics for a while (1 to 3 months).

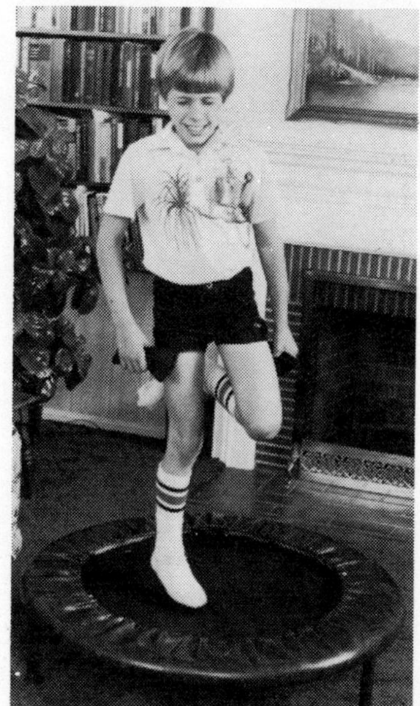

Karl Sneider, hopping on one foot with eyes shut.

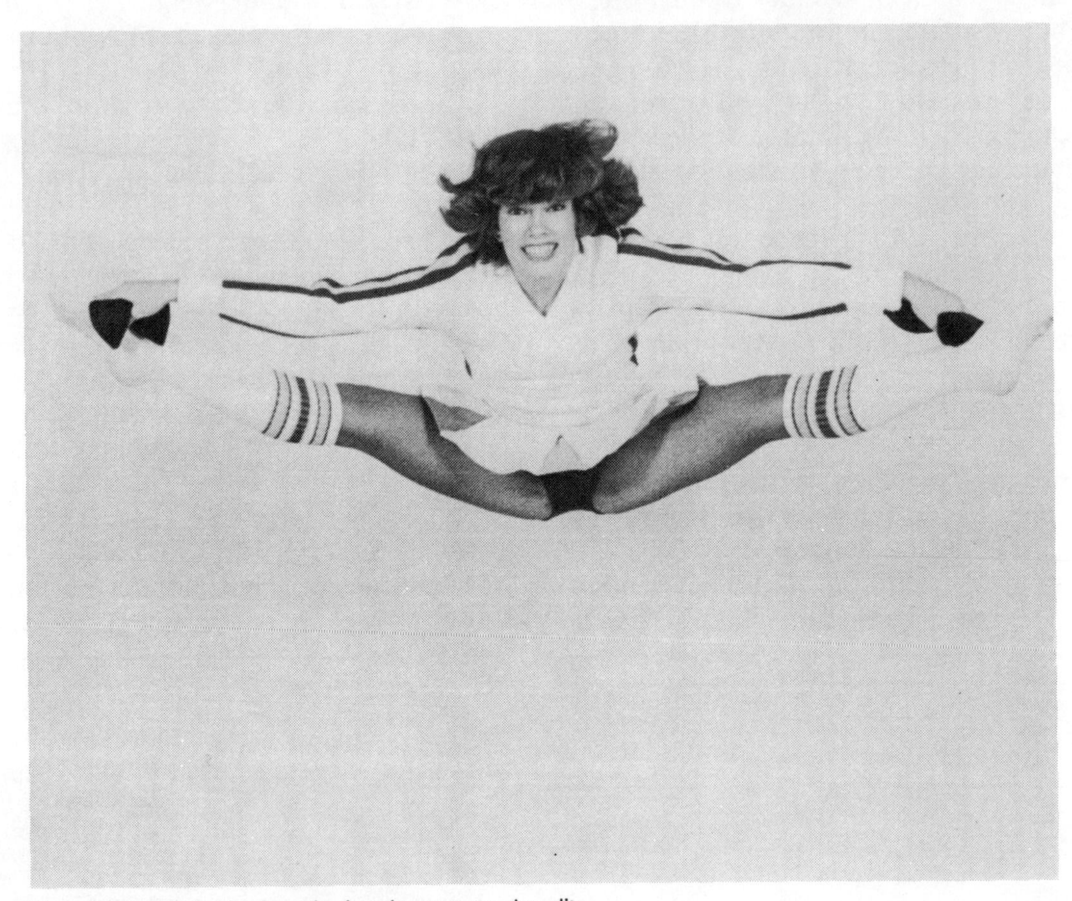

Eileen R. Dennis, cheerleader and writer, demonstrates the splits.

Chapter 7

Cheerleading

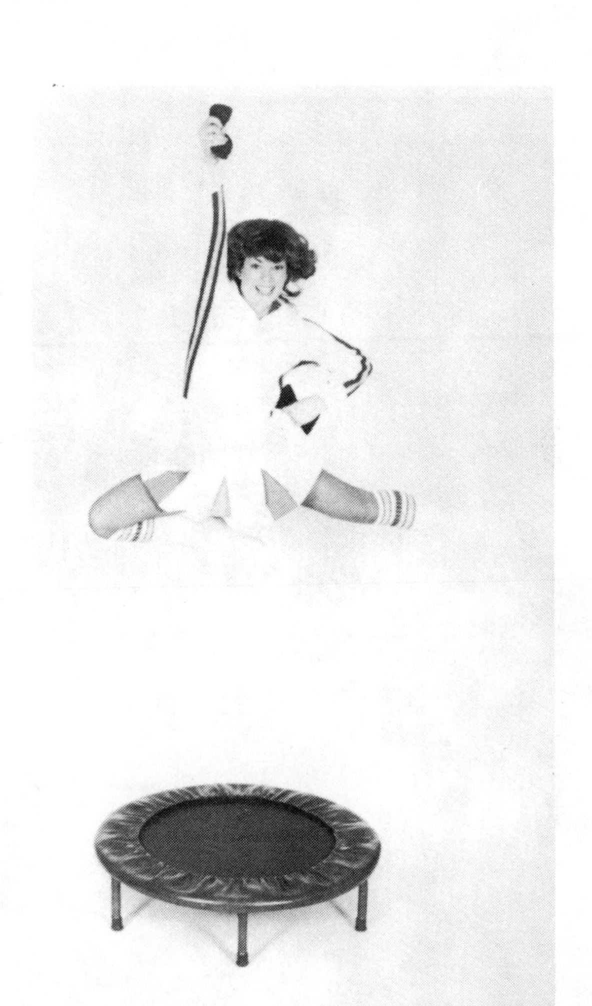

The hurdler.

Improve coordination, timing, conditioning, and help your teams to total athletic success with the following program.

Exercise	Weight	Reps/Time	Sets	Goals
1. Jog Easy	.45 kilo	30 sec.	2	6 sets of each exercise
2. Jump Split (see picture)	.45 kilo	10 reps	2	
3. Single Leg Bounce	.45 kilo	10 reps	2	
4. High Arm Split (see picture)	.45 kilo	10 reps	2	
5. Sprint in Place	.45 kilo	15 secs	2	Add 15 sec. per week
6. Side Raises	.45 kilo	10 reps	2	6 sets of each exercise
7. Bounces (see picture)	.45 kilo	30 sec.	2	Add 30 sec. per week
8. Upright Row	.45 kilo	10 reps	2	6 sets of each exercise
9. Jog Easy	.45 kilo	30 sec.	2	Add 30 sec. per week

Add one set every week till you reach 6 sets. Those who are advanced cheerleaders use the "Daily Dozen" as a program. Add .45 kilo Sanbag weight every month **if** you feel the Sanbags are too light, till you reach 1.36 Sanbags. Sanbagging programs are excellent tools for improving your cheerleading. On your running program, add 15 seconds per week till you do 1½ minutes in the Sprint and 3½ minutes in the Bounce and Jog Easy.

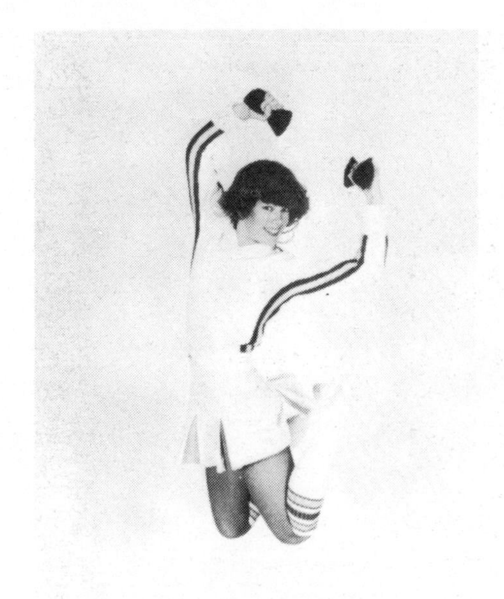

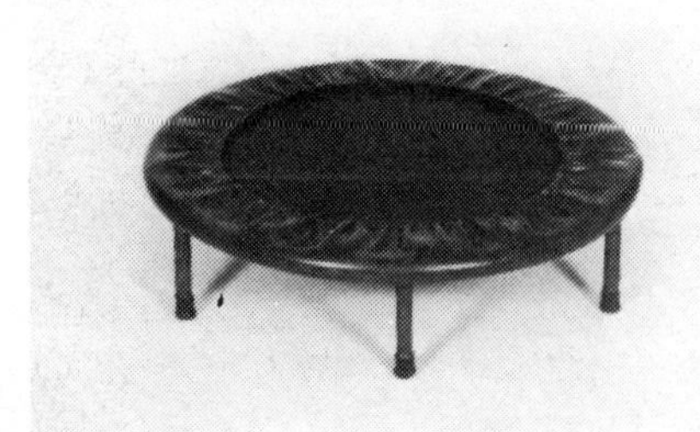

The Side "C".

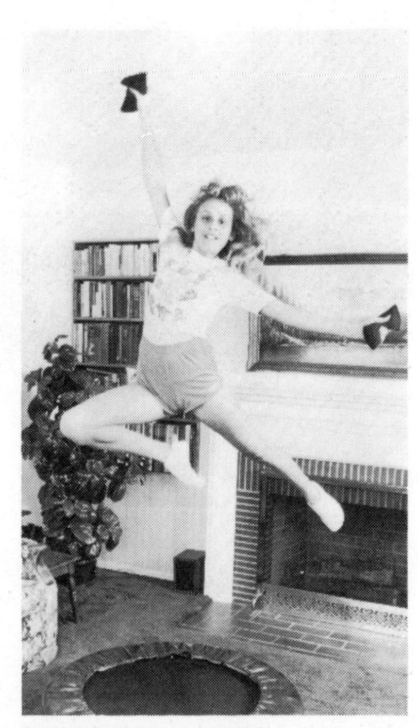

Debbie Sneider, the hurdler.

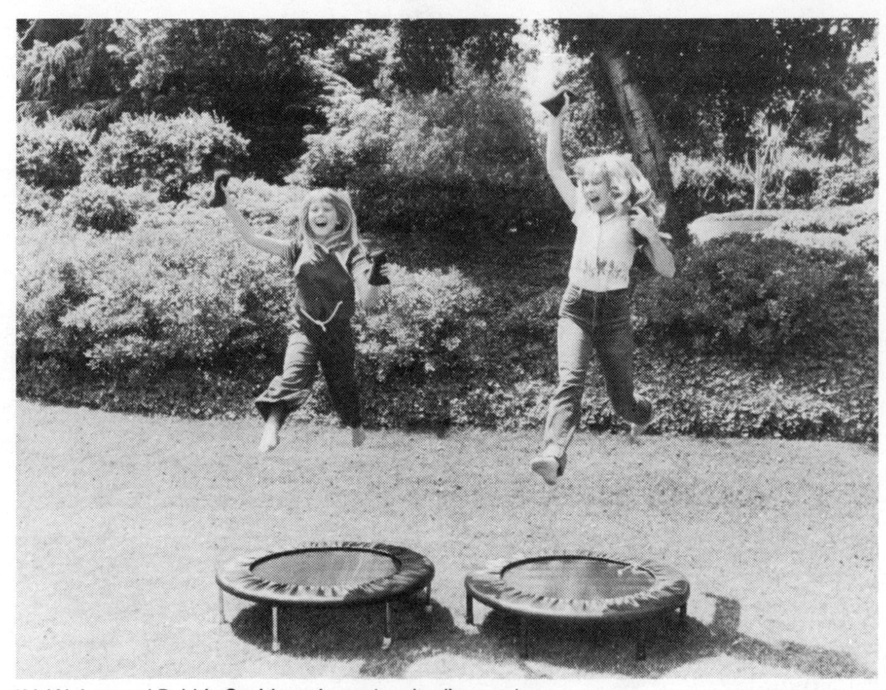

Krisi Nelson and Debbie Sneider enjoy a cheerleading workout.

Chapter 8

Program for Women

SHAPE UP with the new exciting fitness program that's FUN!

These simple movements will trim inches, tone muscles, make you look good and feel great in only 15 minutes a day! The key is **consistency.**

This unique fitness package is for you. You can do the "Big Four" (Lymphatic Bounce, Shuffle, Jog, and Bounce, (Chapter 3) as a warmup. The "Beginner's Modified Program" or the "Daily Dozen" may be the program for you, especially if you are overweight or have back problems. Start with the beginning program in each activity and you will achieve wonderful results.

Perhaps you might enjoy a special program that's just a little more advanced. So, if the "Daily Dozen" are easy for you and you would like a little more advanced program with variations, try the following "Perfect Ten."

In these programs you never use weights heavy enough to hurt you. The Sanbags are soft and pliable. Working with light weights is exhilarating. As you increase your strength with these exercises, you will have a great deal more energy throughout the day.

Will Lifting Weights Develop Huge Muscles?

Much has been written about resistance training for women. We see health clubs and aerobic centers doing very well. One myth that should be dismissed is that women develop large muscles from lifting weights. Not true.

Women need not worry about losing their feminine curves because no matter how many weights they lift, they will never develop the bulging muscles of a Mr. Universe. Since they have only a very small amount of the male hormone testosterone, women just cannot build those huge muscles.

Muscles are what give shape to your figure. Well-shaped and toned muscles mean a well-shaped you! Muscles not used will become loose and flabby.

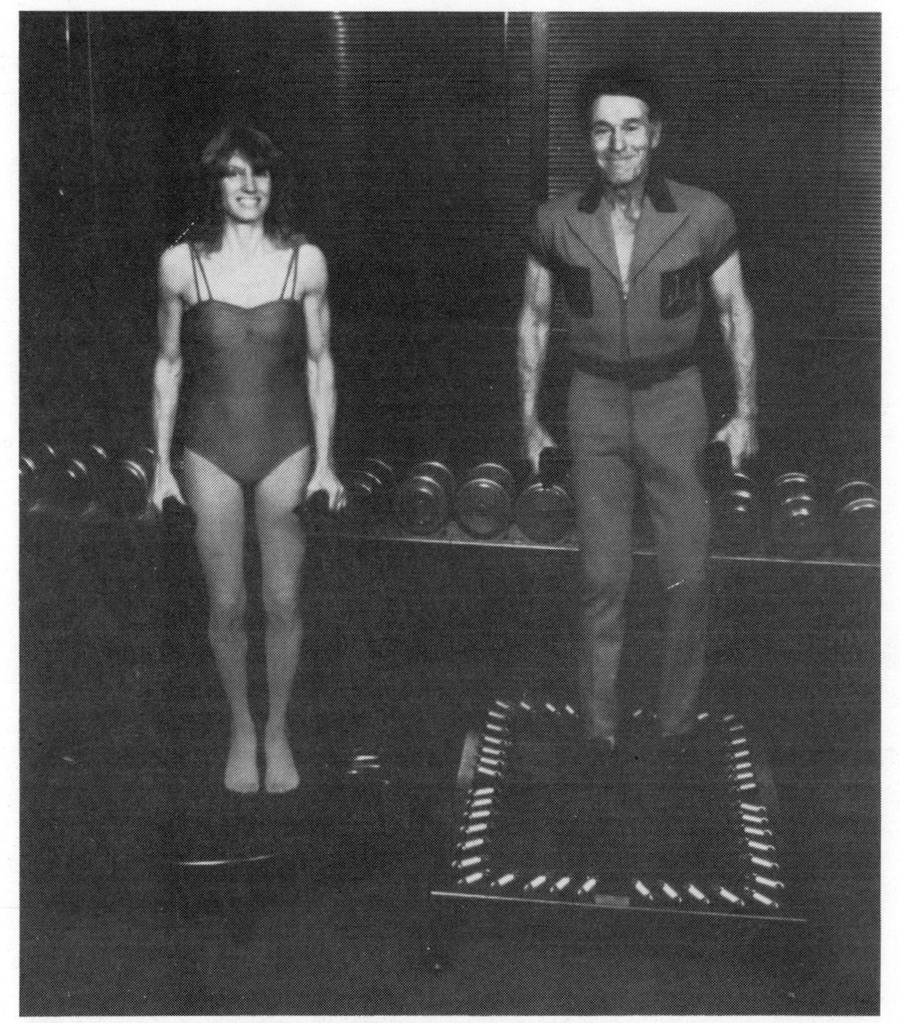

Sarah Sneider and Jack LaLanne demonstrate the lymphatic bounce.

There is nothing better than Sanbagging for conditioning the body and losing weight. Light weight training, Sanbagging, will give you a gentle curve on the upper arm instead of saggy fat. It will build the pectoral muscles supporting the breasts for a rounder, firmer chest. Well-developed muscle may help get rid of "cellulite" and "saddlebags" and actually decreases overall hip measurements.

Some of the comments from ladies I've worked with in our fitness centers are: *"I've gained two inches in my bust line with the Sanbagging exercises" . . . "My dresses are looser in the waist" . . . "I've lost inches in my hips"* . . . etc.

There is a kind of emotional and physical confidence that comes only when one is physically fit. The psychological benefits are just as great as the physical benefits. So, let's get "high" on bounce exercise!

Any Exercise Program Should Have:

1. **Warm-up Period** —The "Big Four" or "Stretching" (Chapter 3)
2. **Work Period** — Your program (Carefully monitor your working heart rate during this period).
3. **Cool Down** — Easy Jog, Stretching, etc.

The exercises that make the heart pump faster, lungs take on greater loads of oxygen, and circulation to carry that oxygen to all parts of the body is the kind of exercise we need.

If you can cut your heart rate by 10 to 15 beats per minute, which is very likely with the Sanbagging program, you will be saving it 15,000 to 20,000 beats per day! The heart, then, will be more efficient and not have to work so hard to pump the blood to your body.

Exercise To Music:

We suggest you exercise to music with a definite beat that will keep you moving at a smooth, fairly fast pace. It's more fun, too!

As you learn the exercises, you can do them to the flow of the music.

What To Wear:

Your clothing should be comfortable and allow you to move without restriction. Women should wear a supportive bra while bouncing.

Helpful suggestions: Those of you who are overweight (10-100 pounds), or out of condition or who have difficulty maintaining balance on the rebound unit, stay with the "Big Four" or the "Beginner's Modified Program" to help gain balance and

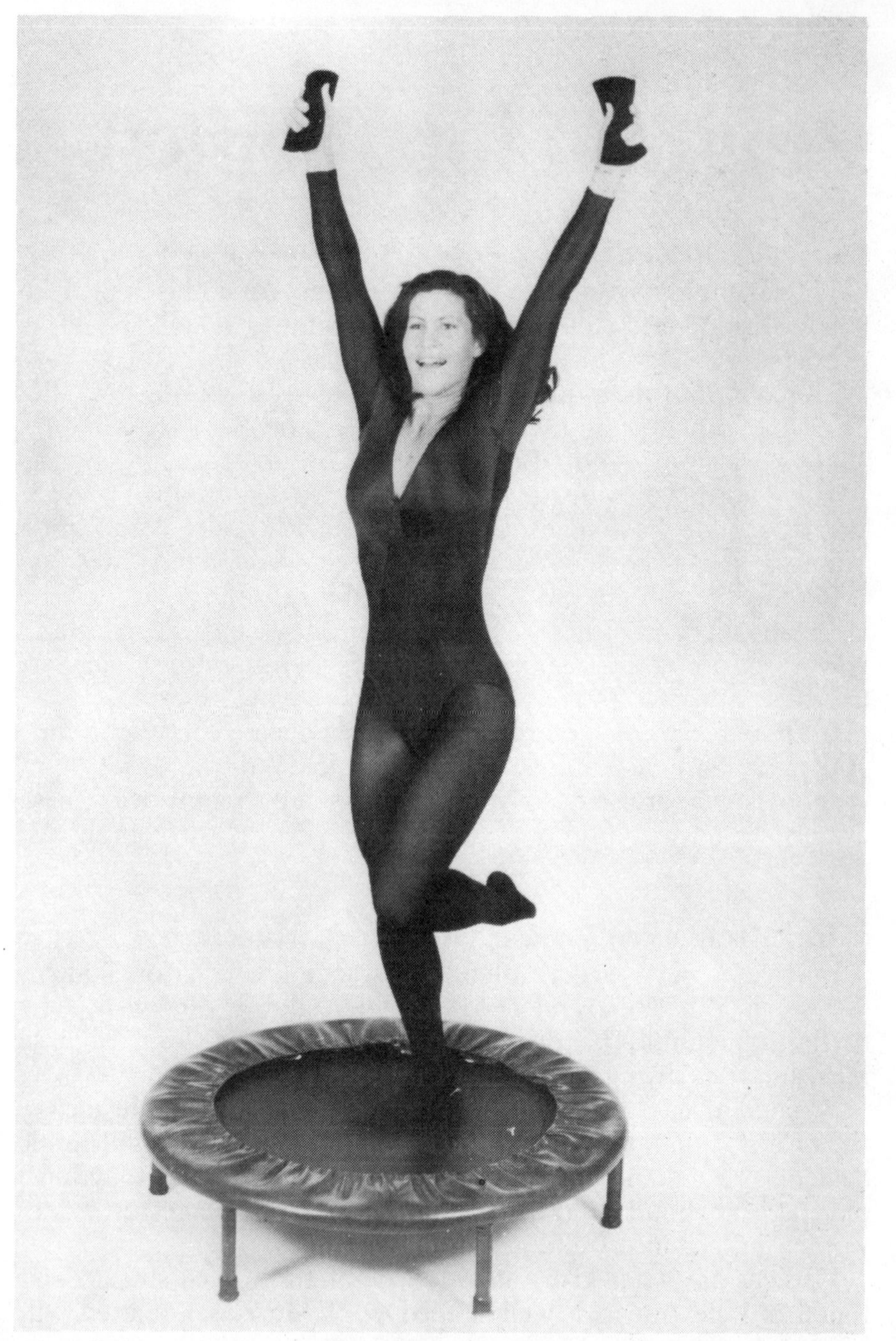

Nancy J. Collins, aerobic dance instructor, gets excellent results from rebound exercise program.

confidence before attempting the "Daily Dozen" program or the "Perfect Ten."

Sanbagging is a wonderful way to shape up in the privacy of your own home. You will not only greatly improve your cardiovascular fitness, you will trim and tone your entire body. Sanbagging is aerobic fitness and weight training combined — a super winning combination.

Here's your beginning program:

THE BIG FOUR

Exercise	Wt.	Reps.			Sets	Goals
		B*	I	A		
1. Lymphatic Bounce	.45 kilo	10 sec.	30 sec.	1 min.	1	Add 1 set every week till you reach 15 minutes total time.
2. Shuffle	.45 kilo	10 sec.	30 sec.	1 min.	1	
3. Jog	.45 kilo	10 sec.	30 sec.	1 min.	1	
4. Bounce	.45 kilo	10 sec.	30 sec.	1 min.	1	

*B — Beginner, I — Intermediate, A — Advanced

Suggested Progression:

Add 1 set every week till you reach 15 minutes total time. One set means one completion of the 4 exercises. To add another set start again from #1 Lymphatic Bounce and continue through #4 Bounce.

For those who are overweight (10-100 pounds) and inexperienced in rebounding here is a modified program:

THE BEGINNER'S MODIFIED PROGRAM

Warm-up: The "Big Four"

Exercise	Wt.	Reps	Sets	Goals
1. Curl	.45 kilo	10	1	3 sets of 25 reps
2. Upright Row	.45 kilo	10	1	
3. Curl & Press	.45 kilo	10	1	
4. Sprint High Knee	.45 kilo	15 sec.	1	2½ minutes
5. Side Raise	.45 kilo	10	1	3 sets of 25 reps
6. Squeeze	.45 kilo	10	1	
7. Jog Easy	.45 kilo	30 sec.		4 minutes

1. Do 10 repetitions in each exercise using .45 kilo Sanbags, add 1 repetition per day till you reach 25.
2. When you reach 1 set of 25 repetitions with .45 kilo Sanbags, then add another set of 10 repetitions till you reach 25 reps. Continue till you reach your goal of 3 sets of 25 repetitions.
3. In the Sprint High Knee add 15 seconds per week till you reach 2½ minutes; in the Jog Easy, add 1 minute per week till you reach 4 minutes.
4. Remember, TRAIN, DON'T STRAIN, go at your own pace.
5. You may go on to the .91 kilo Sanbags if you see that the exercise is too light or when you reach 3 sets of 25 repetitions.

THE PERFECT TEN

Warm-up: The "Big Four"

Exercise	Wt.	Reps.			Sets	Goals
		B*	I	A		
1. Alt. Curl & Press	.45 kilo	10	12	15	1	3 sets of 25 reps. in each exercise
2. Twist	.45 kilo	10	12	15	1	
3. High Bent Elbow Touch	.45 kilo	10	12	15	1	
4. Slalom	.45 kilo	10	12	15	1	
5. Press Up, Out & Front	.45 kilo	10	12	15	1	
6. Alt. Knee Up & Out	.45 kilo	10	12	15	1	
7. Upright Row w/ Front Kick	.45 kilo	10	12	15	1	
8. Windmills	.45 kilo	10	12	15	1	
9. Side Raise & Curl	.45 kilo	10	12	15	1	
10. Clock	.45 kilo	10	12	15	1	

*Beginner, Intermediate, Advanced

1. Using .45 kilo Sanbags, do 10 repetitions in each exercise, add 1 repetition per day till you reach 25.

2. When you reach 1 set of 25 repetitions with .45 kilo Sanbags, then add another set of 10 repetitions, till you reach 25 repetitions. Continue till you reach your goal of 3 sets of 25 repetitions.

3. Remember, TRAIN, DON'T STRAIN. Go at your own pace. A consistent program will produce excellent results.

4. You may go on to the .91 kilo Sanbags if you see that the exercise is too light or when you reach 3 x 25.

The Perfect Ten

Here's the FUN way to shape up, slim down, and stay healthy!!

Suggested warm-up: The "Big Four"

Sarah Sneider

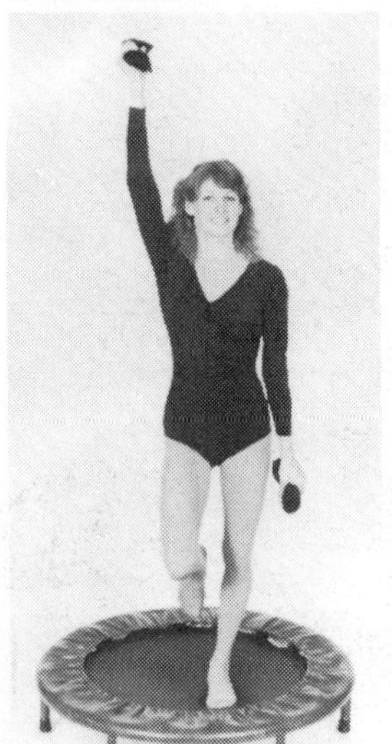

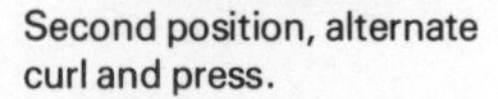

Second position, alternate curl and press.

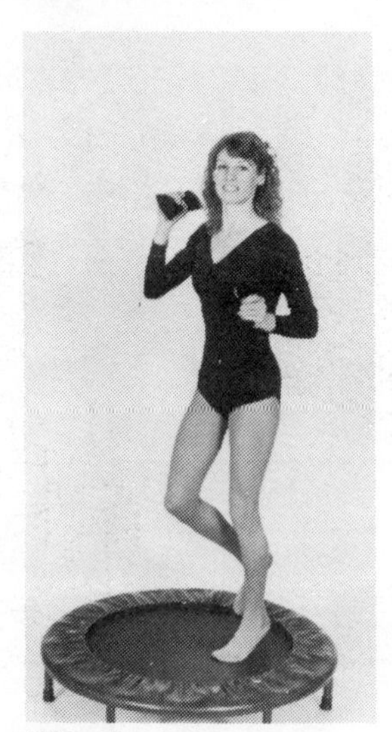

Mid-point.

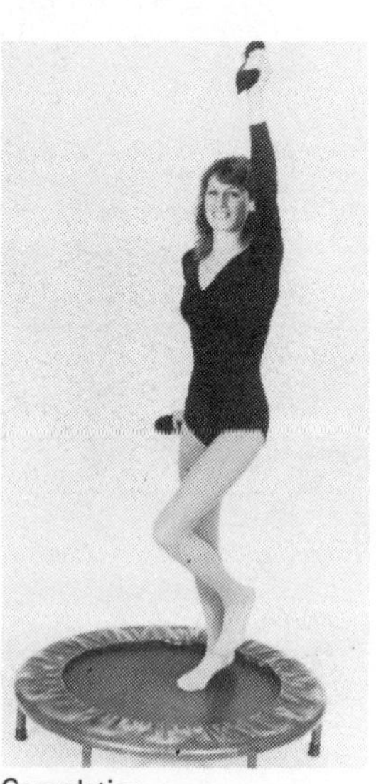

Completion.

1. ALTERNATE CURL AND PRESS

Purpose: Excellent for shaping arms, shoulders, upper back; reduces size in hips and thighs; works entire cardiovascular system (heart, lungs, and arteries).

Beginner:	10 repetitions with each arm
Intermediate:	12 repetitions with each arm
Advanced:	15 repetitions with each arm

Firmly grip your .45 kilo Sanbags in hands; jog or shuffle in the center of the mat. Begin with both Sanbags at shoulders. Push right arm overhead and left arm down at side. Return both Sanbags to shoulders. Now push left arm overhead and right arm down at sides. Continue in a rhythmic pattern.

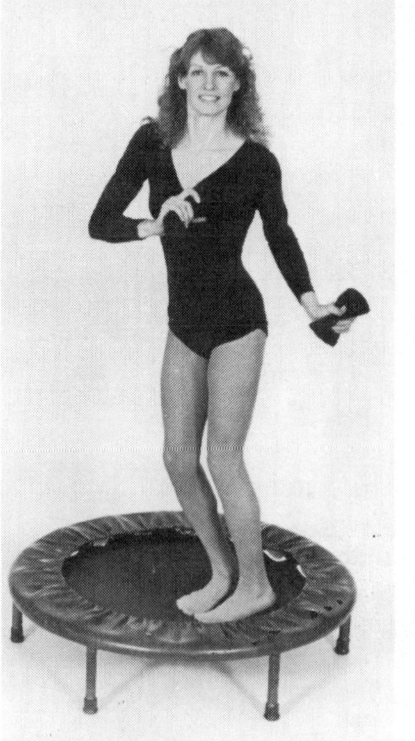

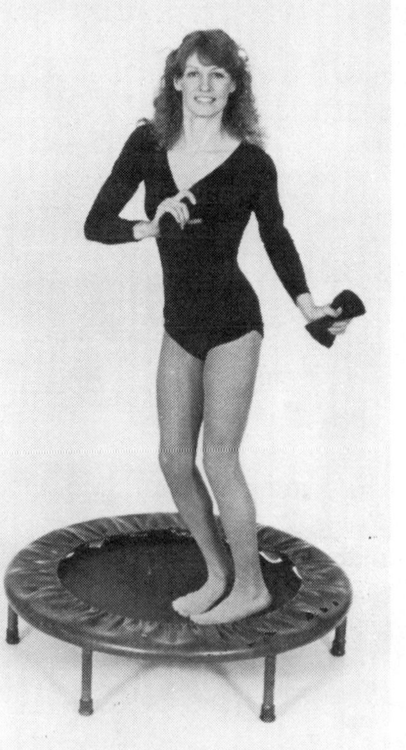

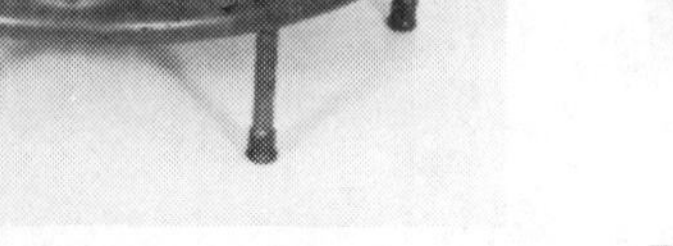

Twist

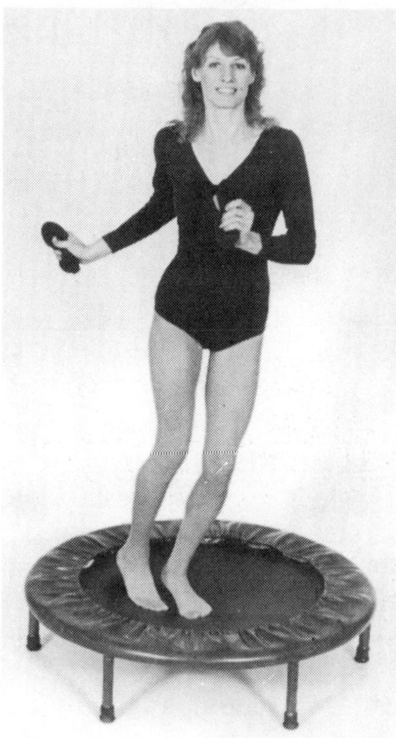

Twist

2. TWIST

Purpose: Excellent for the sides of waist, hips, thighs, forearms, and entire cardiovascular system.

Beginner:	10 repetitions (twisting to both sides counts as 1 repetition)
Intermediate:	12 repetitions
Advanced:	15 repetitions

Firmly grip your .45 kilo Sanbags in hands, center yourself in middle of mat, raise on toes, twist right to left using your arms to balance.

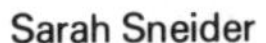

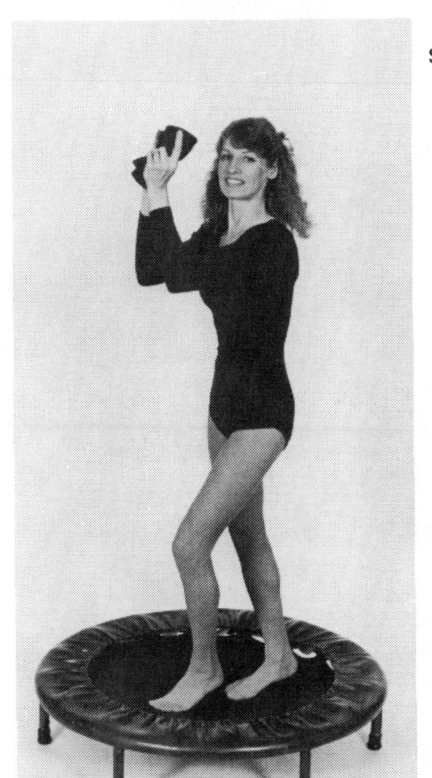
Beginning, high elbow touch.

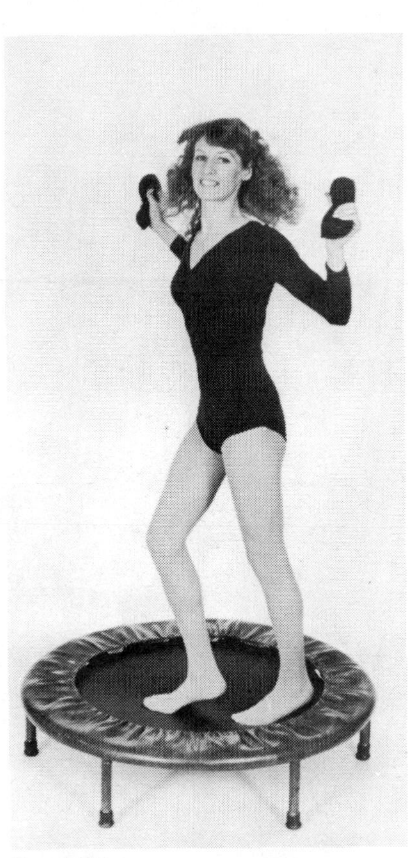
Completion.

3. HIGH BENT ELBOW TOUCH

Purpose: Terrific bust line exercise, excellent for shaping and firming upper back, shoulder, and arms, works entire cardiovascular system.

Beginner:	10 repetitions
Intermediate:	12 repetitions
Advanced:	15 repetitions

Firmly grip your .45 kilo Sanbags in hands, jog, shuffle or bounce in the center of the mat with your elbows at eye level. Start with elbows together and extend to side. Bring back to original position for each repetition.

Lynn Grimditch

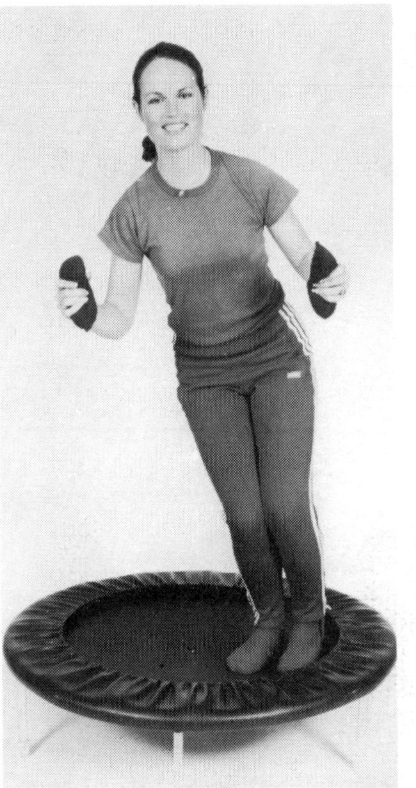
The slalom

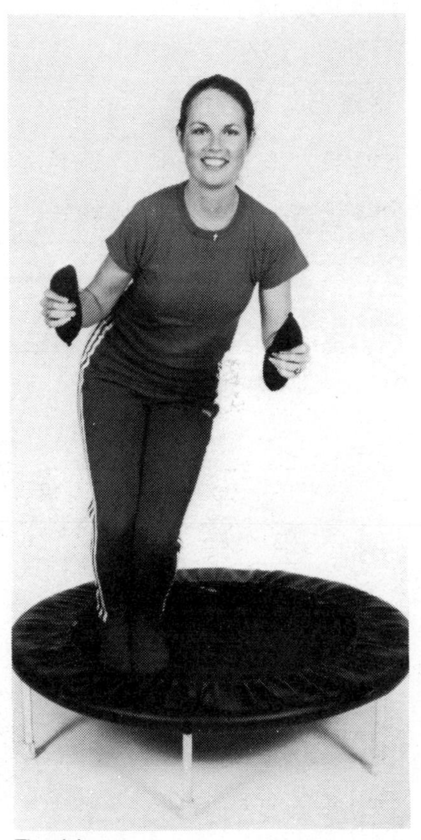
The slalom

4. THE SLALOM

Purpose: Outstanding exercise for thighs, hips and entire cardiovascular system.

Beginner:	10 repetitions
Intermediate:	12 repetitions
Advanced:	15 repetitions

Firmly grip your .45 kilo Sanbags in hands, with knees slightly bent, feet together, bounce side to side.

Sarah Sneider

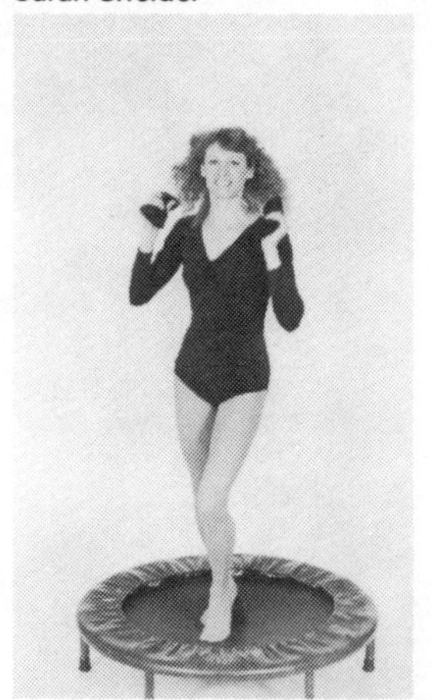

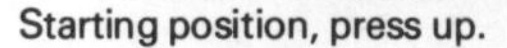

Starting position, press up.

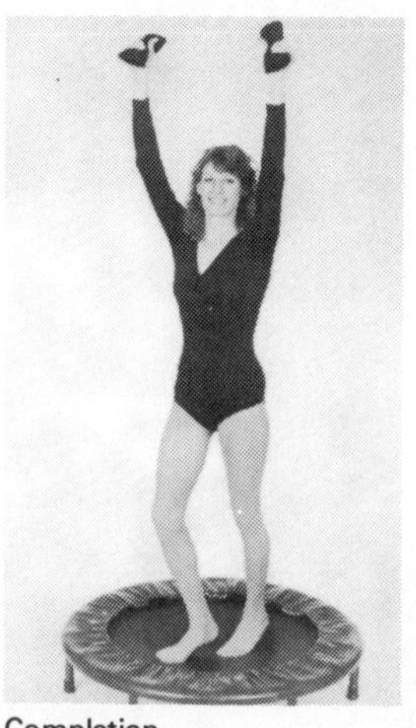

Completion.

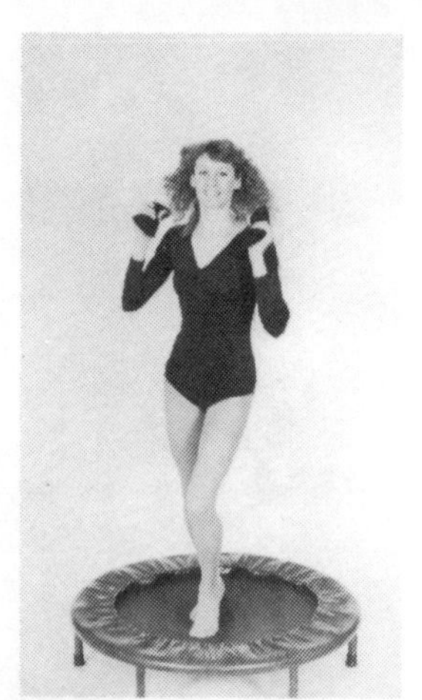

Starting position, press out.

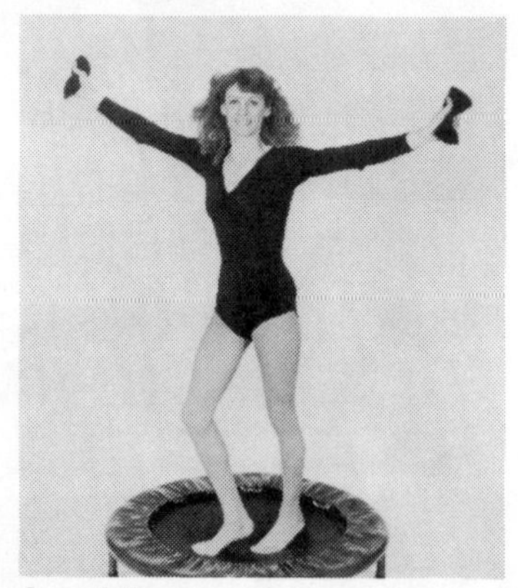

Completion.

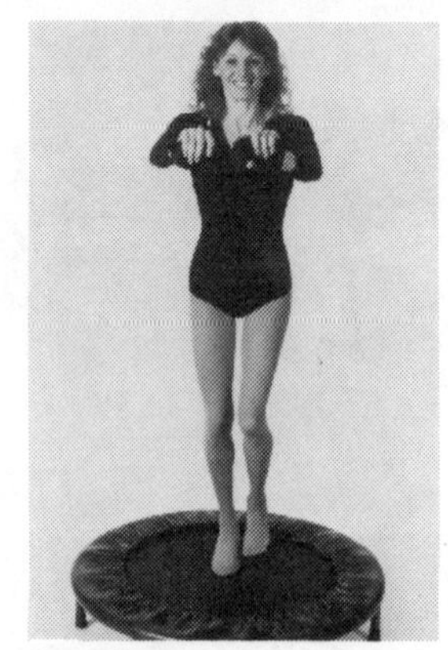

Press front.

5. PRESS UP, OUT & FRONT

Purpose: Excellent for shoulders, bust, arms, entire upper body and entire cardiovascular system.

Beginner: 8 repetitions (pressing up, out and front counts as 1 repetition)
Intermediate: 10 repetitions
Advanced: 12 repetitions

Firmly grip your .45 kilo Sanbags in hands, jog, shuffle, or bounce in the center of the mat. Pull Sanbags to shoulders, push overhead together, bring back to shoulders, now push Sanbags out to sides and bring back to shoulders, then push Sanbags out front and bring back to shoulders. Alternate by pressing overhead, pressing to the side, and pressing to the front.

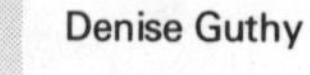

Denise Guthy

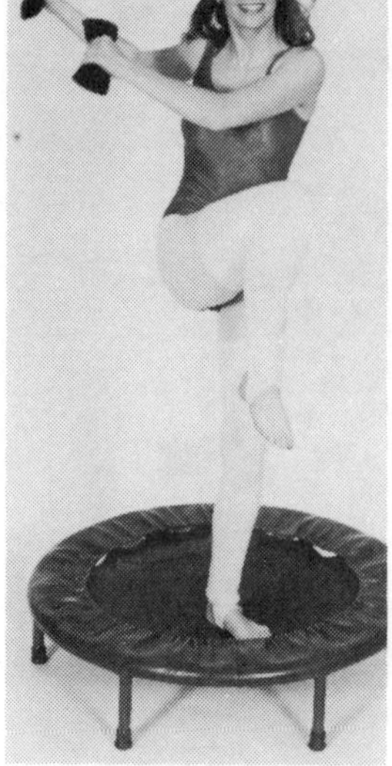

Beginning, alternate elbow to knee.

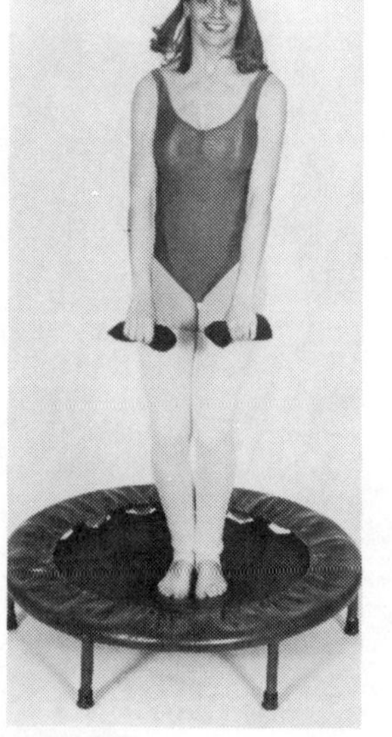

Mid-point.

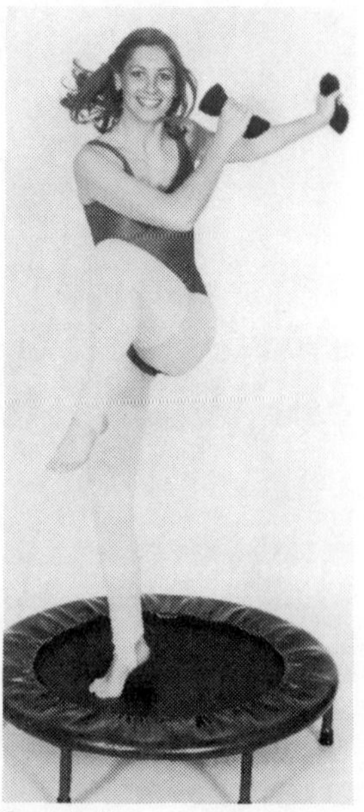

Completion.

6. ALTERNATE KNEE UP WITH ARM CURLS

Purpose: Excellent for hips, thighs, and calves. Shapes arms, firms stomach, and works entire cardiovascular system.

Beginner: 10 repetitions (right and left knee up count as 1 repetition)
Intermediate: 12 repetitions
Advanced: 15 repetitions

Firmly grip your .45 kilo Sanbags in hands. In the middle of mat, bring your right knee up to left elbow, alternate by bringing left knee to right elbow, the palms should be out.

Sarah Sneider

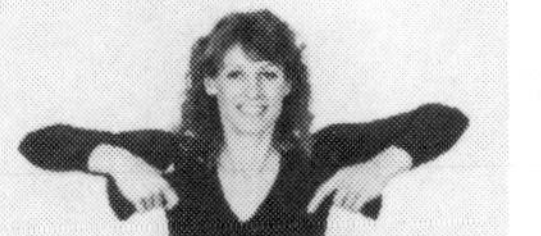

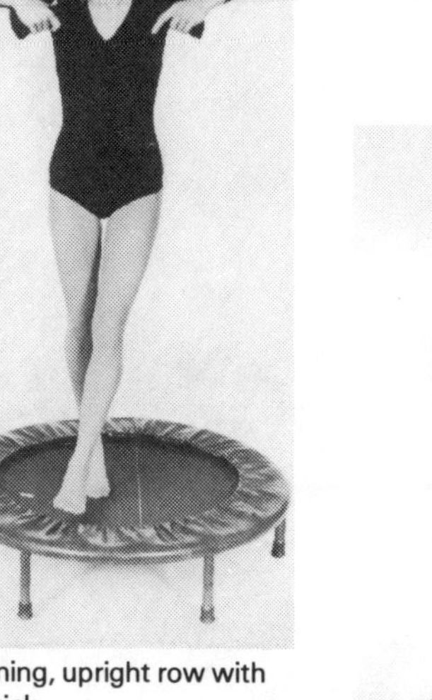

Beginning, upright row with front kick.

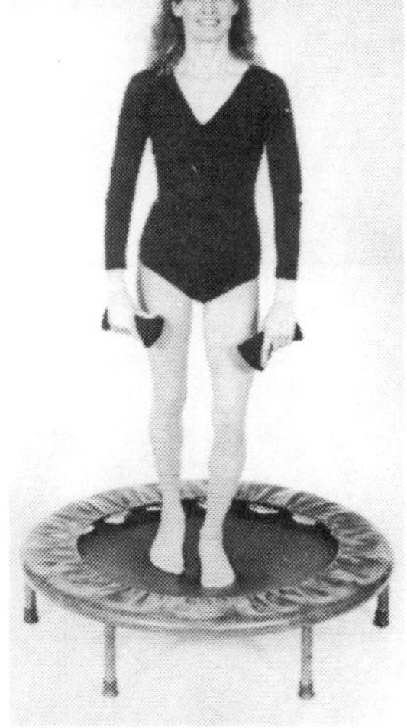

Mid-point.

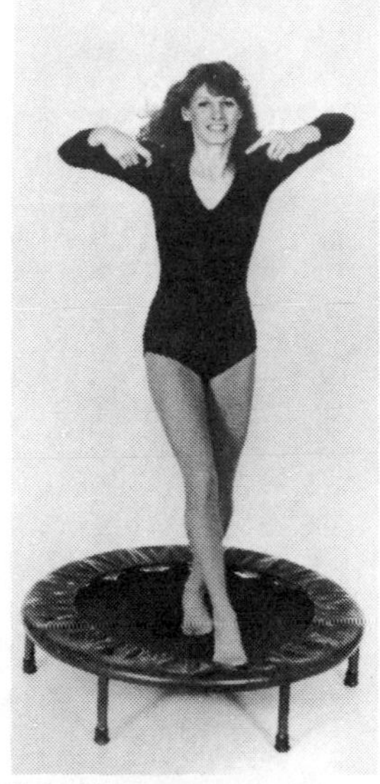

Front kick on opposite leg.

7. UPRIGHT ROW WITH FRONT KICK

Purpose: Excellent for shoulders, upper back, great for hips and thighs, works entire cardiovascular system.

Beginner:	10 repetitions (bringing Sanbags to chin; count as 1 repetition)
Intermediate:	12 repetitions
Advanced:	15 repetitions

Firmly grip your .45 kilo Sanbags in hands. Pull your hands to your chin (both together) with high elbows, while kicking right leg to front. Bounce feet together as you lower Sanbags. Now kick left leg front as you pull Sanbags to chin, lower Sanbags as you bounce feet together. Continue this pattern.

Nancy Collins

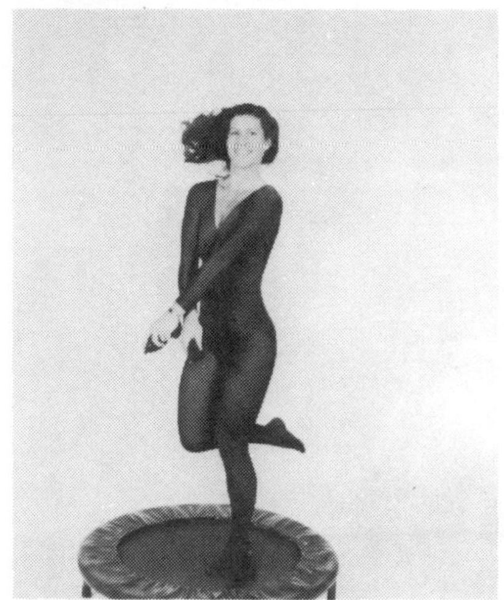

Starting position, windmill.

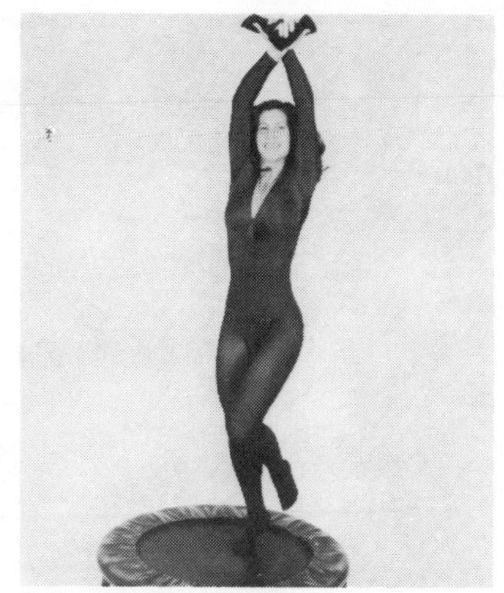

Second position.

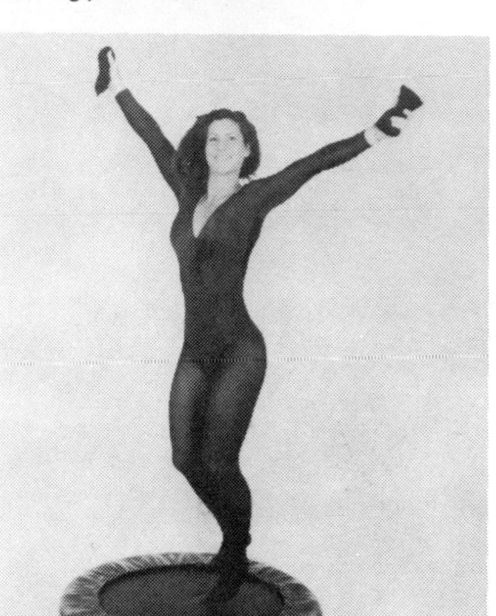

Third position.

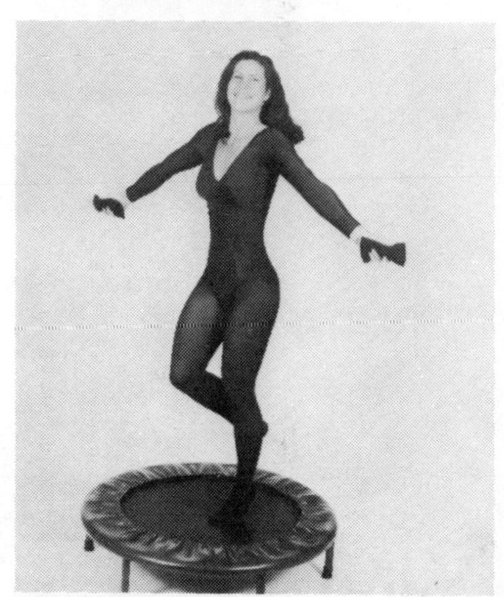

Completion.

8. WINDMILLS

Purpose: Excellent for bust, shoulders, arms, upper back, posture, entire cardiovascular system, plus hips and thighs.

Beginner:	10 repetitions
Intermediate:	12 repetitions
Advanced:	15 repetitions

Firmly grip the .45 kilo Sanbags in hands; jog, shuffle, or bounce in the center of the mat. Now, with your arms straight, make large circles with your arms, rotating your arms in an upward motion.

Lorraine Rapp

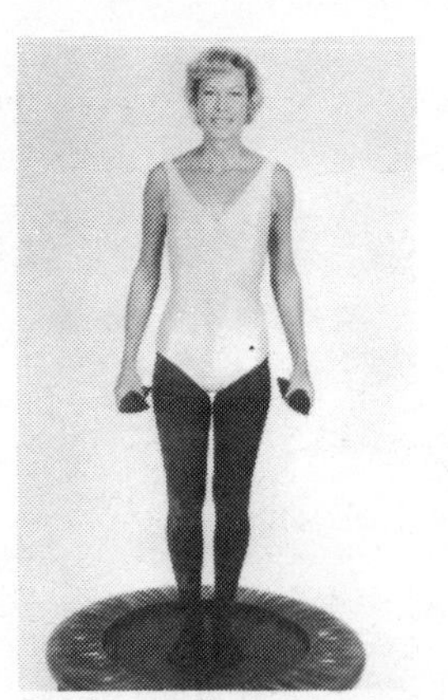

Starting position, side raise.

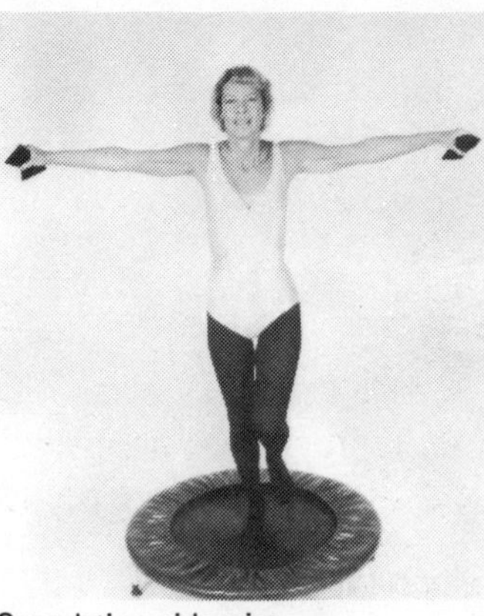

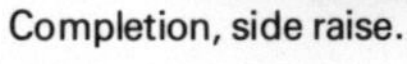

Completion, side raise.

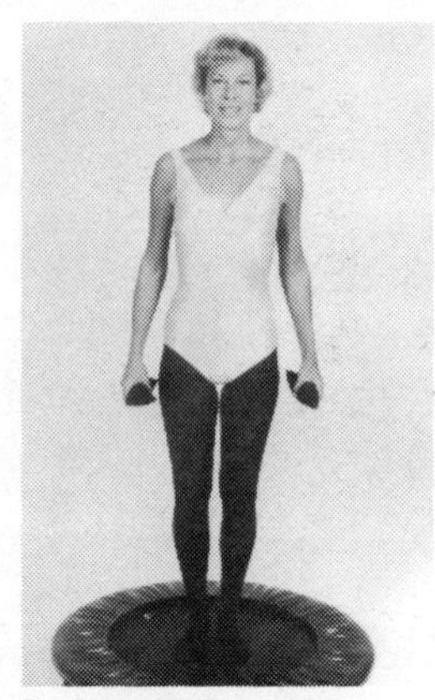

Back to starting position.

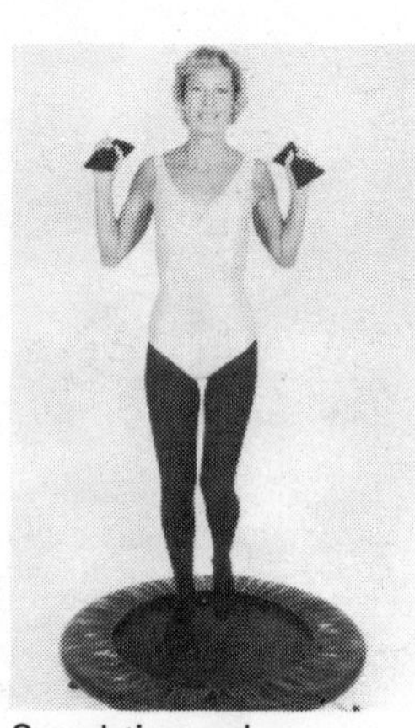

Completion, curl.

9. SIDE RAISE & CURL

Purpose: A very specific exercise for shoulders, arms, and upper back, reduces hips and thighs, works entire cardiovascular system.

Beginner:	10 repetitions
Intermediate:	12 repetitions
Advanced:	15 repetitions

Firmly grip your .45 kilo Sanbags in hands, jog, shuffle, or bounce in the center of the mat. Raise the Sanbags with straight arms to at least shoulder level, without bending your elbows, and then let them back down to your sides again. Now, bending your elbows, bring Sanbags to your shoulders and then back down. Repeat this pattern.

Nancy Collins

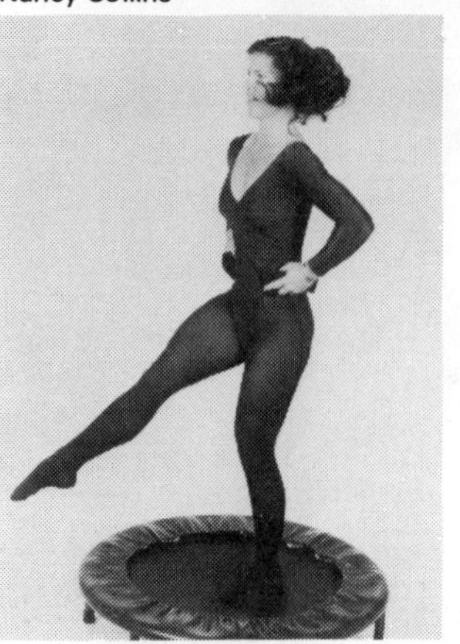

First turn of the clock.

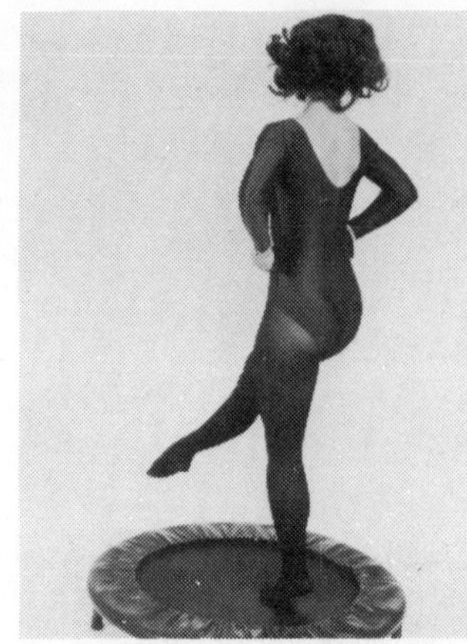

Low kick to front, turning on mat.

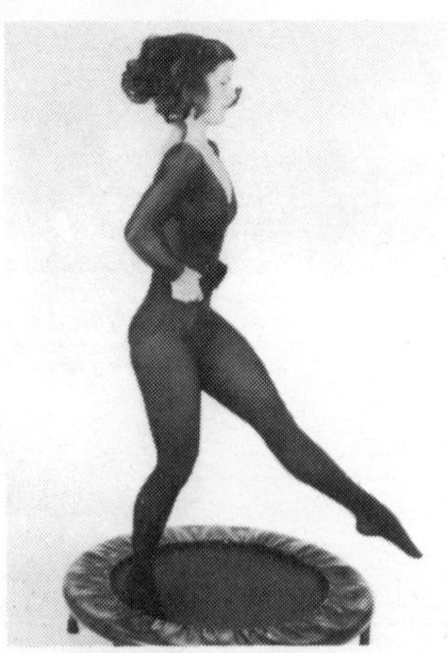

Continue to turn on mat.

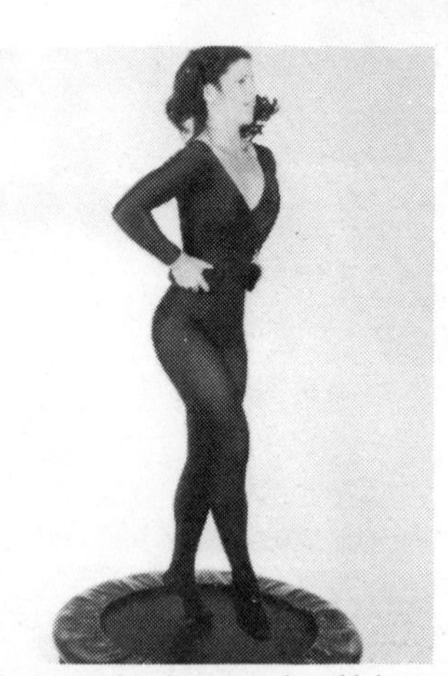

Feet together between low kicks to front.

10. CLOCK

Purpose: Great warm down exercise, works hips and thighs, too.

Beginner:	10 repetitions (Right and left alternate kick front counts as one repetition)
Intermediate:	12 repetitions
Advanced:	15 repetitions

Firmly grip .45 kilo Sanbags in hands. Start with both feet together bounce in middle of mat, with straight leg kick right leg front, bounce both legs together, then turn slightly and kick left leg front. As you turn around mat alternate right and left kicks to the front. Hold Sanbags in hands on hips.

You may enjoy combining several programs. For instance, begin by warming up with the "Big Four," do 1 set of the "Daily Dozen," then 1 set of the "Perfect Ten," then 10-12 minutes of Dance'n Bounce routines (See Chapter 12). Total time: approximately 20 minutes.

Or some of you may prefer doing one program in the morning, another in the evening. Either way you will benefit greatly. Strive for consistency, that is, EVERY day. As you reach your goal of 15-20 minutes per day, you will see fantastic results!

Other Mat Exercises:

There are literally dozens of exercises that can be done on your rebound mat while you are seated, on your back or on your hands and knees as well. As you can see, your rebound unit is extremely versatile! Here are just a few suggestions to get you started:

HIP ROLLS

Lynn Grimditch

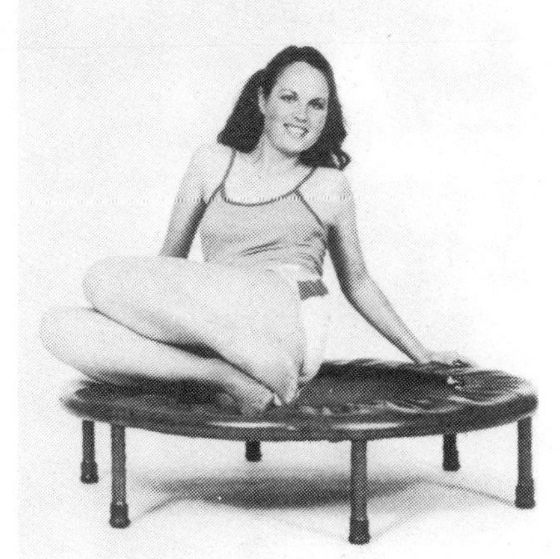

Hip roll to right.

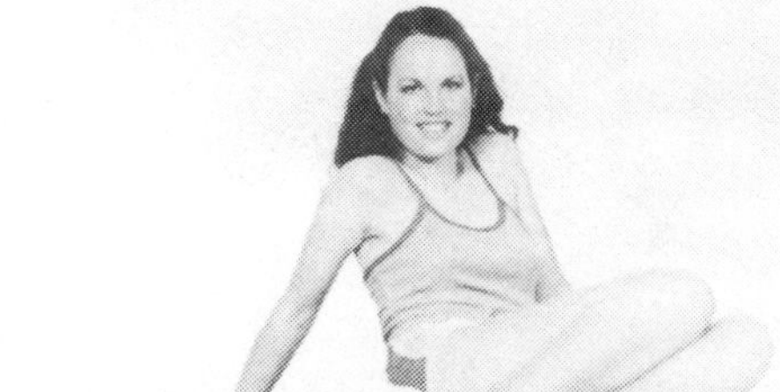

Hip roll to left.

Sit on mat, draw knees to chest, lean back on buttocks and rest on arms. Now, roll hips to left side, then roll to right, swinging knees up and over. Do ten rolls to each side.

BICYCLE

Lynn Grimditch

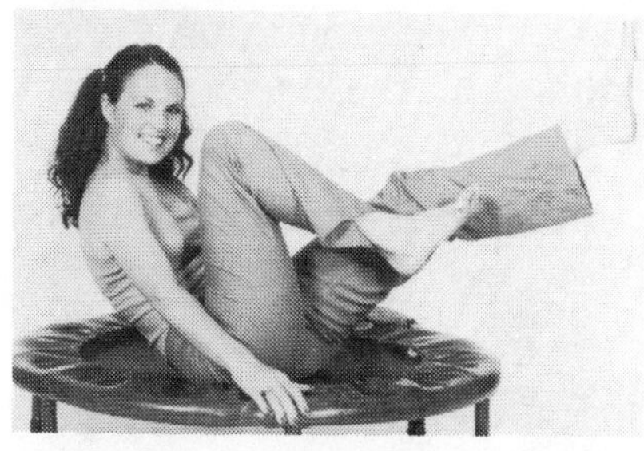

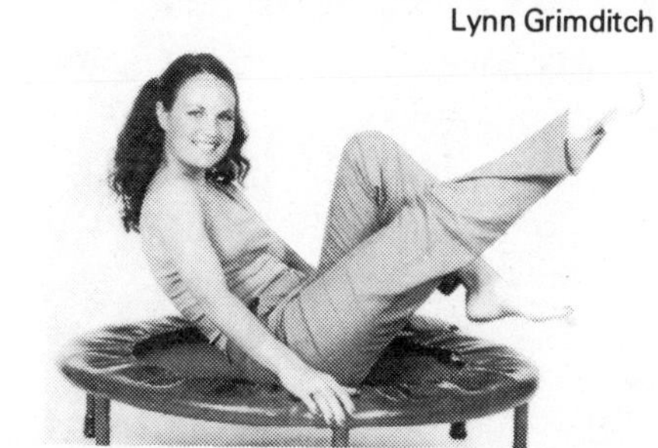

Sitting on mat, lean back on buttocks and rest on arms. Bend right and left leg alternately to "pedal" 10 times.

HYDRANT SIDE

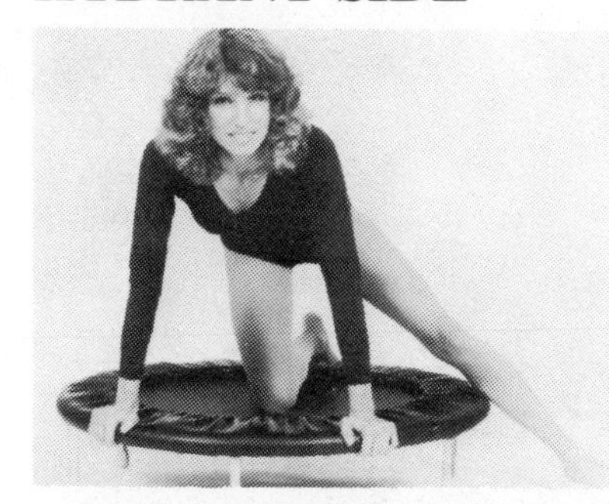

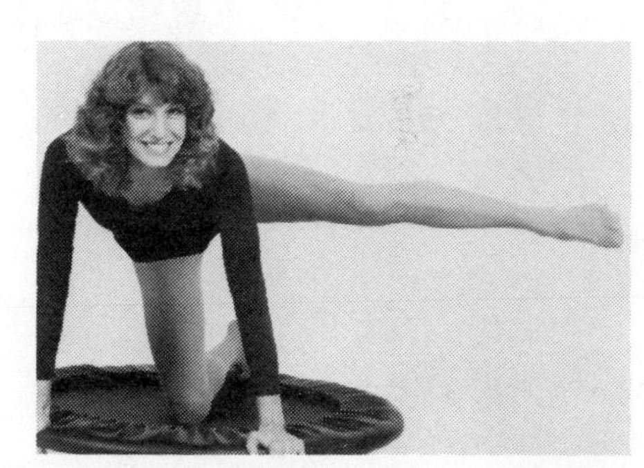

Begin on hands and knees. Keep back straight. Now raise left leg and lower back to floor. Raise 10 times. Repeat on right side.

HYDRANT BACK

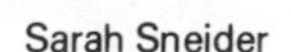

Sarah Sneider

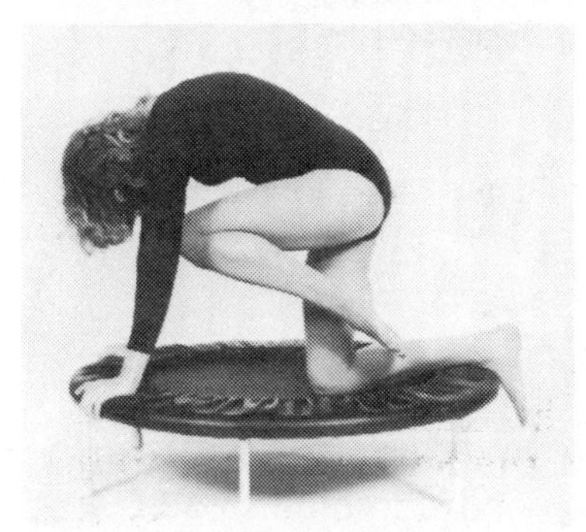

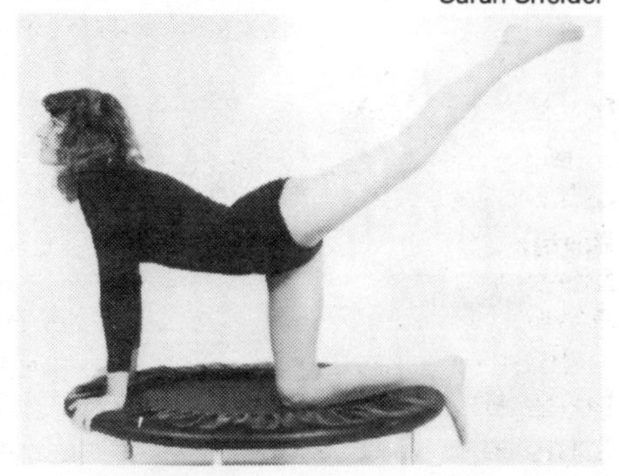

Begin on hands and knees. Begin left knee to chin, lowering head. Then, kick left leg back and up, keeping leg straight, arch back, and raise head. Do 10 times, repeat right side.

Exercises For Pregnancy

It is so very important to be in good physical condition during pregnancy. If your doctor gives permission, these exercises are designed to help you become strong and physically fit for carrying and delivering your baby. Exercising during pregnancy will also give you a lot more confidence at the time of delivery. These exercises will help you gain good muscle tone for regaining your figure after birth as well.

Be sure to ask your doctor if there is any reason why you should not do these exercises during the early months of pregnancy.

CROSSOVER WITH SQUAT

Robin J. Morelli, former cheerleader, mother-to-be

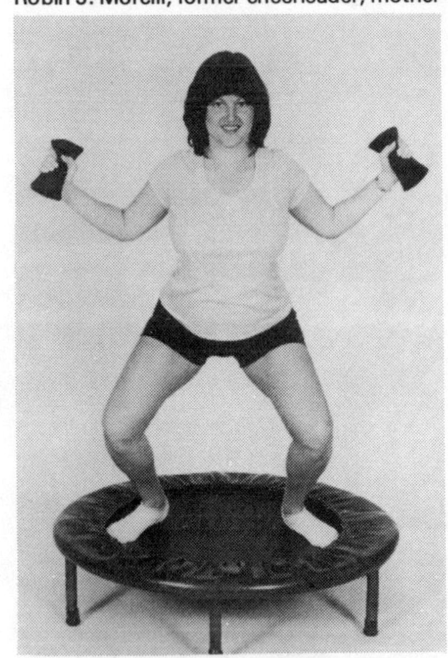

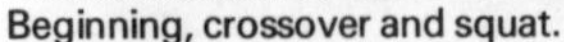

Beginning, crossover and squat.

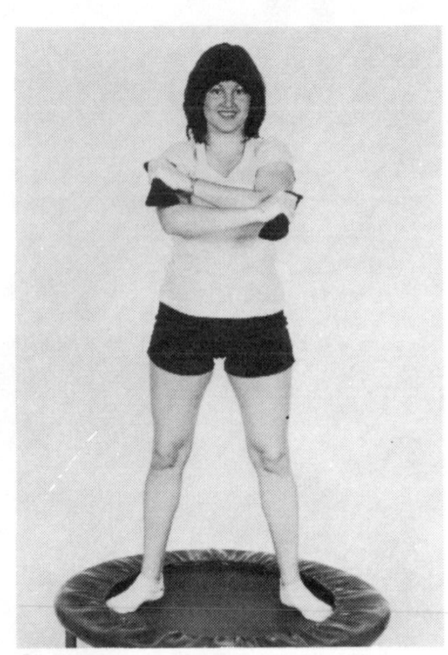

Completion.

With .45 kilo Sanbags in hands, standing on mat, squat partially down. Bend elbows slightly in front of face, hug yourself with Sanbags. Return to standing position. Squat again. Alternate right hand over left hand, then next repetition left hand over right hand. Do 10 times.

PELVIC ROCK

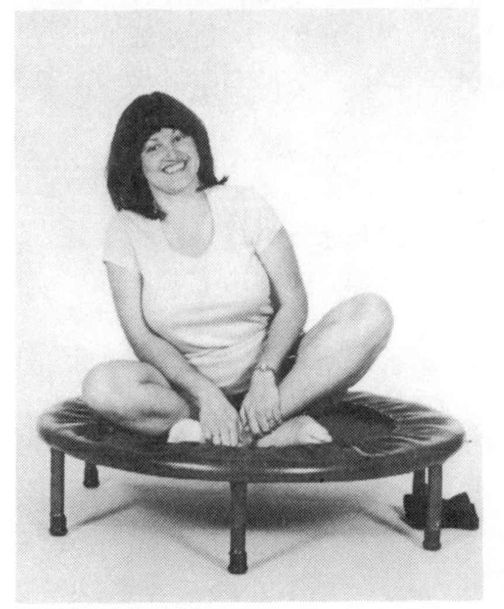

Pelvic rock to right.

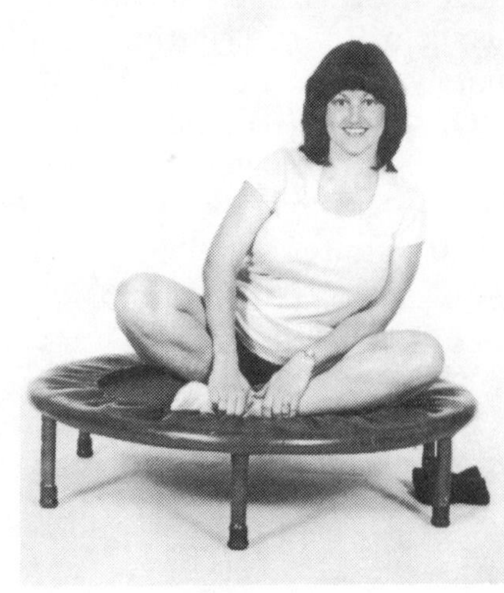

To left.

Sit on mat, legs crossed. Rock to right, rock to left. Rock 25 times.

BACK ARCH

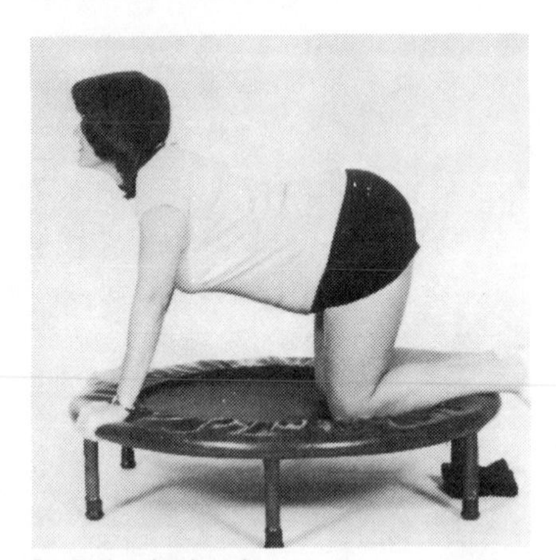

Beginning, back arch.

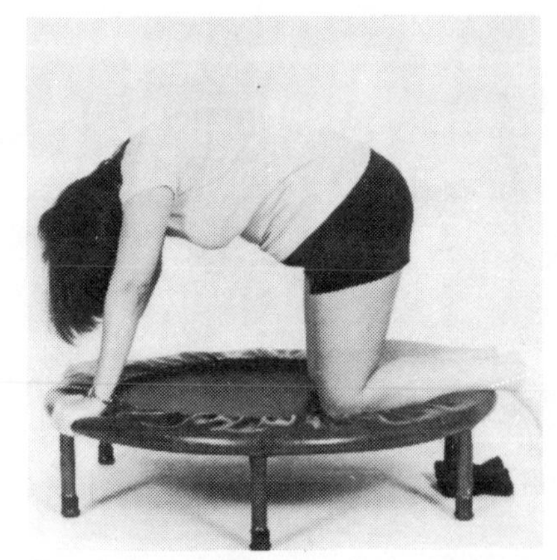

Completion.

On hands and knees, arch your back as high as you can, then lower. Repeat 10 times.

JOG EASY

Robin Morelli

The jog easy.

Hold .45 kilo Sanbags in hands. Knees are higher than a walk. Swing arms keeping elbows high. An easy rhythmic jog. Jog 3 minutes.

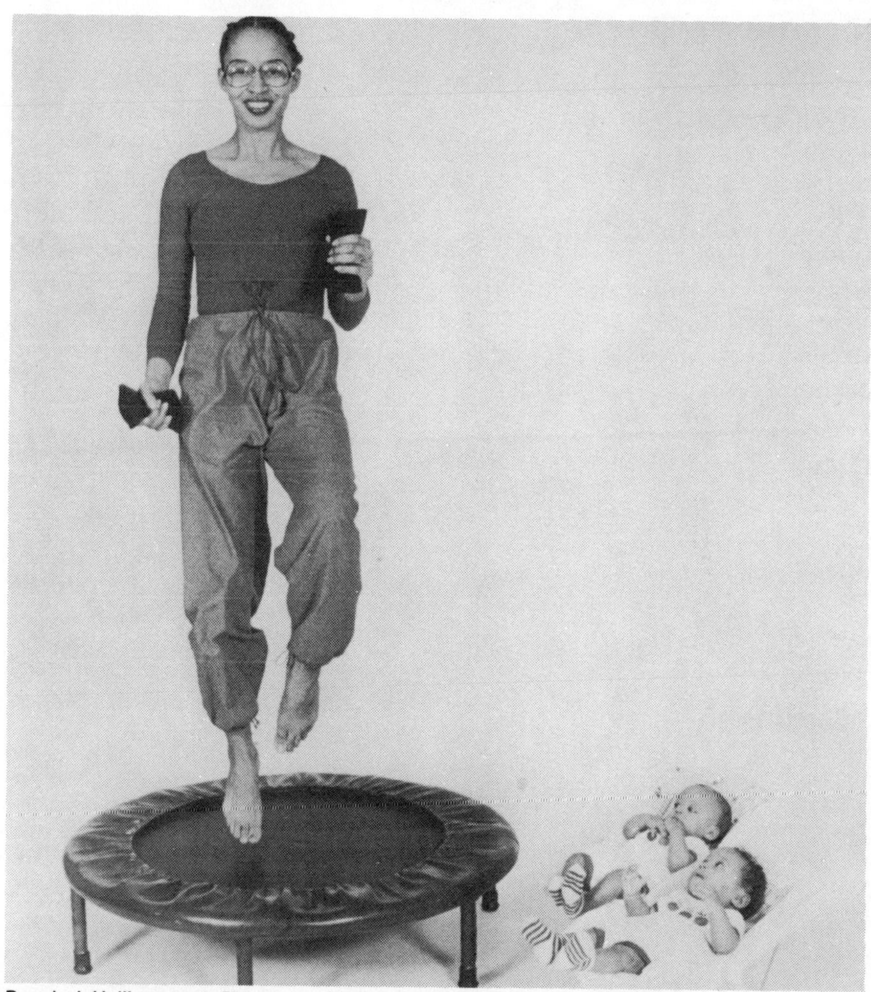

Brenda J. Hollingsworth-Pickett Jr., dancer, martial artist, with 4-month-old twin daughters, Akilah Nayo and Eshe Nayo. Demonstrably, rebound exercise and "sitting" go together.

After The Baby:

After birth, Sanbagging is your most convenient form of exercise to regain your shape and maintain fitness. You will not have to spend time away from the baby traveling to a spa or exercise class. Your Sanbagging program can be right in your own living room.

Check with your doctor to see when it is all right for you to begin. Start with the "Big Four" and move on to the "Daily Dozen" as you progress.

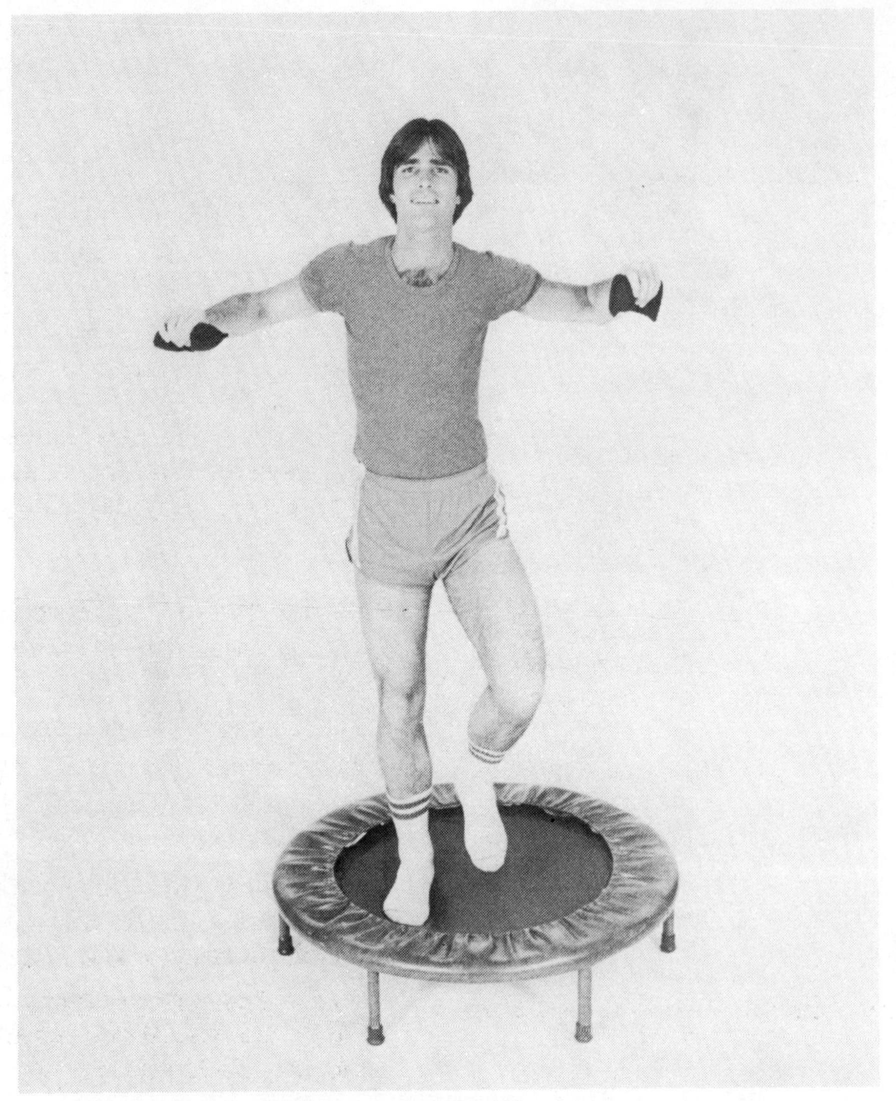

T.J. McCavitt shows mid-point of crossover (see page 46).

Chapter 9

Program for Men

Ten to fifteen minutes of Sanbagging will increase your total health for years to come! Your critical years of helping your family, business, or your church depends on your being in excellent health.

Sanbagging on your rebound unit can truly be a most desirable activity. The brief 10-15 minutes per day can help you feel better, lose inches in your hips and thighs and achieve overall health. Sanbagging is your program for the office, home, or recreation center. In my work as executive fitness director in the fitness centers, I have found remarkable improvement with Sanbagging.

Begin with the "Big Four" as a groundwork for a wonderful fitness program. Sanbagging while jogging on your rebound unit adds that extra dimension that is missing in your running program: total body development. Most people who jog develop the legs, lungs and the heart, but neglect upper body development. Sanbagging will develop your shoulders, chest, arms, upper back, forearms, calves, and you won't lose any of the precious cardio-respiratory fitness you are seeking. Try this very basic program.

CAUTION: A physical exam is recommended before beginning any exercise program.

BEGINNERS: Individuals who are overweight by 10 to 100 pounds, out of condition, or who have used a rebound unit for one month or less.

INTERMEDIATE: Those who have used a rebound unit for at least one month and whose resting heart rate is 60-80 beats per minute.

ADVANCED: Individuals who have jogged at least one mile per day, whose resting pulse is 40-65 beats per minute, or who have used their rebound unit for three months or more.

THE BIG FOUR

(Adult Men)

Exercise	Wt.	Time (Secs.)			Sets			Goals		
		B*	I	A	B	I	A	B	I	A
1. Lymphatic Bounce	.45 kilo	10	30	45	1	2	3	8	10	12 to 15 Sets
2. Shuffle	.45 kilo	10	30	45	1	2	3	8	10	12 to 15 Sets
3. Jog	.45 kilo	10	30	45	1	2	3	8	10	12 to 15 Sets
4. Bounce	.45 kilo	10	30	45	1	2	3	8	10	12 to 15 Sets

*B — Beginner, I — Intermediate, A — Advanced

Add one set in each category every week till you reach your goal, leave seconds the same. Work out every day. Add Sanbag weight every thirty days till you reach 1.36 kilo Sanbags.

Rules for Sanbagging Success

1. Start with the .45 kilo Sanbags in your hands, squeezing firmly.

2. Remember, if you are overweight, check with your doctor to make sure it is okay for you to exercise.

3. For the beginner, easy does it, don't get carried away. Start with only 10 seconds in each exercise.

4. Monitor your pulse with 6 second checks (Chapter 2). Try not to work over double resting pulse rate in the first month. Example: Resting Pulse, 70; Double Resting is 140.

5. The key is **consistency.** Try to do these at least 5 days a week for best results. Work up to 8 sets for beginners, 10 sets for moderate, 12-15 sets for advanced.

The "Big Four" done daily will add so much to your day. You can do this in your own bedroom first thing in the morning. Set some goals for yourself by watching your diet, you can lose inches in the right places with this program. You will truly enjoy this painless activity. Compared to jogging, this program is pure delight on the joints and helps you to develop the upper body, too.

THE DAILY DOZEN PROGRAM FOR ADULT MEN

Beginning Program

Suggested Warm-up: The "Big Four"

Exercise	Wt.	Reps/Time	Sets	Goals
1. Curl	.45 kilo	10	1	3 x 25 with 1.36 kilo Sanbags
2. Press	.45 kilo	10	1	
3. Upright Row	.45 kilo	10	1	
4. Tricep Press	.45 kilo	10	1	
5. Squeeze	.45 kilo	10	1	
6. Curl & Press	.45 kilo	10	1	
7. Side Raise	.45 kilo	10	1	
8. Crossover	.45 kilo	10	1	
9. Sprint High Knee	.45 kilo	15 sec.	1	Add 10 sec. per week till reach 2½ min.
10. Press Up & Out	.45 kilo	10	1	3 x 25 with 1.36 kilo Sanbags.
11. Pullover	.45 kilo	10	1	
12. Jog Easy	.45 kilo	30 sec.	1	Add 30 sec. per week till reach 8 min.

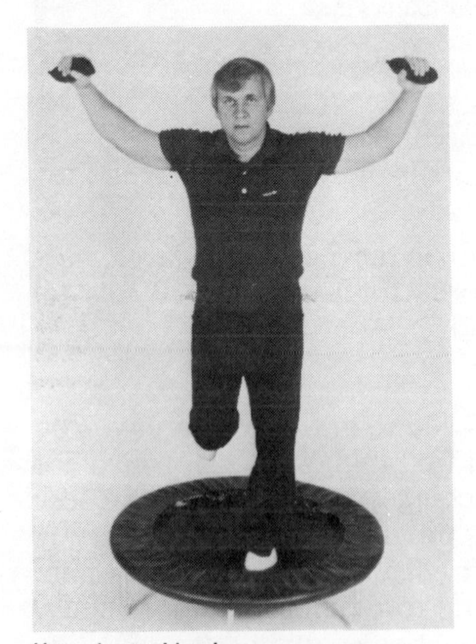

Harry shows side raise.

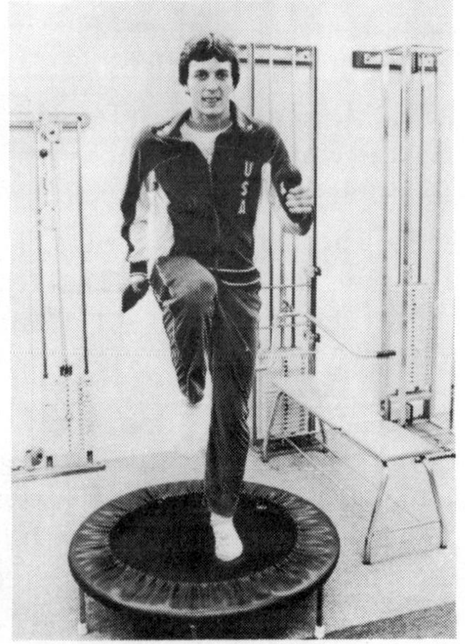

Kenny Sutton, sprint high knee.

1. Suggested beginner's program: Using .45 kilo Sanbags, do 10 repetitions in each exercise, add 1 rep. per day till you reach 25.
2. When you reach 1 set of 25 repetitions with .45 kilo Sanbags, then add another set of 10 repetitions, till you reach 25 reps. Continue this till you reach 3 sets of 25 reps, go on to the .91 Sanbags only if you see that the exercise is light or when you reach 3 x 25.
3. Remember, these resistance exercises can be done by shuffling, jogging, or bouncing. Suggested for beginners is the easy jog while doing these exercises.
4. Your goal is to work up to 3 x 25 with each exercise using the 1.36 kilo Sanbags.
5. Easy Jog and Sprint High Knee: Start with 30 seconds per day Easy Jog and 15 seconds in High Knee Sprint. Your goal is 2½ minutes High Knee Sprint and 8 minutes Easy Jog.
6. If you are overweight and have not had a physical or feel tired, check with your doctor before embarking on a program.

The key to your success is GOALS. Set a goal that you would want to weigh. Put a 3 x 5 index card near your mirror where you can look at that figure every morning. Resolve that you will get there by watching your diet. A consistent program like Sanbagging with the "Daily Dozen" will get you there so much quicker than a haphazard program. You will be doing your family a favor by staying in shape. You are needed on your job. You are made to succeed, it's up to you, **so do it!**

Modified Program For Adult Men

A modified program for you who may be in a hurry or have very little time would look like this:

THE BIG FOUR

Exercise	
1. Lymphatic Bounce	Use .45 kilo Sanbags, start with 10 seconds a day each exercise, add 10 sec. every three days in each exercise till you work up to the following.
2. Shuffle	
3. Jog	
4. Sprint	Lymphatic Bounce, 2 min.; Shuffle, 3 min.; Jog, 4 min.; Sprint, 2 min. TOTAL: 11 min.

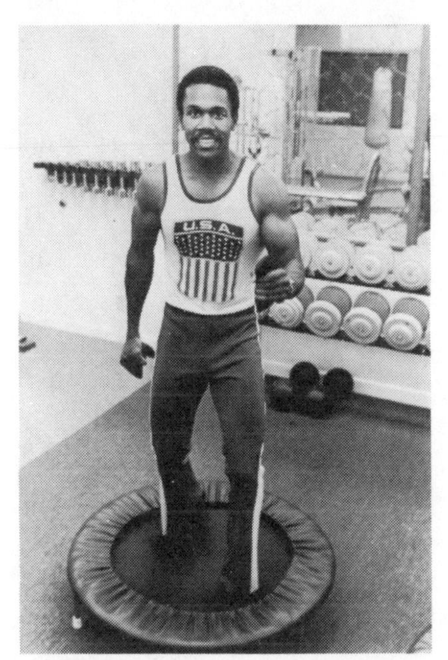

Hainsley L. Best Jr., champion body builder and gymnast, demonstrates the shuffle (page 46).

SANBAG RESISTANCE PROGRAM

Exercise	
1. Curl & Press	Do 10 reps in each exercise, add 1 repetition per day till you reach 25. Add .91 kilo Sanbags after you reach 25 reps, then 1.36 Sanbags after that.
2. Side Raise	
3. Pullover	
4. Sprint High Knee	Start with 10 seconds, add 10 seconds per day till you reach 2 minutes.

You can do these two programs together or separately.

Try these programs when you are feeling tense. Many executives, salesmen, teachers, etc. can do these right in their offices. You owe it to yourself to keep in shape mentally as well as physically. Try this program and you will see a difference in your attitude for the rest of the day.

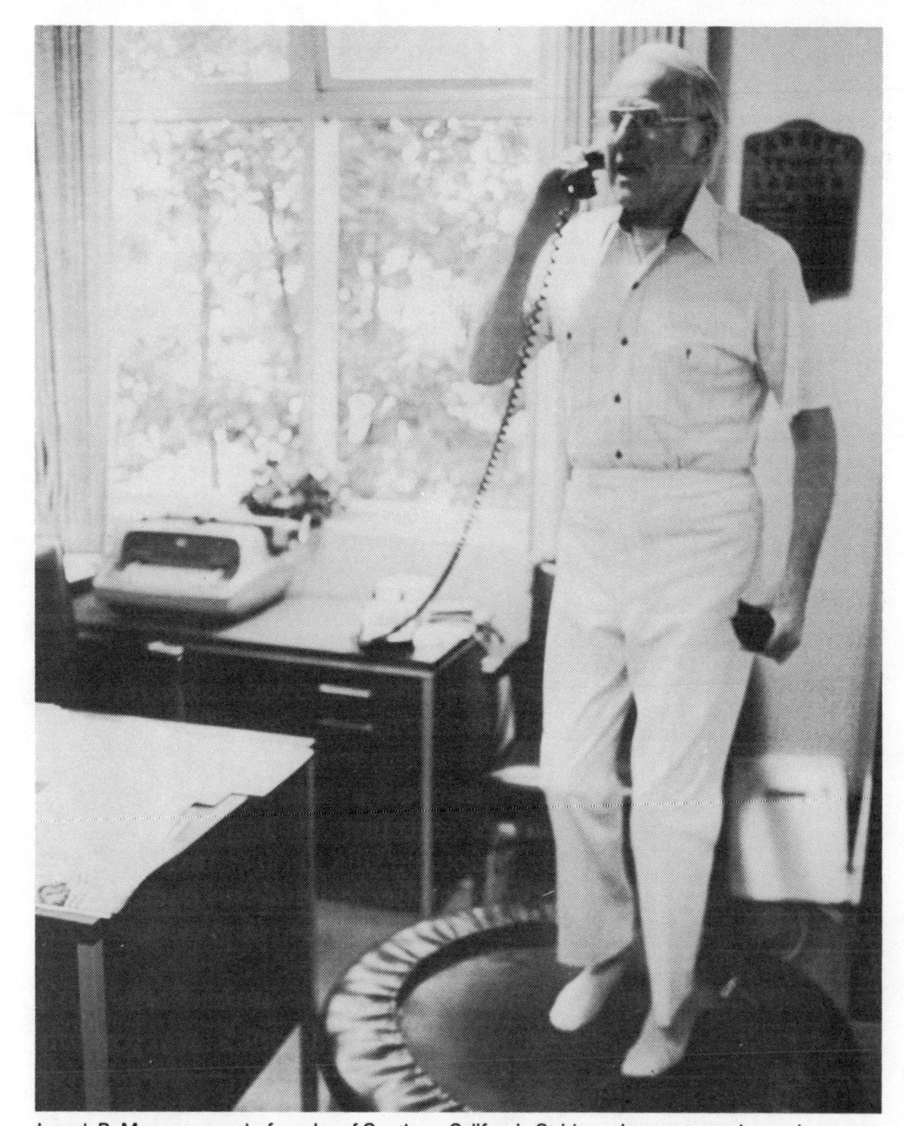

Joseph R. Mangan, coach, founder of Southern California Striders, demonstrates how a busy executive can conduct business and keep in shape simultaneously.

Many of my closest friends are putting this program to the test right in their office and finding they don't need that extra coffee or martini. You can even conduct business on your phone while you are doing this program with the telephone in one hand and a .45 kilo Sanbag in the other.

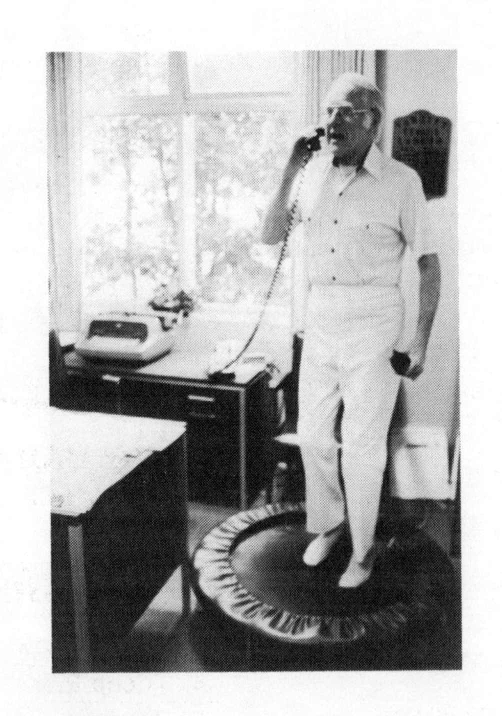

Chapter 10

For Men and Women 55 Plus

Who want to feel really good

There is a wonderful saying: "With age there comes wisdom."

You are being very wise if you take care of your health. There is much wisdom in using a Sanbag program in your exercise picture. As we age, we lose some of our strength, endurance and coordination. You will be surprised how much you will retain if you start the simple program that is outlined here. I have a number of amazing specimens of health in our fitness centers, people in their sixties and seventies. They are vigorous, happy and carrying right body weight — because they **exercise every day.** They are consistent in their program.

The "Big Four" will help you to feel better no matter what your age. Start that positive health habit today. You may increase your life by 10, 20 or 30 years.

CAUTION: A physical exam is recommended before beginning any exercise program.

THE BIG FOUR FOR 55 + MEN & WOMEN

Exercise	Wt.	Time	Sets	Goals
		B* I A	B* I A	B*I A
1. Lymphatic Bounce	.45 kilo	10 - 20 - 30 sec.	2 - 4 - 6 to 10	6 10 15 sets
2. Shuffle	.45 kilo	10 - 20 - 30 sec.	2 - 4 - 6 to 10	
3. Jog Easy	.45 kilo	10 - 20 - 45 sec.	2 - 4 - 6 to 10	
4. Sprint	.45 kilo	10 - 20 - 30 sec.	2 - 4 - 6 to 10	

*B — Beginner, I — Intermediate, A — Advanced

BEGINNER: Has not exercised in months.
INTERMEDIATE: Occasional exercise, has used rebound unit 1-2 months.
ADVANCED: Jogger (1-3 miles), has worked out regularly on rebound unit.

1. Use .45 kilo Sanbags in hands; if they become too light after 1 month, go on to the .91 kilo Sanbags.
2. Start with 10 seconds in each position, add 10 seconds per week.
3. Those of you already in good shape, start with 4 sets of each exercise a day until you work up to 10 sets in each position.
4. Regular joggers, swimmers, cyclists, etc., those advanced, may start at 1 minute in each position, add 15 seconds per day, work up to 5 minutes in each position.

THE BIG FOUR MODIFIED PROGRAM FOR 55 +

This Modified Program Will Bring Excellent Results

Modify the "Big Four" program by doing the Lymphatic Bounce **only** up to 3 minutes by starting with ten seconds, and adding 10 seconds each day. The same can be done with the other exercises. You can split up the routine by doing two exercises in the morning and two at night. I would encourage you to be consistent at least once a day if you are to improve.

THE DAILY DOZEN FOR 55 + MEN AND WOMEN

Suggested Warm-up: "The Big Four"

Exercise	Wt.	Reps/Time	Sets	Goals
1. Curl	.45 kilo	10	1	You can work up to as many as 6 sets of 10 with 1.36 kilo Sanbags
2. Press	.45 kilo	10	1	
3. Upright Row	.45 kilo	10	1	
4. Tricep Press	.45 kilo	10	1	
5. Squeeze	.45 kilo	10	1	
6. Curl & Press	.45 kilo	10	1	
7. Side Raise	.45 kilo	10	1	
8. Crossovers	.45 kilo	10	1	
9. Sprint High Knee	.45 kilo	10	1	2½ minutes
10. Press Up & Out	.45 kilo	10	1	6 sets of 10 with 1.36 kilo Sanbags
11. Pullover	.45 kilo	10	1	
12. Jog Easy	.45 kilo	10	1	8 minutes

1. Add 1 set of 10 reps on each exercise till you reach 6 sets.
2. Add to Sanbag weight every month if possible till you reach 1.36 kilo Sanbags.

3. Add 10 seconds on the Sprint High Knee every 3 days till you reach 2½ minutes.

4. Add 30 seconds on the Jog Easy every three days till you reach 8 minutes.

THE MODIFIED PROGRAM FOR 55+ BEGINNERS

Men and Women

Exercise	Wt.	Reps/Time	Sets	Goals
1. Lymphatic Bounce	.45 kilo	10 sec	1	2 minutes with 1.36 kilo Sanbags
2. Jog Easy	.45 kilo	10 sec	1	4 minutes with 1.36 kilo Sanbags
3. Curl & Press	.45 kilo	10 sec	1	3 x 25 with 1.36 kilo Sanbags
4. Pullover	.45 kilo	10 sec	1	3 x 25 with 1.36 kilo Sanbags
5. Sprint High Knee	.45 kilo	10 sec	1	2 minutes with 1.36 kilo Sanbags
6. Shuffle	.45 kilo	10 sec	1	4 minutes with 1.36 kilo Sanbags

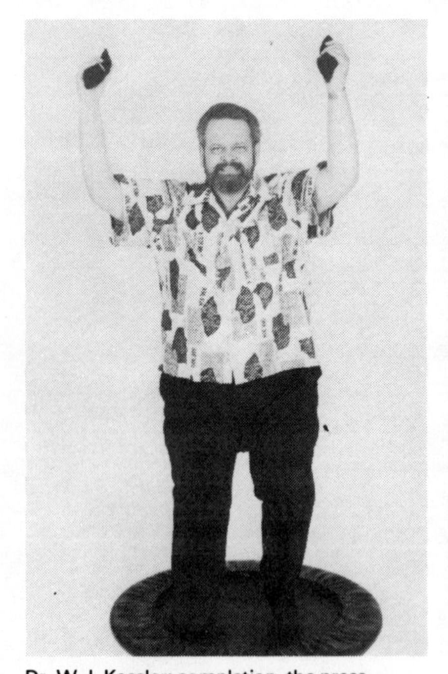

Dr. W.J. Kessler; completion, the press.

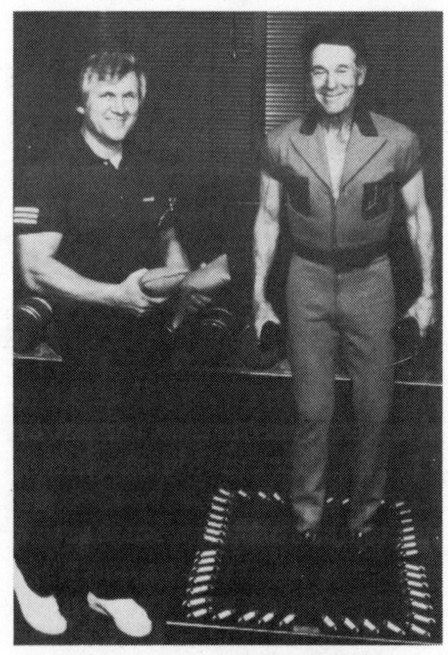

Harry, Jack LaLanne; lymphatic bounce.

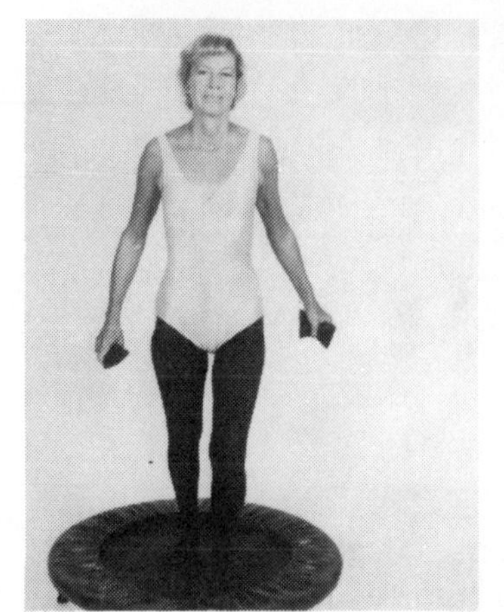

Lorraine Rapp demonstrates the lymphatic bounce.

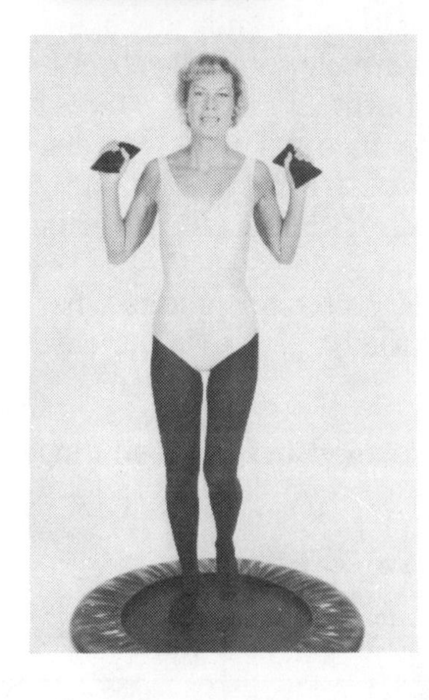

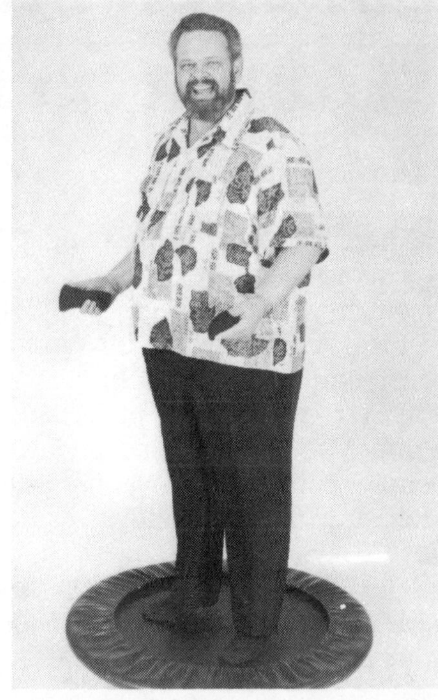

Dr. William J. Kessler, doctor of chiropractic, minister, Worldwide Church of God, demonstrates curl in men's modified program. Sanbagging enabled Dr. Kessler to drop his resting pulse from 90 to 70.

1. Work up to 1 set of 25 in Curl & Press and Pullover.

2. After you reach a set of 25, then add another set; when you reach 3 sets of 25 reps, then add to your Sanbag weight every thirty days until you reach your goals.

3. Add 10 seconds per week in each of the other exercises till you reach your goals.

4. This program can be done twice a day if it is too easy for you.

5. Try to set a goal of working out **every day** if possible.

Chapter 11

For Men and Women 70 Plus

We strongly suggest this Sanbagging program for you. It is very easy on the joints. There is excellent body toning with the light Sanbags. You need not worry about the program being too strenuous; it is much easier than jogging or weightlifting.

You may find the .45 kilo Sanbags a little heavy. If you do, use tennis balls, shoes, or wadded up sweat socks. The most important thing you can do is get started. You will have a lot of surprises in store (physiologically and psychologically speaking) with this excellent program. Try it and see.

CAUTION: A physical exam is recommended before beginning any exercise program.

PROGRAM FOR THE 70 + BEGINNERS

Exercise	Wt.	Reps/Time	Sets	Goals
1. Lymphatic Bounce	.45 kilo	10 sec.	2	Work up to 6 minutes a day total in all exercises combined.
2. Curl & Press	.45 kilo	10 reps.	2	
3. Shuffle	.45 kilo	10 sec.	2	
4. Jog Easy	.45 kilo	10 reps.	2	

Add one set every week till you reach six minutes total. Add Sanbag weight only if you feel you need it. Your goal is to get all around circulation and fitness. Eventually you can add more exercises from the "Daily Dozen" as you get stronger. Every week you can add one exercise from the "Daily Dozen" to your program, within a short time you can be doing the complete program.

A word of caution here as in all the other programs: "Haste makes waste." Be patient with your progress. Monitor your pulse and check your working heart rate (See Chapter 2), have FUN, and if in doubt check with your family doctor.

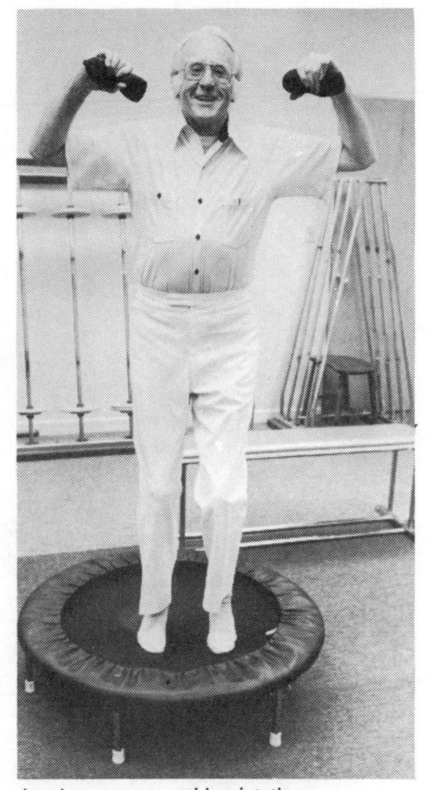

Joe demonstrates mid-point, the press.

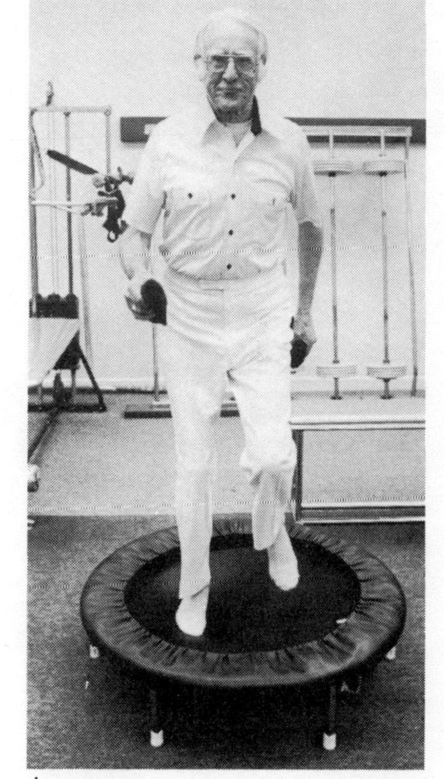

Jog easy.

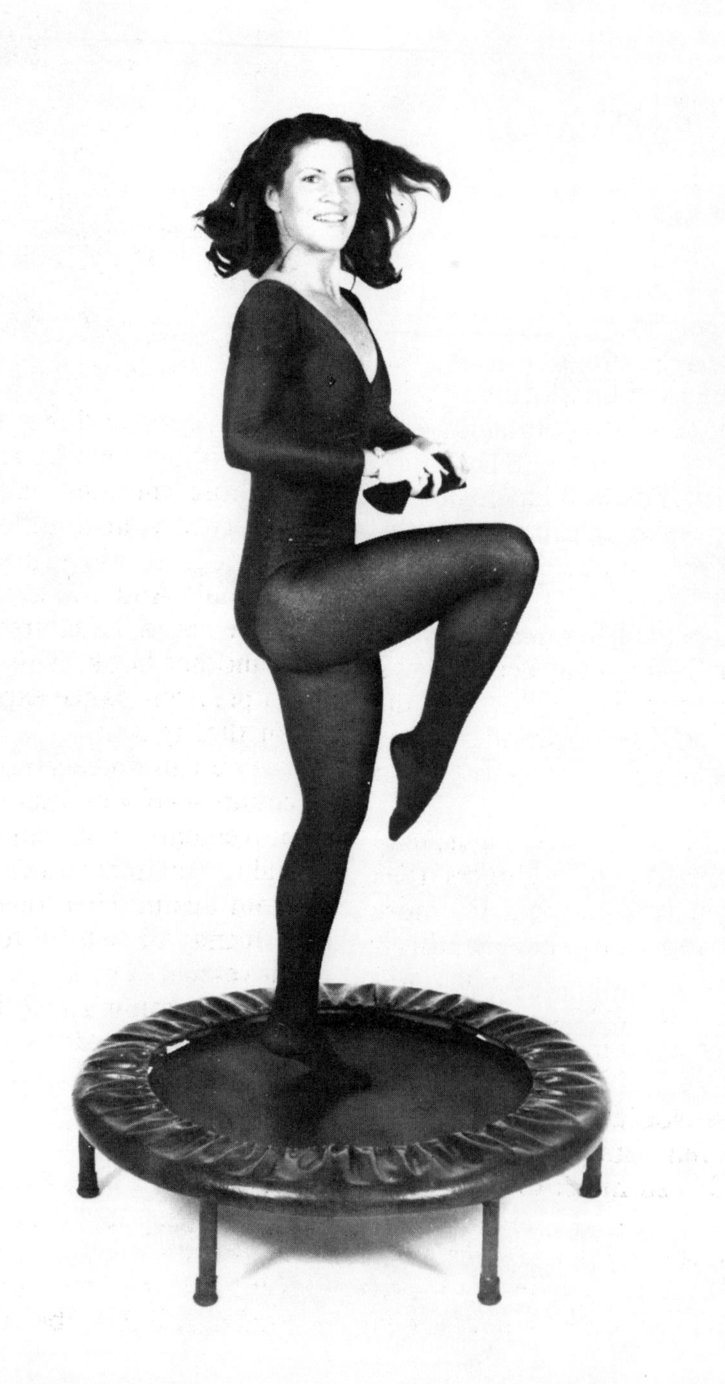

Chapter 12

Dance 'n Bounce

No Dance Experience Necessary!

If you've never like to exercise, this FUN program is for you!

Super fun, terrific variety and excellent conditioning with your beautiful Sanbag program. Dance yourself into total fitness in 15-20 minutes a day!

There is so much fun getting in shape while dancing. You certainly have heard of all the popular crazes in dance: aerobic, jazz, disco, etc. Many of these movements can be done on your rebound unit with your small Sanbags.

These dance movements may be done without Sanbags, but there is a greater fitness benefit with Sanbagging because you have resistance along with your movement. This will shape the upper body and improve fitness in a much shorter period of time. This all can be done in the privacy of your own home if you so desire.

If you are not in good condition, or are a little overweight, may we recommend the basic ladies' program for beginners (See Chapter 4). If you have been using your rebound unit for more than two months, and are in fairly good physical condition, this is for you. Those who are positively addicted to rebounding will have a blast with the following. So let's get started.

There are literally hundreds of dance movements that can be done on a rebound unit. However, we are limiting this chapter to only 21 **basic** dance movements so you would **try** this program. These are all very simple movements even younger girls can do.

Please try them — a little variety adds so much to your daily program. And dancing is FUN!

I suggest that after you have learned several dance steps from the book, you write them down on a 3 x 5 card or note pad, and place it near your stereo or radio for easy reference. You can then

Sarah Sneider leads a group in aerobic dancing.

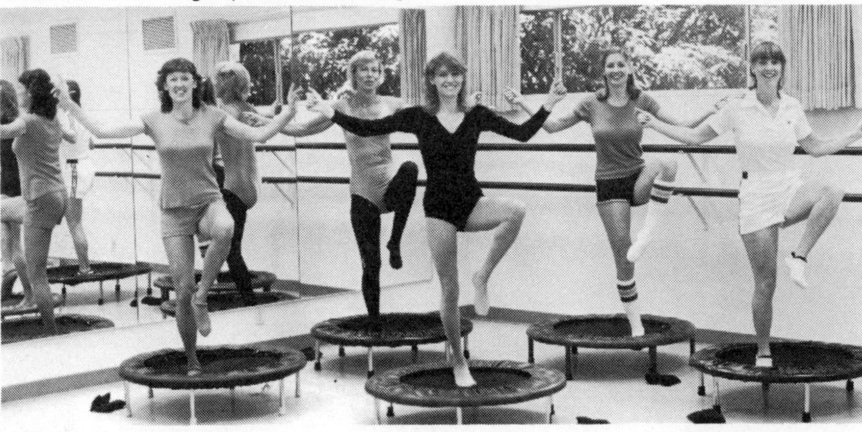

quickly glance down for another movement. It will make your 15-20 minute workout so much more fun.

Those minutes will pass so quickly because you've added variety to **your** routine. It's **your** personal program that you have choreographed to fit **you.** Each workout can be so different and original! And you are getting in shape as well.

We could, of course, picture many more dance steps, but that is another book. This is intended for the in-home audience with no previous dance experience. We've tried to keep it very simple for that reason.

You can do each movement through 4 counts, 8 counts, or 12 counts — if you desire. You can mix or match any of these dance movements. You can turn in circles: Do 4 counts turning to the right, 4 counts to the back, then on to the left and back to the front again. Then reverse, turning to the left first.

It may be helpful to count 1, 2, 3, 4, 5, 6, 7, 8 for an 8-count movement. Or, if the movement is 2 counts, such as knee hops, you can count 1 & 2 & 3 & 4.

After you've done a few of these movements, you will probably create many of your own. Turn on some peppy music, be creative, and HAVE FUN!!

SUGGESTED PROGRAM:

I suggest for your daily program: a warm-up with The Big Four, then one set of The Daily Dozen and one set of The Perfect Ten, and then ten minutes of dance movements with or without Sanbags. Remember to cool down with an easy jog or the clock.

Marsha Whitley, women's athletic director.

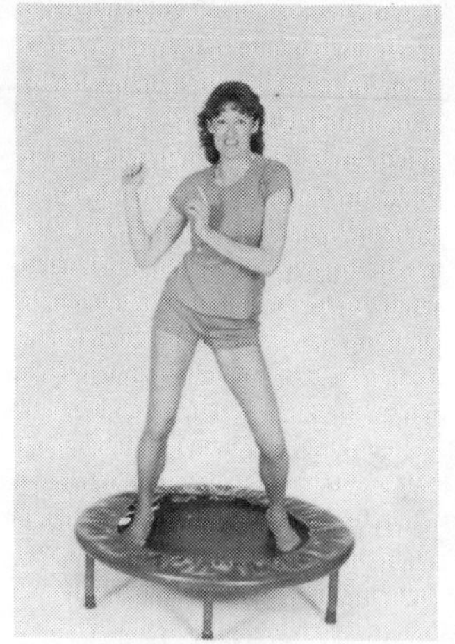

1. Sway hips to right.

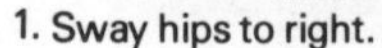

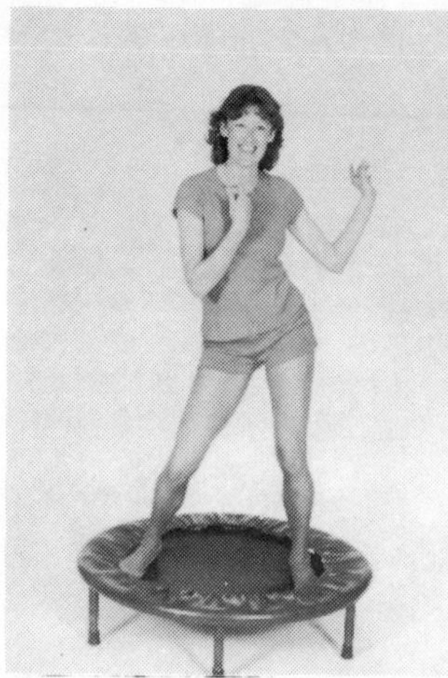

2. Sway hips to left.

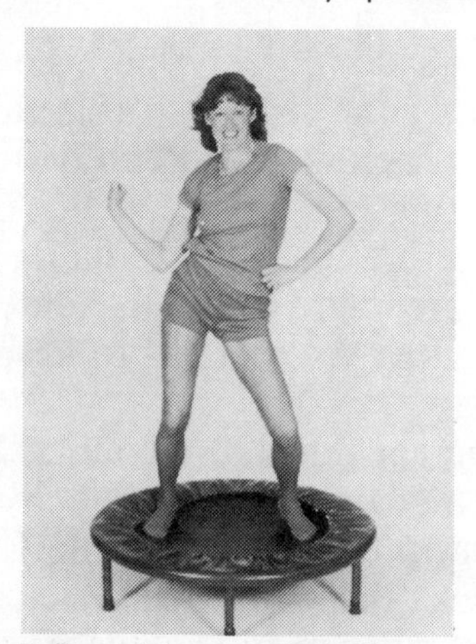

5. Sway right, touch right elbow to right hip.

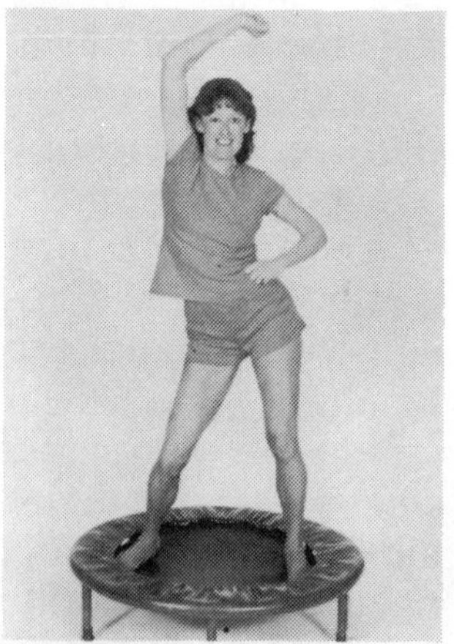

6. Sway left, extend right arm above head.

1. HIPS SWAY WITH HAND PUNCHES

Basically good for the waist.

SP (Starting Position): Stand in center of mat, feet together, arms in jogging position. Count

1. Sway hips to R, as arms swing to R.
2. Sway hips to L, as arms swing to L.
3. Repeat #1.
4. Repeat #2.
5. Sway hips to R, touch R elbow to R hip.
6. Sway hips to L, extend R arm above head.
7. Repeat #5.
8. Repeat #6.

Repeat entire sequence 4 times.

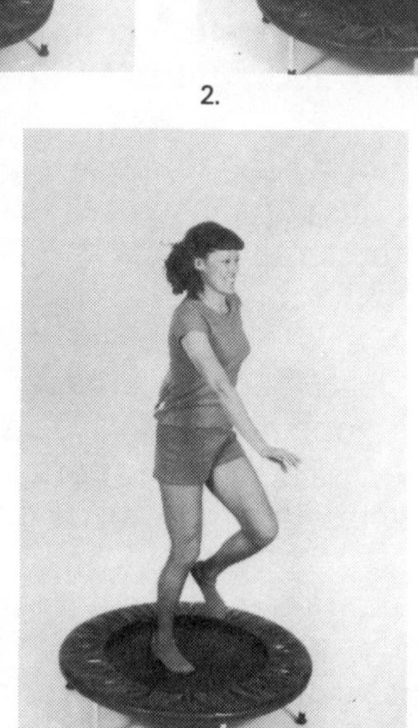

1.

2.

3.

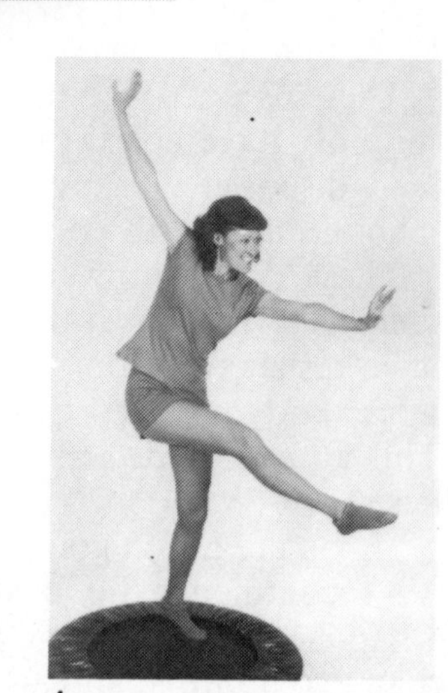

4.

2. JOG, 2, 3, KICK FRONT

Good for the hips, thighs and abdominals.

SP: Stand in center of mat, arms in jogging position.
Count

1. Jog R foot.
2. Jog L foot.
3. Jog R foot.
4. Kick L foot to front.

5, 6, 7, 8. Beginning with L foot: Jog L, R, L, Kick R foot to front.
Repeat entire sequence 4 times.

Variation: Jog, 2, 3, Kick **Side** instead of Kick Front.

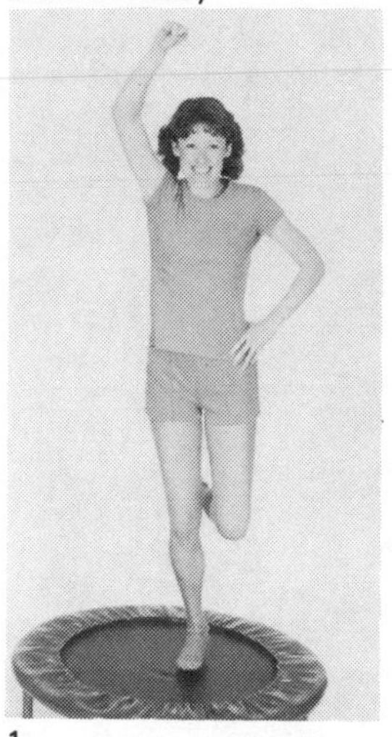

1.

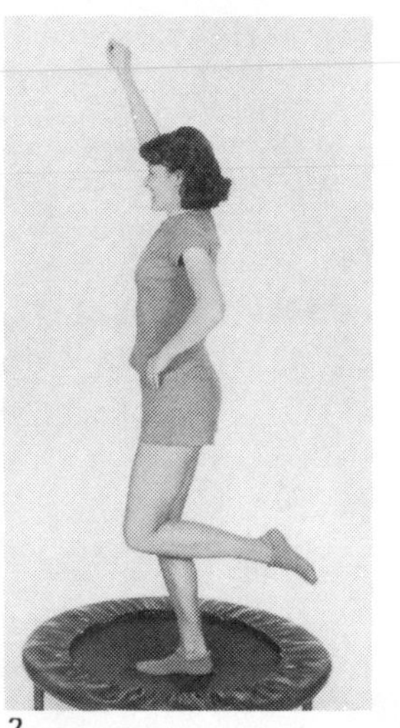

2.

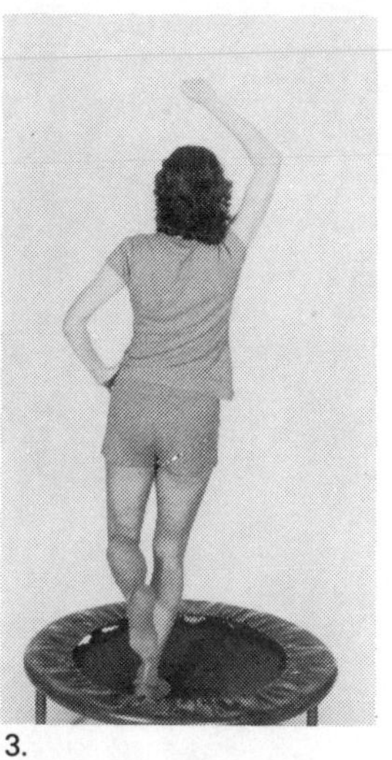

3.

Hop right foot, turning in full circle to right.

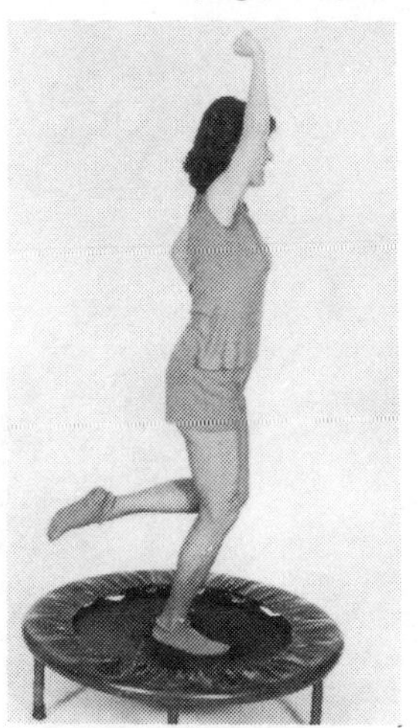

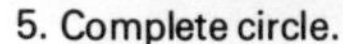

5. Complete circle.

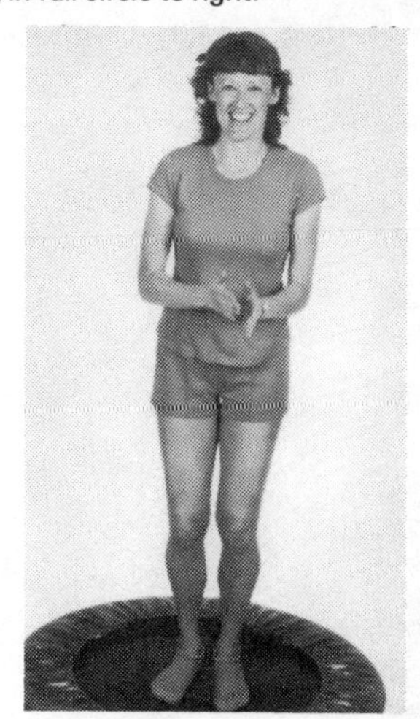

7., 8. Clap twice front. Repeat on left foot.

3. CIRCLE HOP & CLAP

Excellent for ankles and calves.

SP: Stand in center of mat, L hand on hip.

Count

1, 2, 3, 4, 5, 6. Hop R foot, turning in full circle to R. L hand on hip, with R hand make little circles overhead (takes 6 beats).

7, 8. Clap twice front.

Repeat on L foot turning in full circle to L (takes 6 beats), then clap twice front (takes 2 beats).

Repeat entire sequence 4 times.

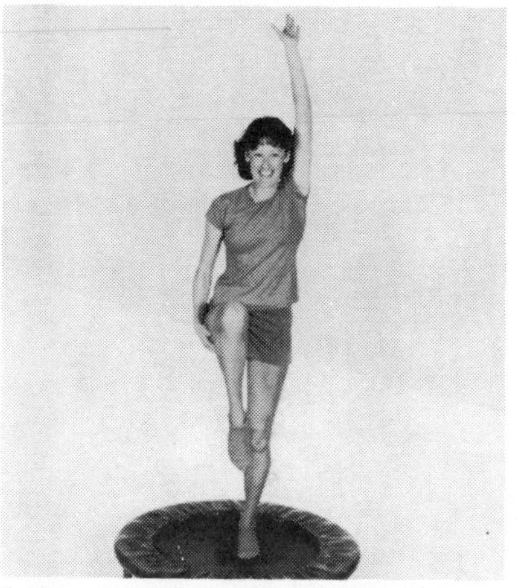

1. Hop on right foot, raise left knee, right arm overhead.

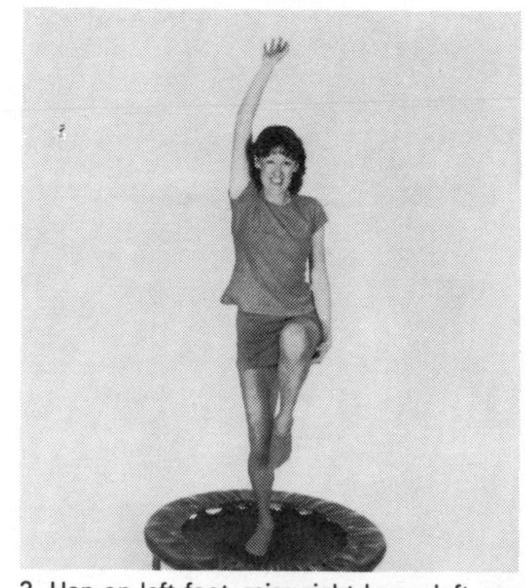

3. Hop on left foot, raise right knee, left arm overhead.

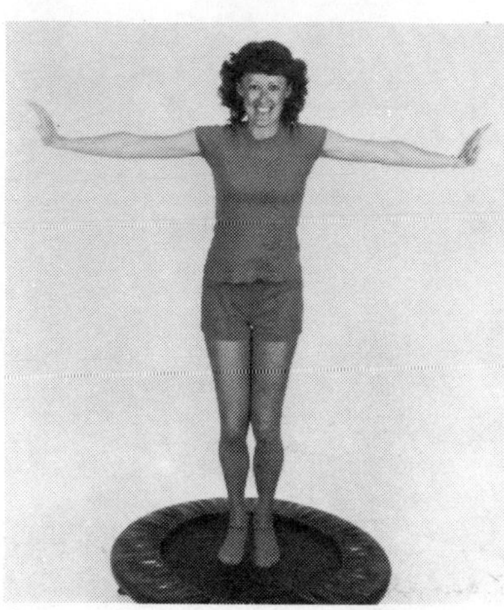

4.

5.

Turn full circle, arms extended to sides.

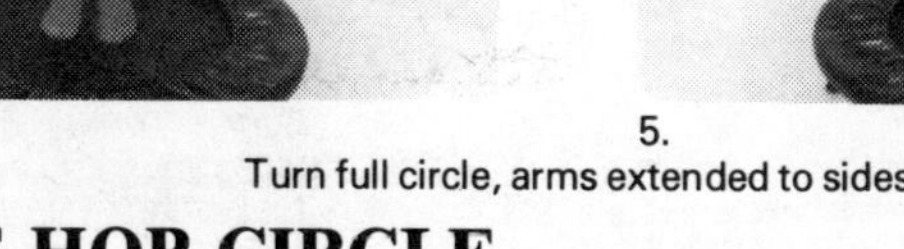

4. KNEE HOP CIRCLE

For the thighs and hips.

SP: Stand in center of mat, arms at side.

Count

1. Hop on L foot, raising R knee, bring L arm overhead.
2. Return to SP.
3. Hop on R foot, raising L knee, bring R arm overhead.
4. Return to SP.

5, 6, 7, 8. Turn in full circle R with arms out to sides.

Repeat entire sequence 4 times. Alternate by circling to L.

NOTE: If using Sanbags, lift bags only to shoulder level instead of overhead on Knee Hops.

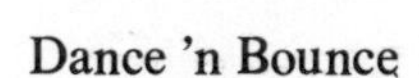

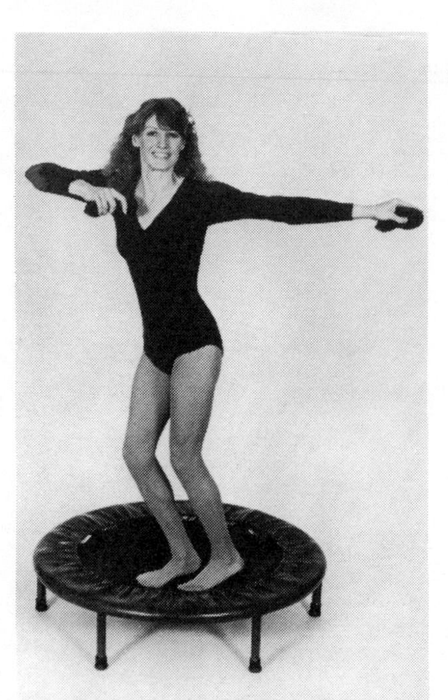

Sarah Sneider

1.

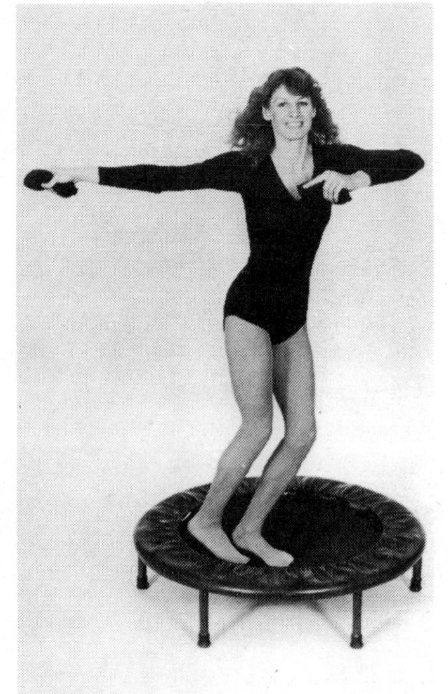

2.

5. BODY TWIST

Trims upper sides of the waist.
SP: Stand in center of mat.
Count
1. Twisting body to R, bring R arm across chest, extend L arm out at side.
2. Twisting body to L, bring L arm across chest, extend R arm out at side.

Repeat at least 4 times.

Barbara Egbert, physical education instructor, author.

1.

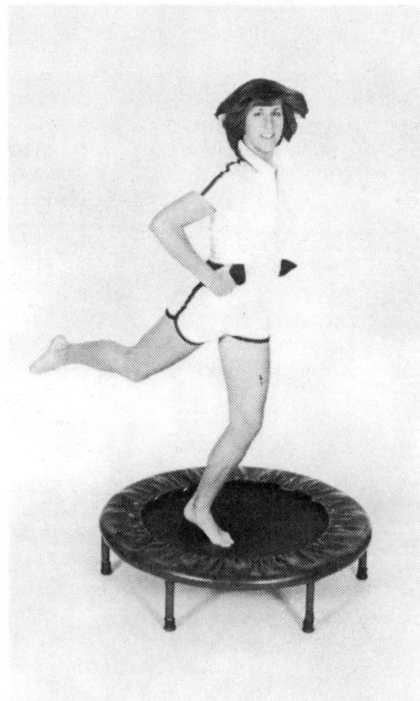

2.

6. FRONT & BACK KICK

Trims the thighs, works calves and strengthens lower back.
SP: Stand in center of mat, hands on hips.
Count
1. Hop on L foot, raising R knee.
2. Hop again on L foot, kicking R leg back.

Hop 7 times on L foot, raising R knee and kicking R leg back, switch to R foot on 8th beat and repeat kicks on L leg.
(Count: 1, 2, 3, 4, 5, 6, 7, Switch.)
Repeat entire sequence 2 times.

Sarah Sneider

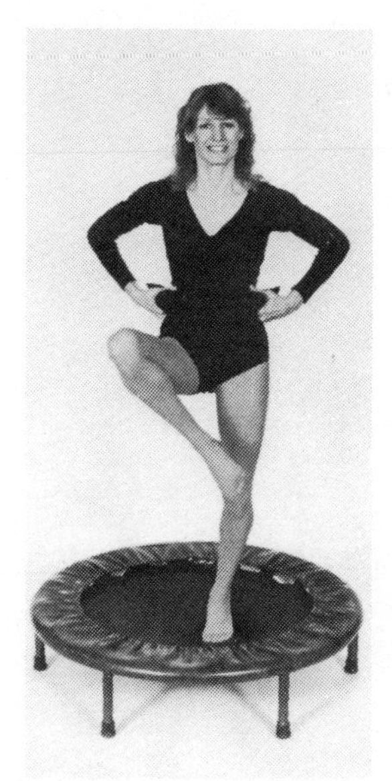
1.

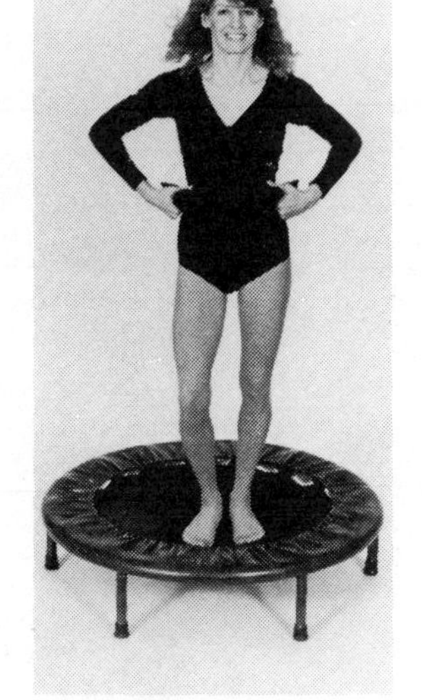
2.

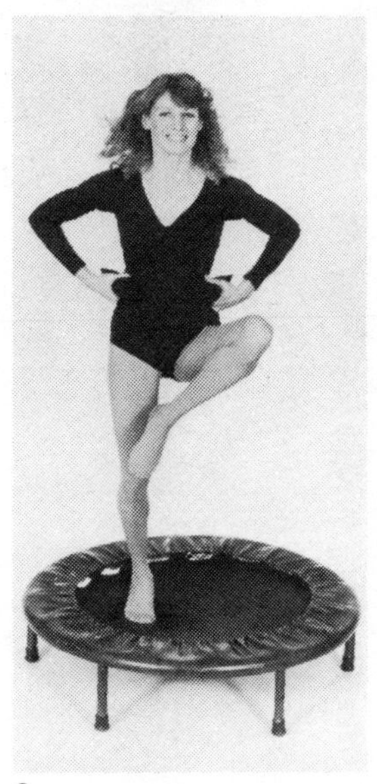
3.

7. INNER THIGH LIFT

Firms inner thighs.

SP: Stand in center of mat, hands on hips.

Count

1. Hop on L foot, bringing R foot to left knee, R knee out.
2. Bounce feet together.
3. Hop on R foot, bringing L foot to right knee, L knee out.
4. Bounce feet together.

Repeat 8 times.

NOTE: If not using Sanbags, snap fingers on each hop, arms out at sides, elbows slightly bent.

Nancy Collins

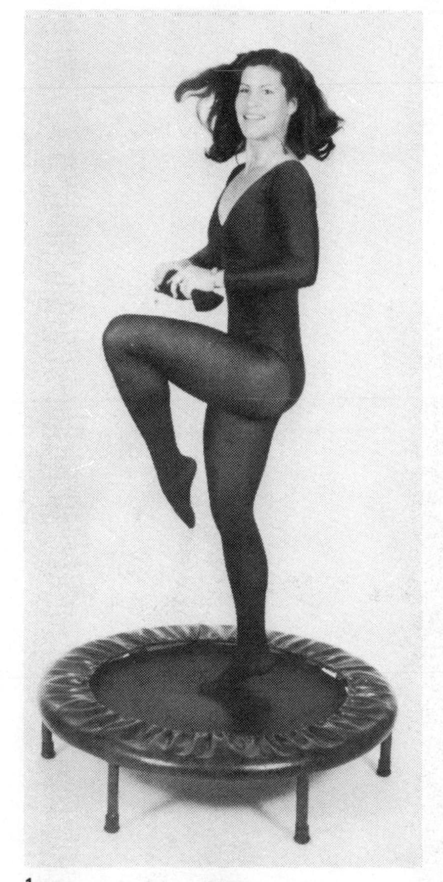
1.

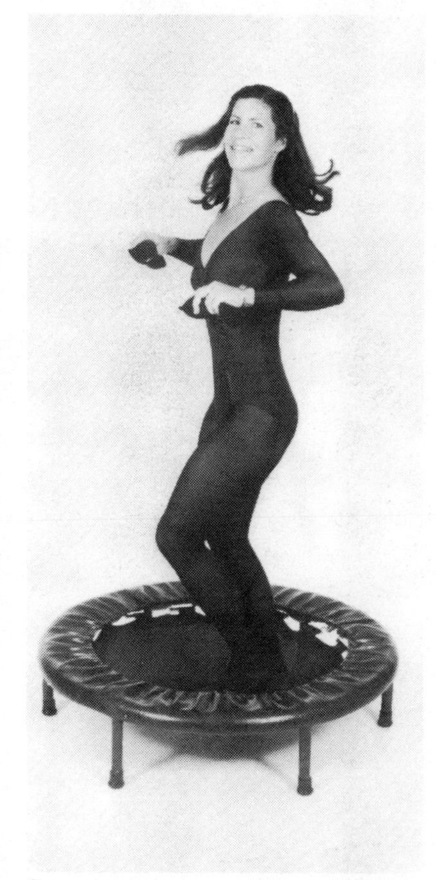
2.

8. POPCORN HOPS

Trims thighs and hips — strengthens lower back.

SP: Stand in center of mat, with arms at sides.

Count

1. Hop on R foot, raising L knee. Touch hands to knee on each hop.
2. Return L foot to mat between each hop.

Hop 4 times on R foot, raising L knee, then hop 4 times on L foot raising R knee. Repeat entire sequence 2 times.

Variation: do above. Then hop 2 times on R foot, raising L knee, returning L foot to mat between each hop. Repeat on opposite leg.

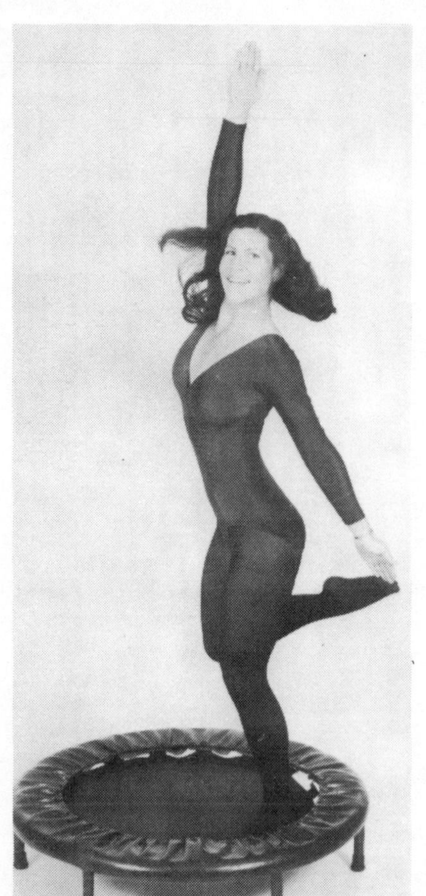

1.

Nancy Collins

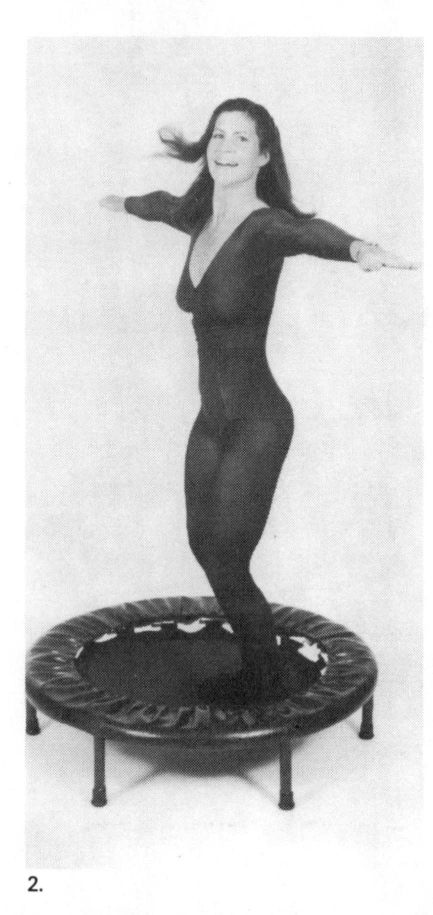

2.

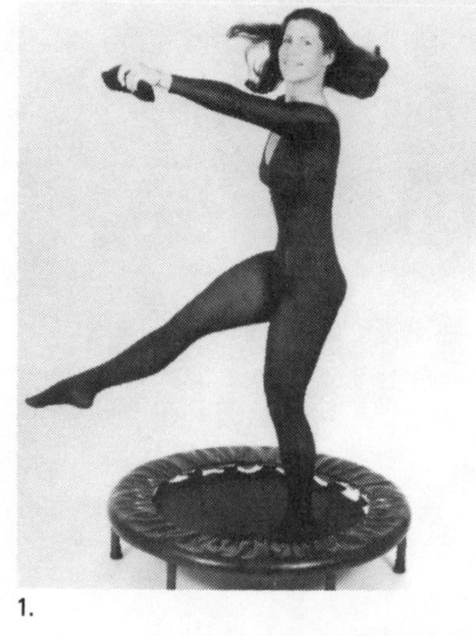

1.

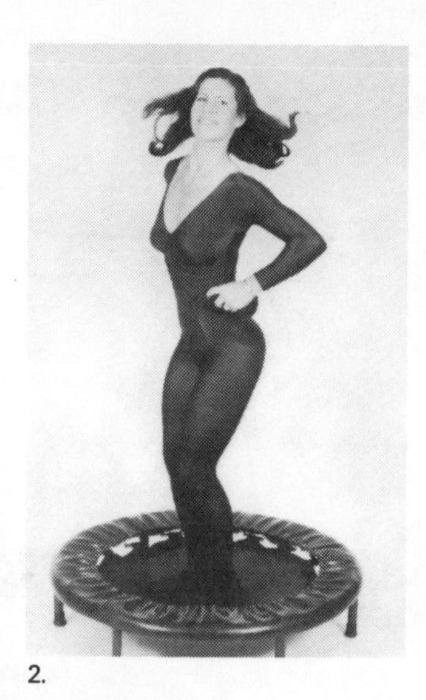

2.

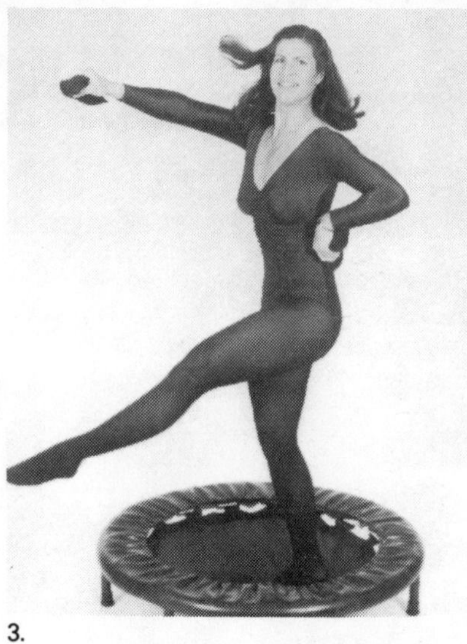

3.

9. HOPSCOTCH

For the inner thighs and hips.

SP: Stand in center of mat, hands out to sides at shoulder level.

Count

1. Hop on L foot, touch L hand to R foot in back. Extend R arm overhead.
2. Return to SP.
3. Hop on R foot, touch R hand to L foot in back. Extend L arm overhead.
4. Return to SP.

Repeat 8 times.

10. KICK & PUNCH

For the ankles and calves; firms abdominals and trims hips and thighs.

SP: Stand in center of mat, arms in jogging position.

Count

1. Hop on L foot, kick R leg to front. Punch L hand to front.
2. Bounce feet together.
3. Hop on R foot, kick L leg to front. Punch R hand to front.
4. Bounce feet together.

Repeat 8 times.

Nancy Collins

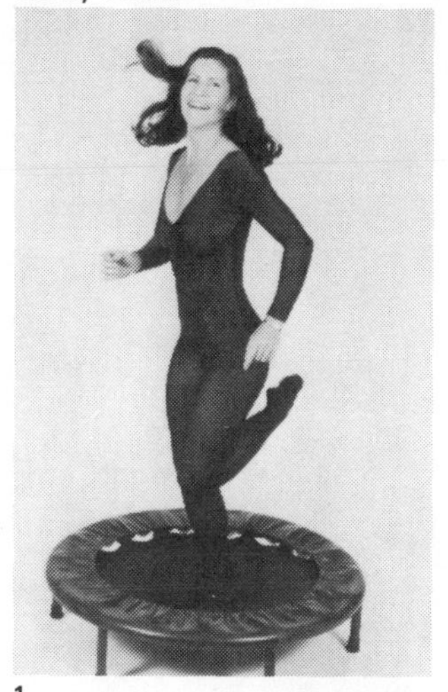
1.

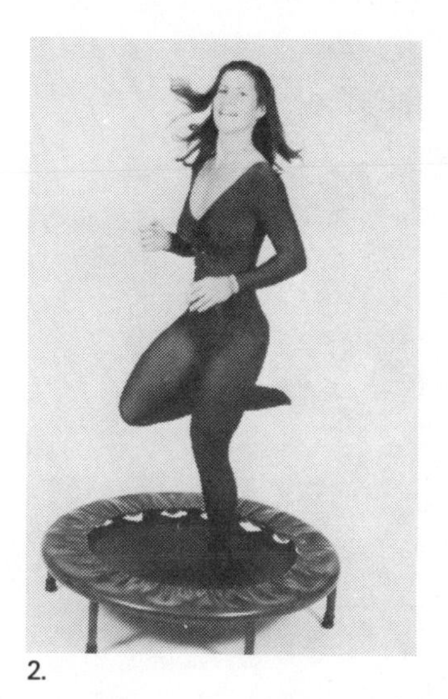
2.

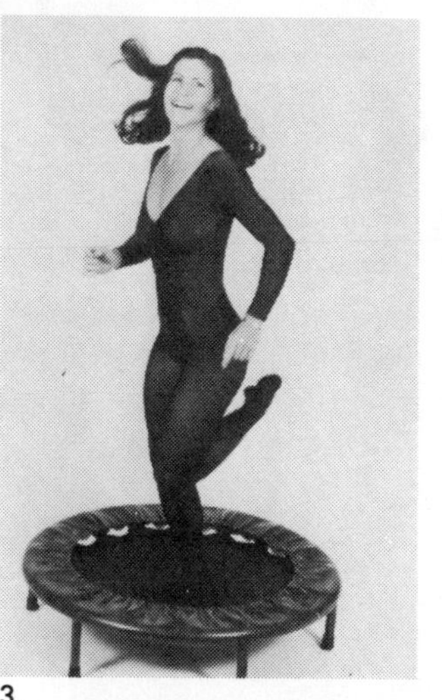
3.

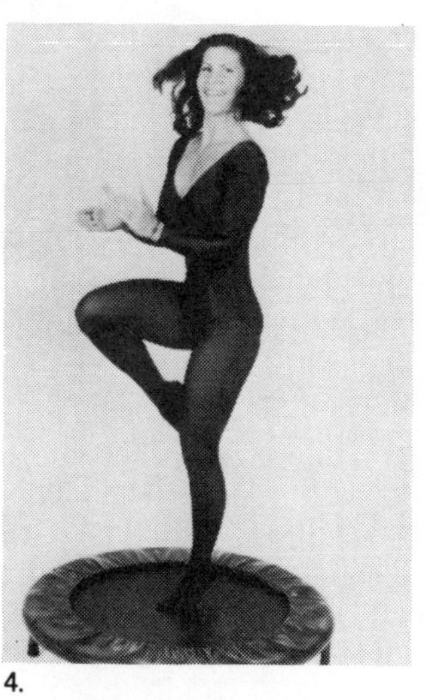
4.

11. JOG, 2, 3, KNEE HOP

Trims hips and thighs; firms abdominals.

SP: Stand in center of mat, arms in jogging position.

Count
1. Jog R foot.
2. Jog L foot.
3. Jog R foot.
4. Hop on L foot lifting R knee high.

5, 6, 7, 8. Then, Jog L, R, L, hop on R foot lifting L knee high.

Repeat 4 times as you turn to left for 4 counts, back (4 counts), right (4 counts), and front (4 counts).

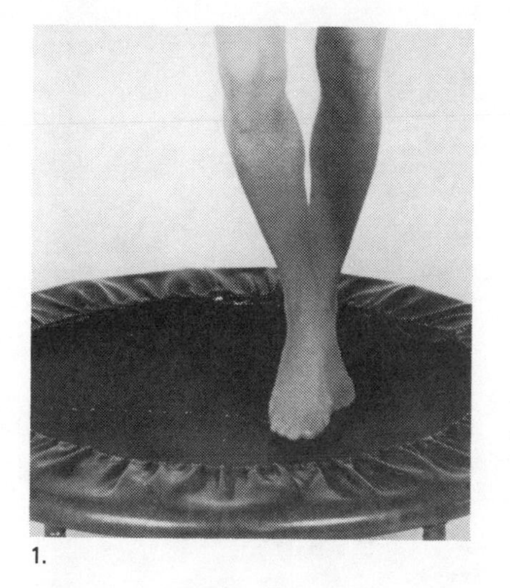
1.

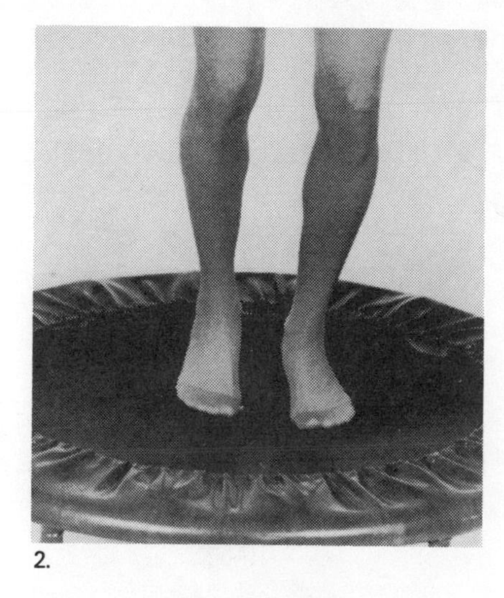
2.

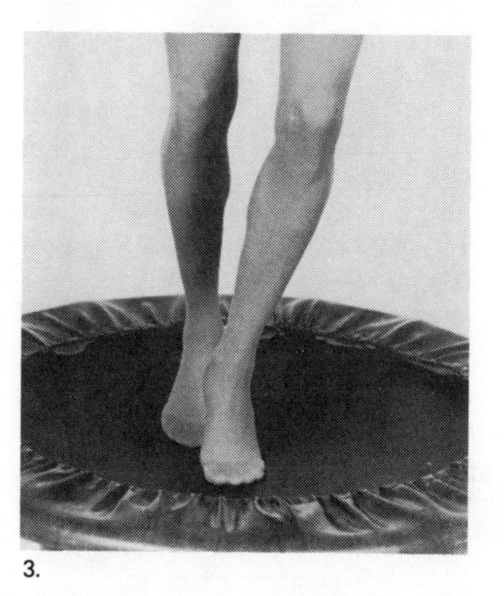
3.

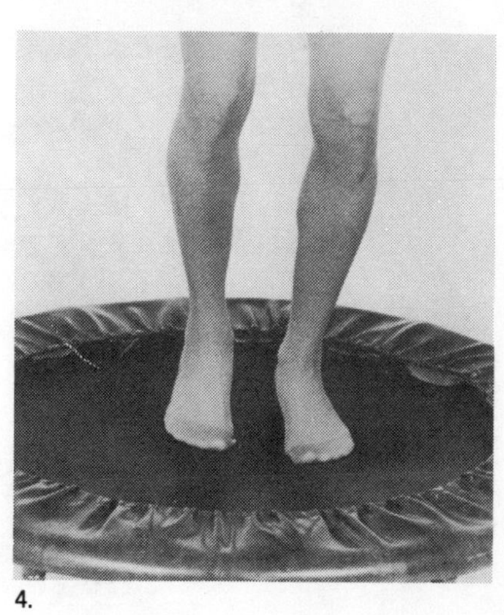
4.

12. STEP-TOUCH

Another one for the hips and thighs.

SP: Stand in center of mat, hands on hips.

Count
1. Touch R toe about 6″ to front.
2. Bring it back to place.
3. Touch L toe about 6″ to front.
4. Bring it back to place.

Repeat sequence 8 times.

Variation: Step-Touch with arms swinging side to side in front.

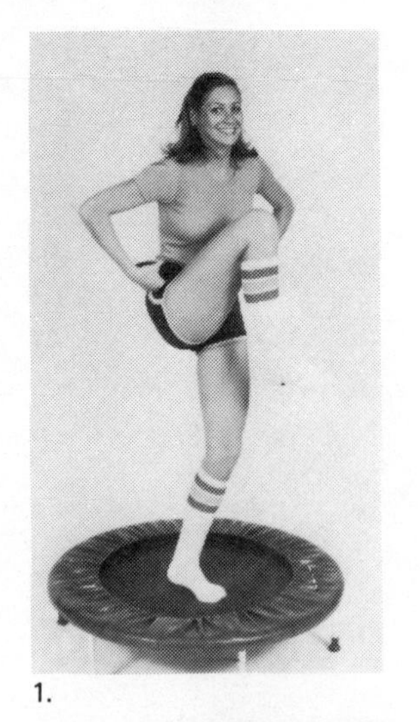

1.

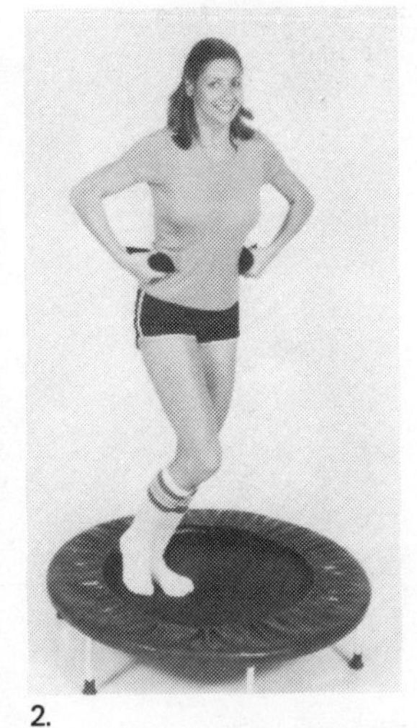

2.

Denise Guthy

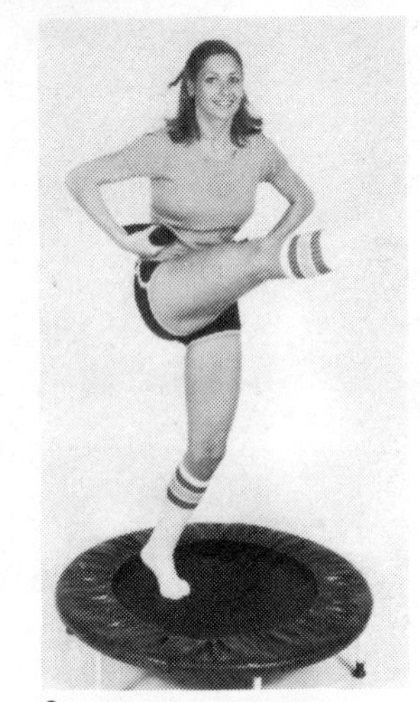

3.

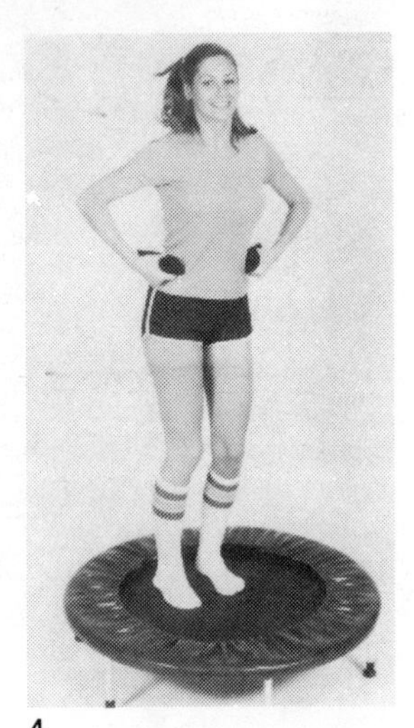

4.

13. PREP & KICK

Firms abdominals, strengthens lower back, works ankles, calves, hips and thighs.

SP: Stand in center of mat, hands on hips.

Count

1. Raise R knee while hopping on L foot.
2. Bounce feet together.
3. Kick R leg while hopping on L foot.
4. Bounce feet together.

5, 6, 7, 8. Repeat with L leg.

Repeat entire sequence 4 times.

Sarah Sneider

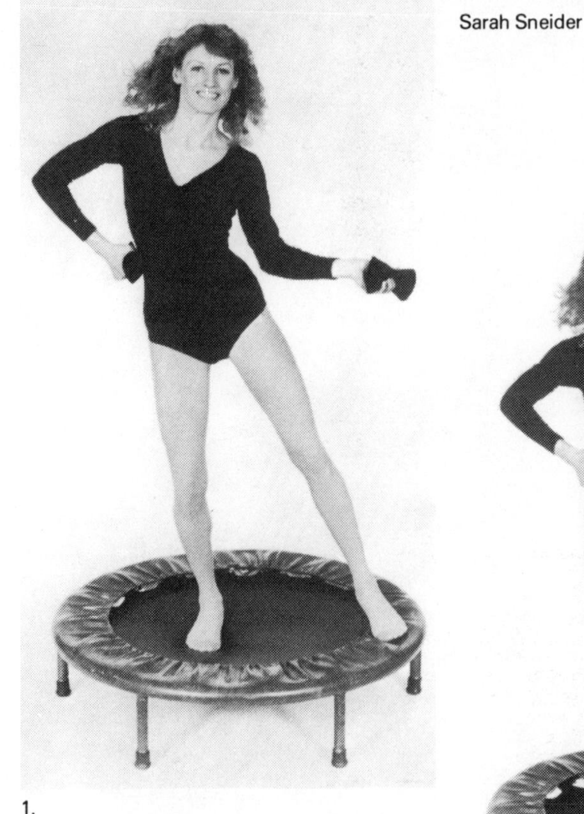

1.

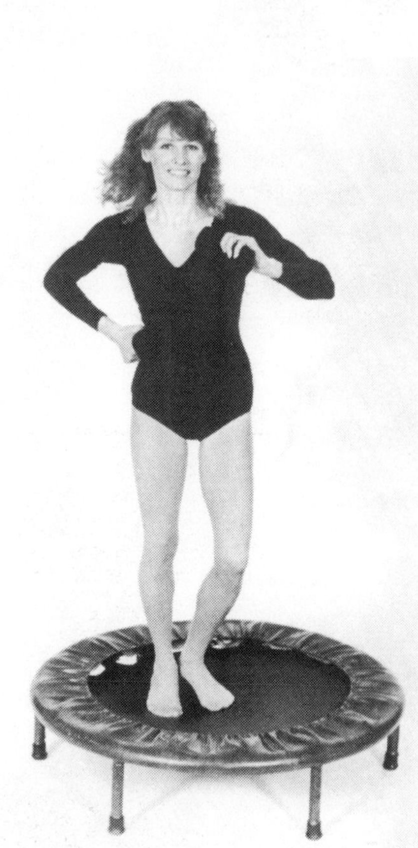

2.

14. KICK SIDE WITH ELBOW BENDS

Trims waist and firms outer and inner thighs.

SP: Stand in center of mat, right hand on hip, L hand at shoulder.

Count

1. Kick or touch L leg to side as you extend L hand out to side from elbow.
2. Return to SP

Kick or touch 4 times, repeat on other side.

Repeat entire sequence 4 times.

Variation: Kick 3 times L side, then bounce twice feet together. Kick 3 times R side, then bounce feet together.

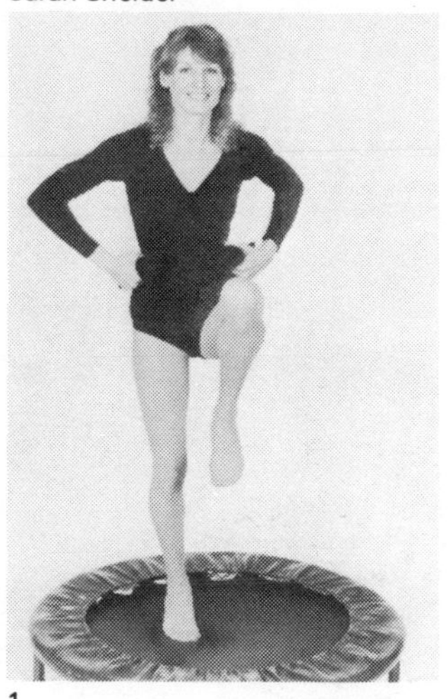
1.

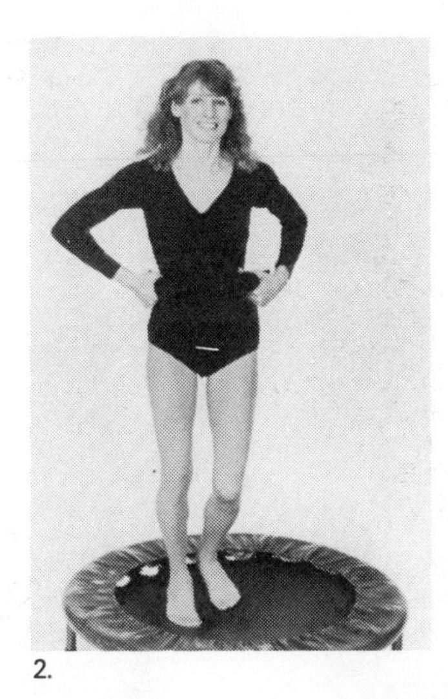
2.

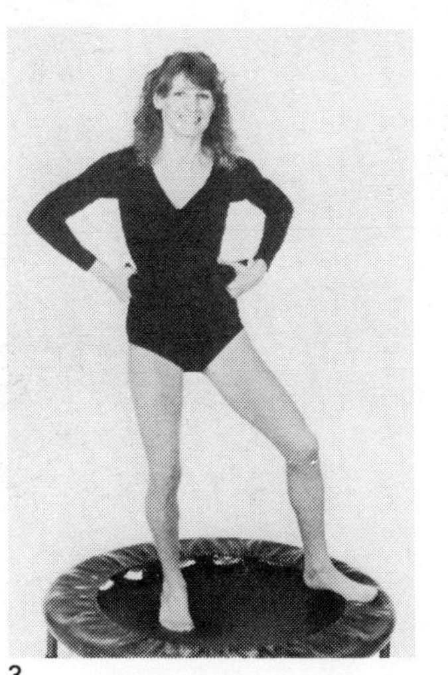
3.

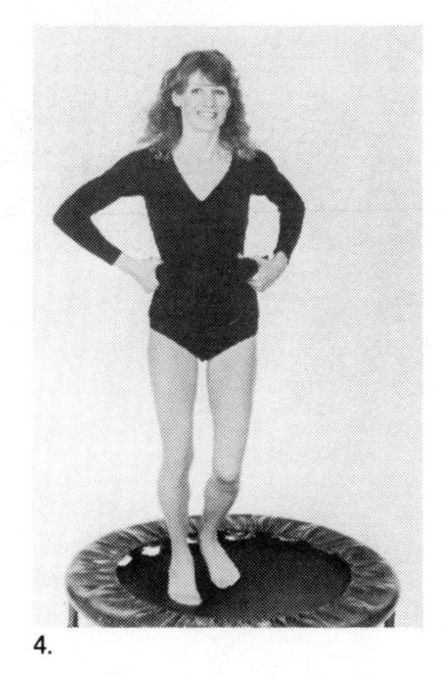
4.

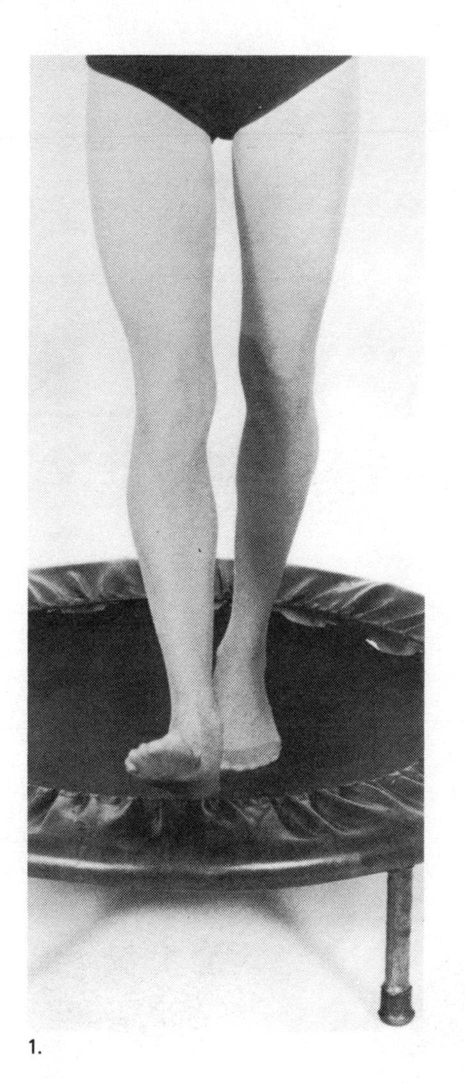
1.

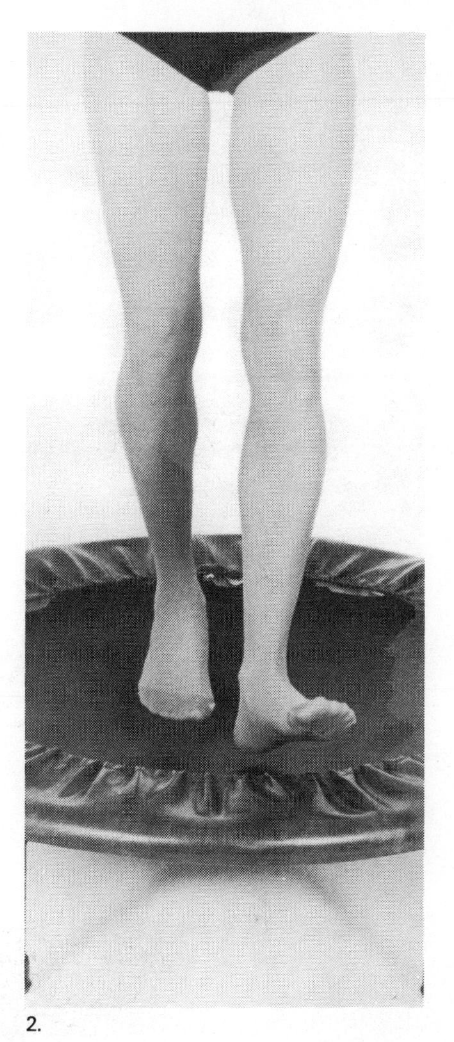
2.

15. KNEE HOP, SIDE TOUCH

Firms abdominals, trims hips and thighs.
SP: Stand in center of mat.
Count
1. Hop on R foot, raising L knee.
2. Bounce feet together.
3. Kick or touch L foot to side.
4. Bounce feet together.

5, 6, 7, 8. Repeat other side.
Repeat entire sequence 4 times.

16. MEXICAN HAT BOUNCE

Good for ankles, calves, hips and thighs.
SP: Stand in center of mat, hands in jogging position or on hips.
Count
1. Bounce R heel front.
2. Bounce L heel front.

A quick shuffle-step bounce. Bounce R, L, R, L.
Repeat 16 times.
Variation: Bounce L, R, L, L; then bounce R, L, R, R.

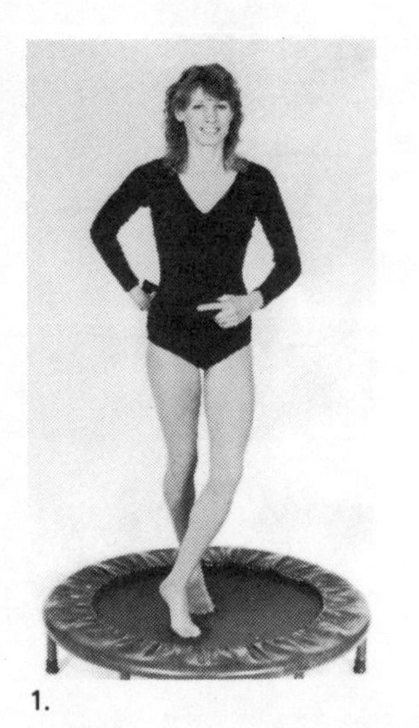

1.

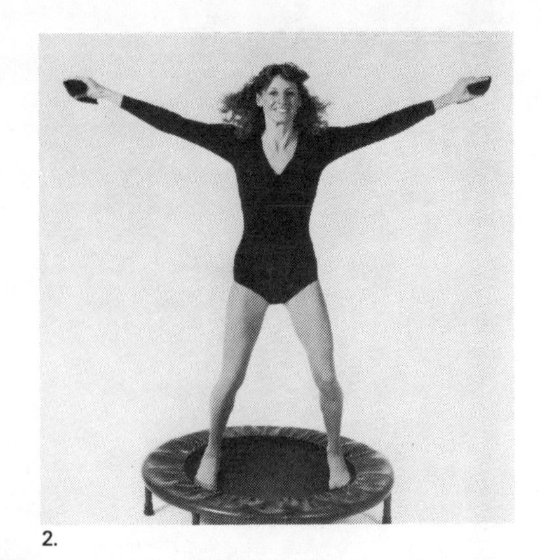

2.

3.

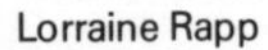

Lorraine Rapp

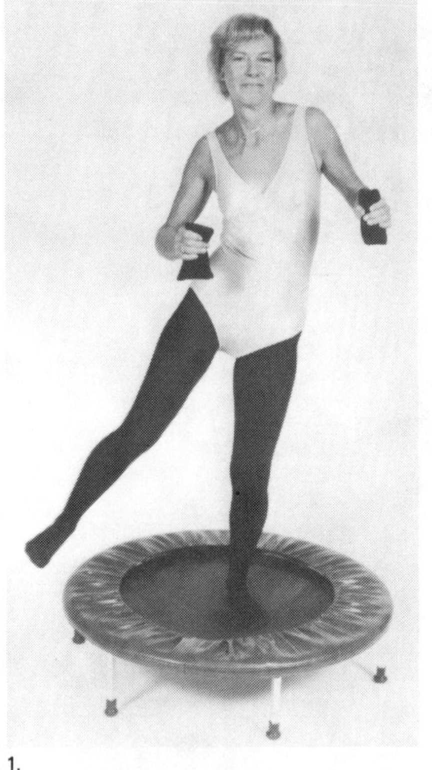

1.

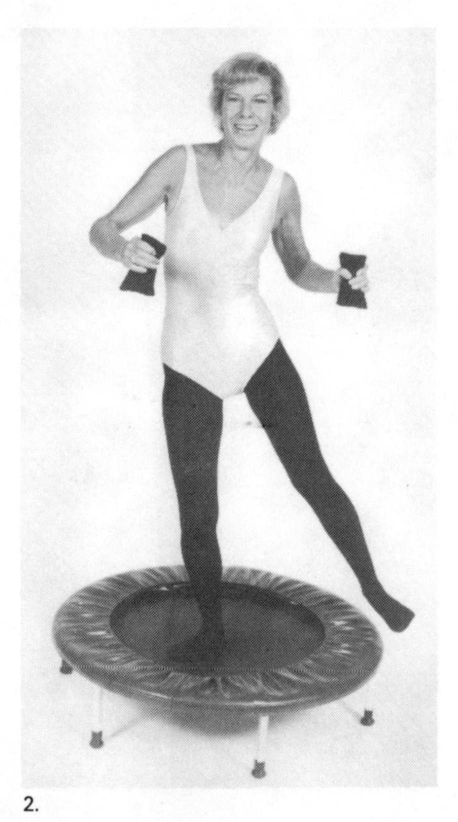

2.

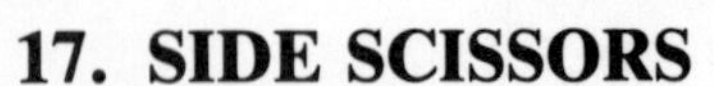

17. SIDE SCISSORS

Firms inner and outer thighs and hips; works the ankles.
SP: Stand in center of mat.
Count
1. Bounce crossing L leg over R leg, bringing L hand to front, R hand to back.
2. Bounce legs apart, bringing hands out at sides.
3. Bounce crossing R leg over L leg, bringing R hand in front, L hand in back.
4. Bounce with legs apart, bringing hands out at sides.
   Repeat 8 times.

18. SIDE KICKS

Trims sides of waist and firms inner and outer thighs.
SP: Stand in center of mat with arms at sides.
Count
1. Hop on L leg, kicking R leg to side.
2. Hop on R leg, kicking L leg to side.

Repeat 8 times.
Variation: Hop L, R, L, L, then hop R, L, R, R, kicking opposite leg to side with each hop.

Debbie Smith, rebound exercise enthusiast.

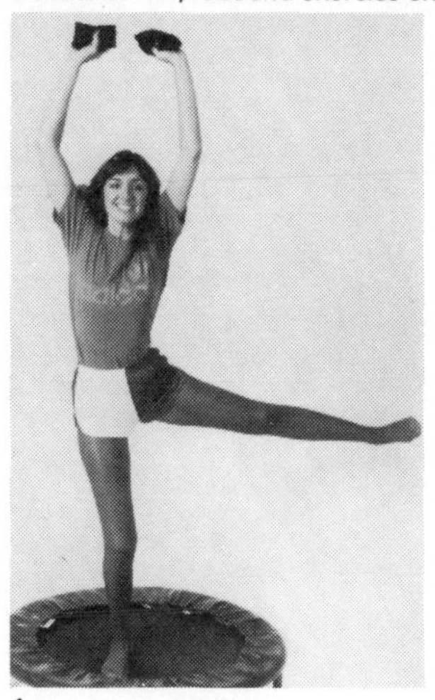

1.

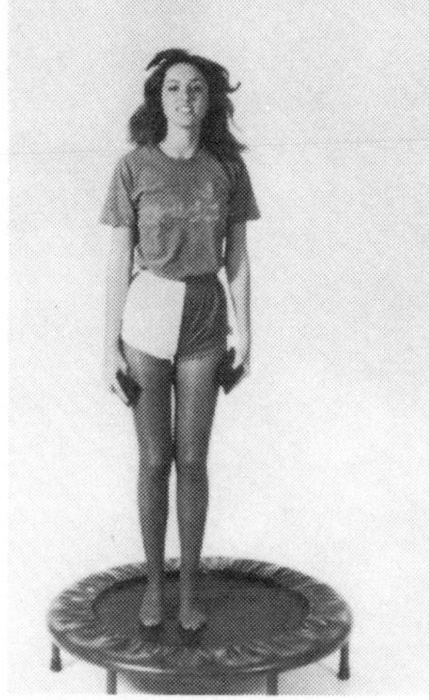

2, 3, 4.

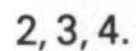

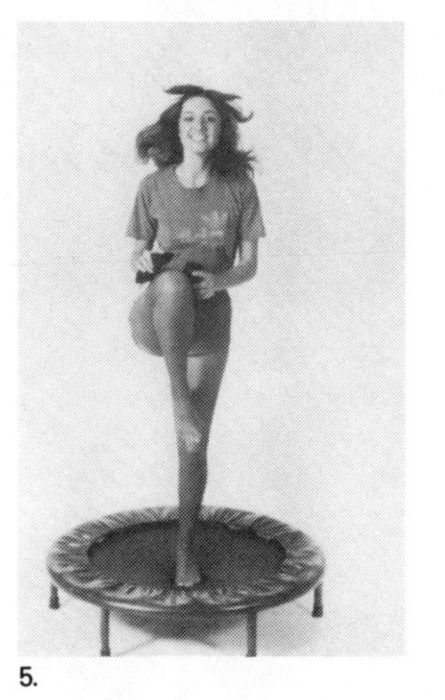

5.

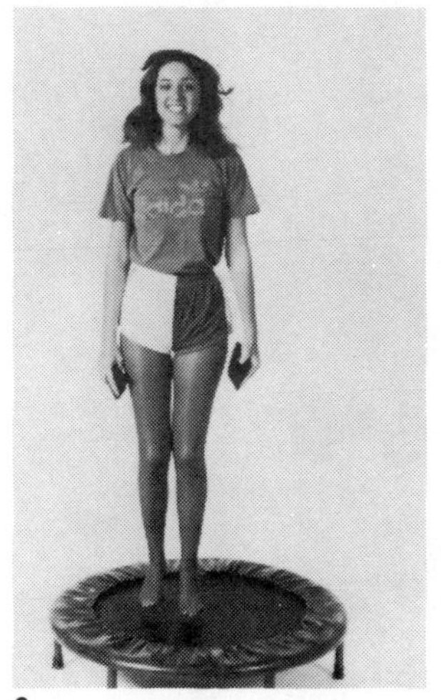

6.

19. KICK, BOUNCE 3, KNEE HOPS

Firms inner and outer thighs; works the abdominals.

SP: Stand in center of mat, hands on hips.

Count

1. Kick L leg to L side.
2, 3, 4. Bounce feet together 3 times.
5. Raise R knee, hopping on L foot.
6. Return R foot to mat.
7. Raise L knee, hopping on R foot.
8. Return L foot to mat.

Repeat 4 times, alternate kicking R and L leg to side.

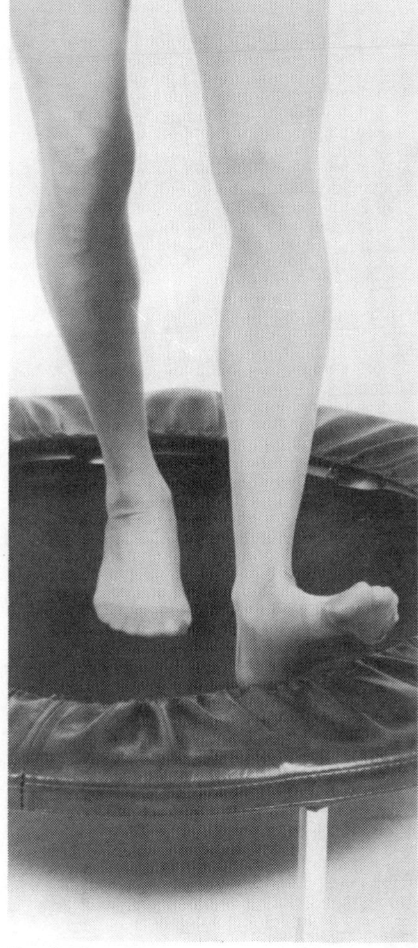

Hop, heel to mat.

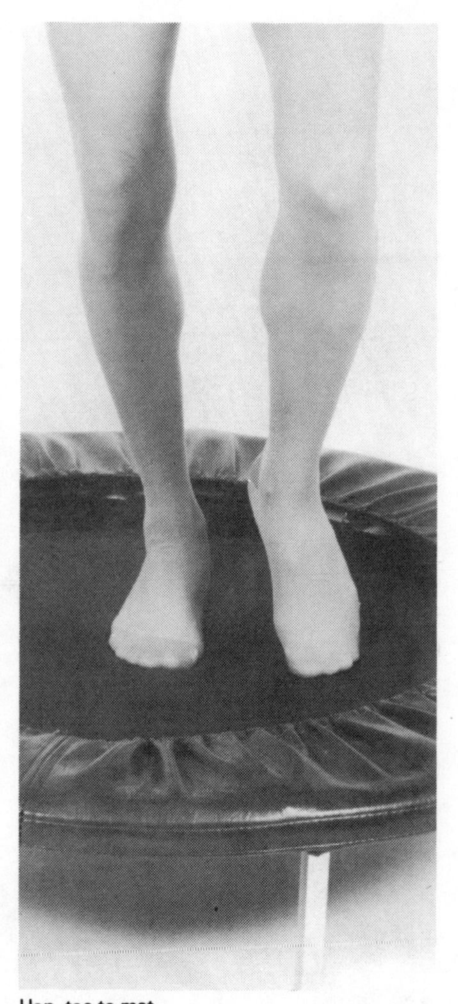

Hop, toe to mat.

20. HEEL-TOE BOUNCE

Great for the ankles.

SP: Stand in center of mat, hands on hips.

Count

1. Hop on R foot touching L heel to mat.
2. Hop again on R foot touching L toes to mat.

Repeat 4 times on R foot, 4 times on L foot.

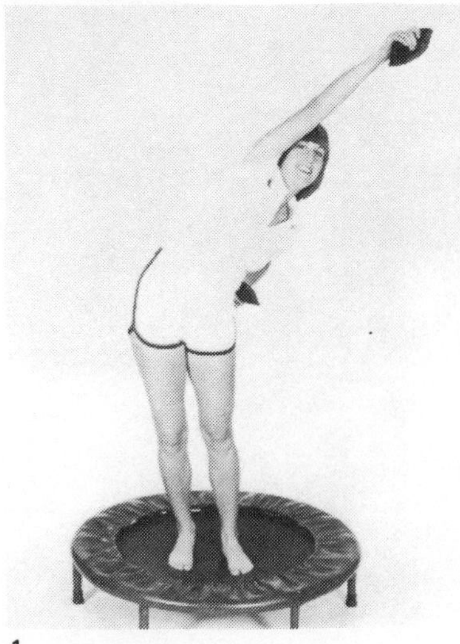

1.

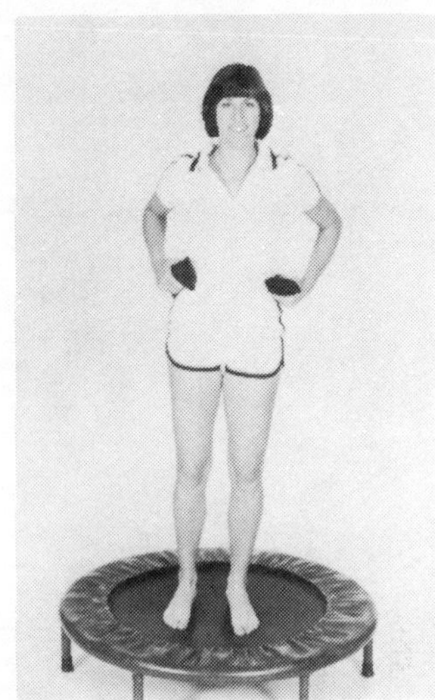

2.

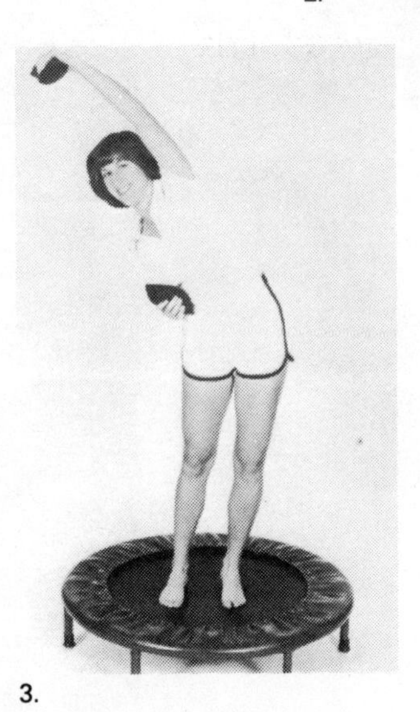

3.

21. WAIST PUNCHES

Excellent to trim the waist.

SP: Stand in center of mat, hands on hips.

Count

1. Punch R arm overhead with slight bend at waist.
2. Return to SP.
3. Punch L arm overhead with slight bend at waist.
4. Return to SP.

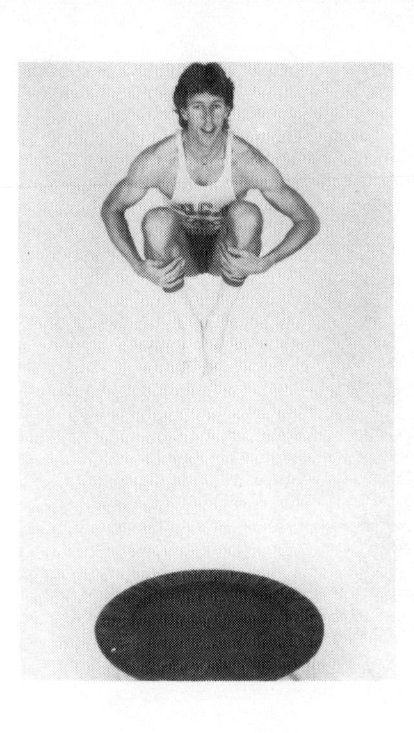

PART TWO

The athlete of any sport — seeking Olympic standards of performance.

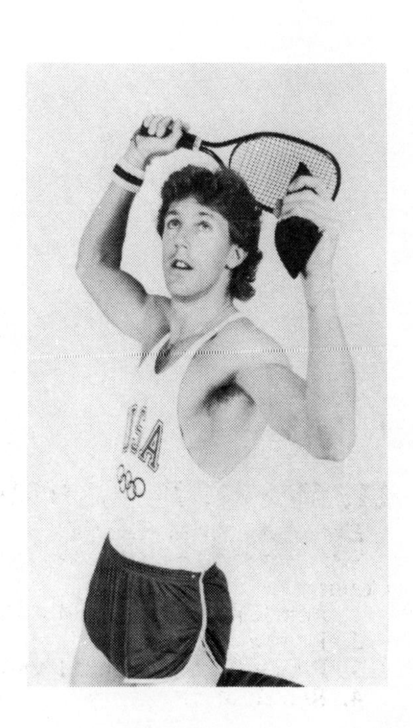

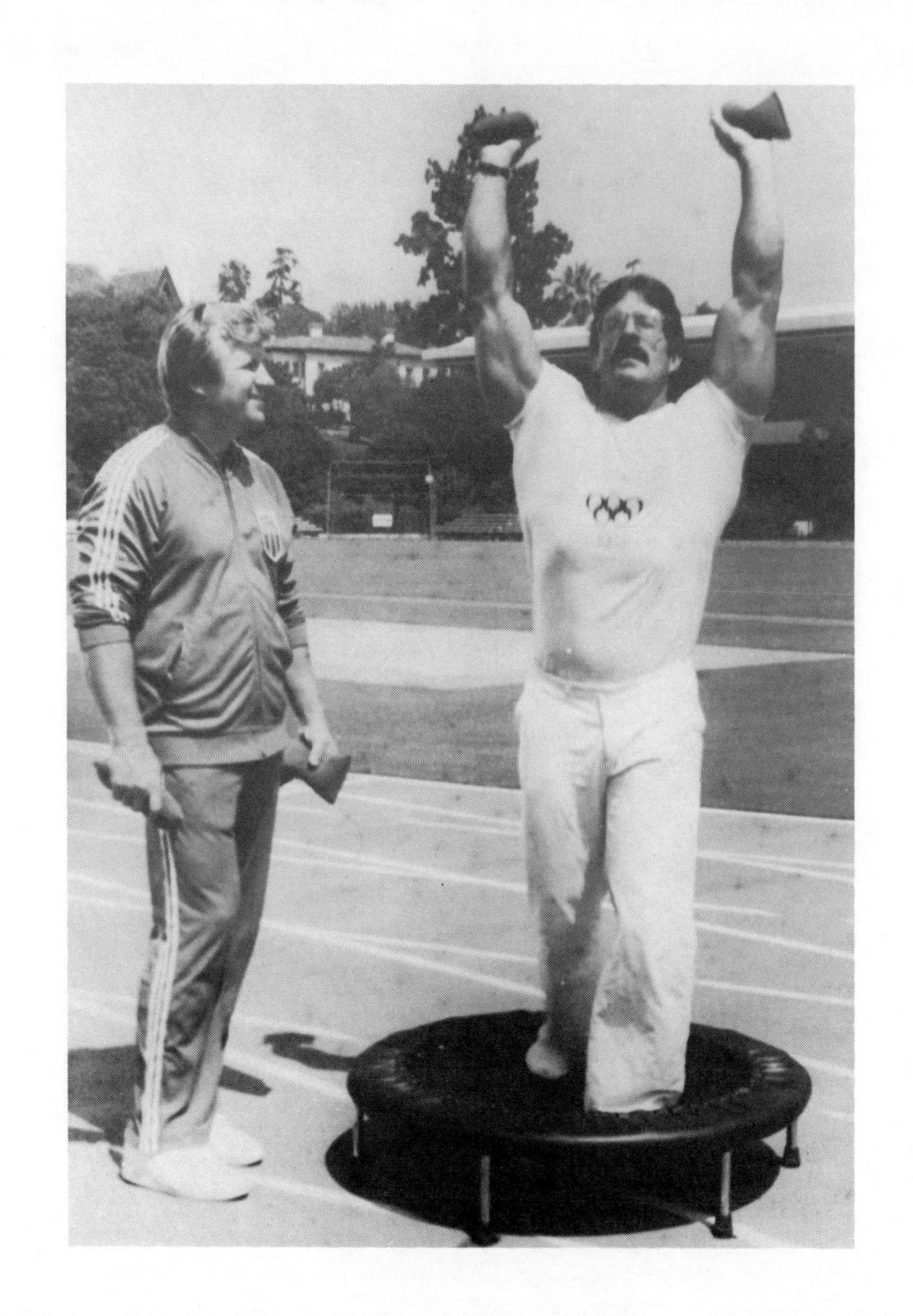

Chapter 13

Be a Superstar in Your Sport

With resistive rebounding

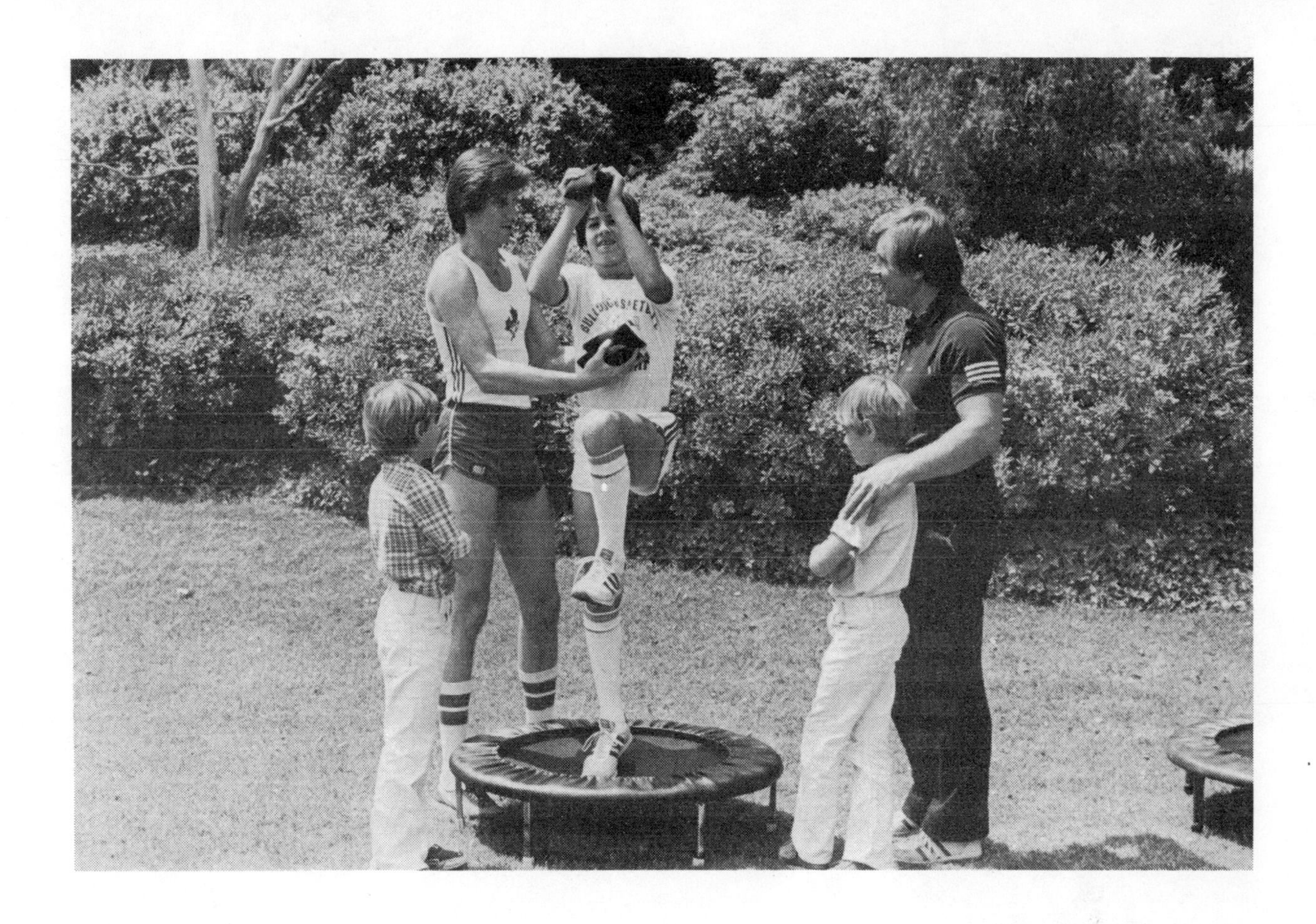

Athletic success can be yours with this program of Sanbagging. It includes what every sports training program needs: conditioning, strength, explosiveness, coordination, agility, flexibility, variety, brain-eye development, and much more. The most important thing you can do as an athlete is try this remarkable breakthrough in sports training.

In my work as a coach and trainer to many world class athletes and a number of very famous Olympic stars, I have been using this program of Sanbagging with remarkable results. One young man who won a silver medal in the high jump told me that trampolining was used extensively in his program that broke the world record in the high jump. This young man has had three achilles tendon operations and he felt that using the small rebound unit and Sanbagging was just right for his program of rehabilitation.

Young women who are training with their Sanbag routines are improving their racquetball game, vertical jump in volleyball, their tennis strokes, and more. There are many athletes under my care who wouldn't let a day go by without doing these incredibly simple but effective exercises we have mentioned.

For Men and Women

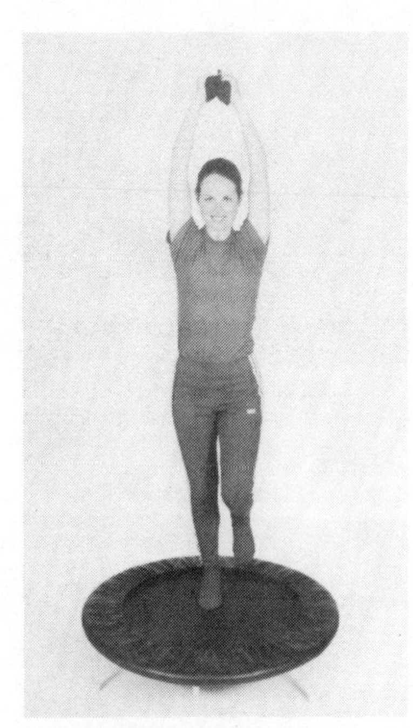

Lynn Grimditch, completion, tricep press.

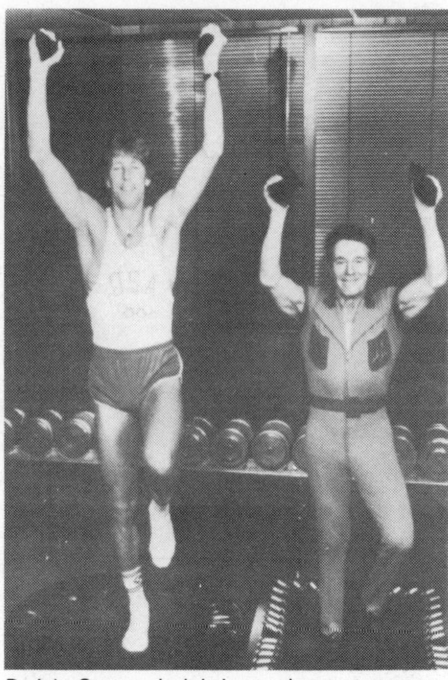

Dwight Stones, Jack LaLanne demonstrate completion of press.

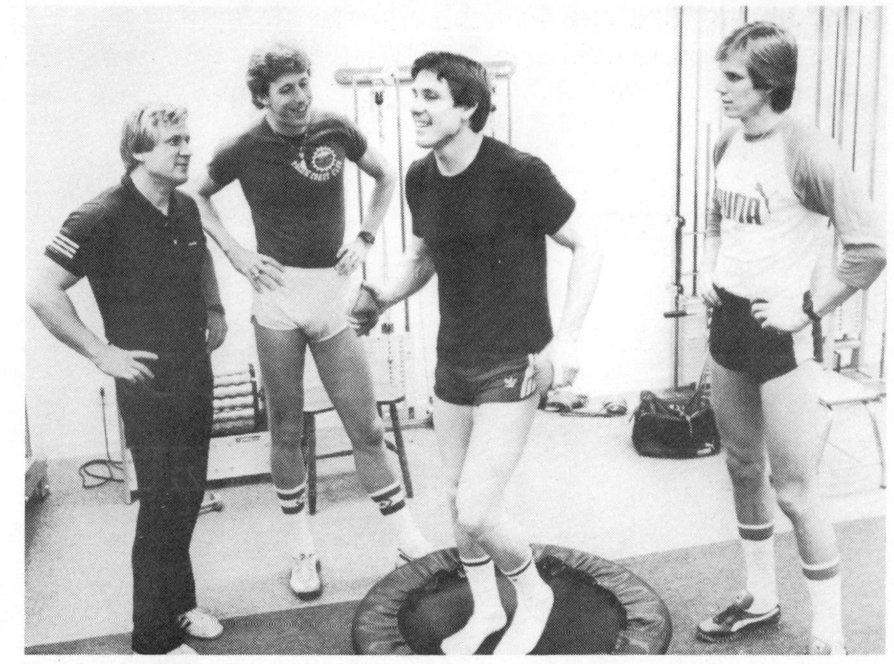

Harry Sneider, Dwight Stones, Dan Ripley and Greg Joy enjoy workout. Stones and Joy are both high jump champions; Ripley is former world pole vault record holder. All three are Olympics competitors. (See page 139.)

These programs are for men and women both. You can **adapt** the resistance if you are a younger female (.45 kilo Sanbags) or if you are a powerful male (lineman, weight lifter, etc.) then you can add more resistance (1.36 Sanbags). The key to your program is that you can **adapt** the Sanbag weight that is comfortable. The following programs are general programs for all ages, both sexes. So let's start our journey to real athletic success!

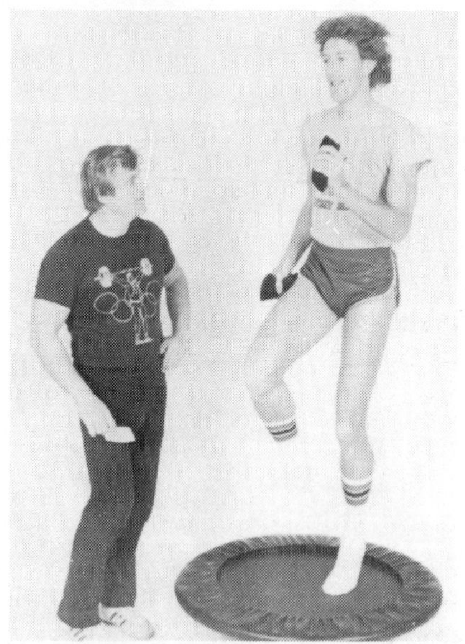

Dwight Stones, jogging on rebound unit, with Harry looking on.

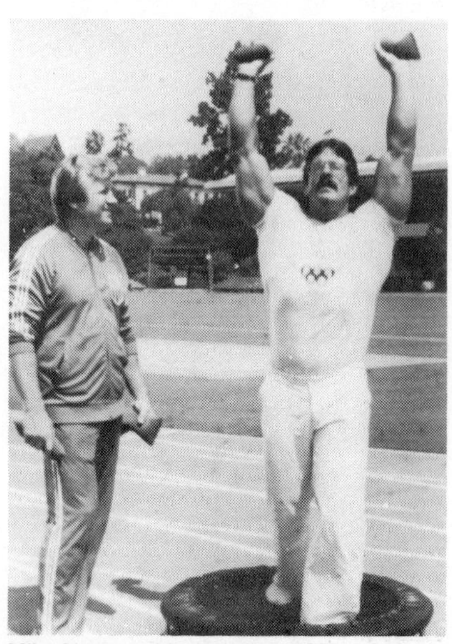

Mike Mentzer, Mr. Universe, 1979, and body builder, with author.

Sanbagging Exercise For All Sports

All these sports techniques can be developed with your daily program of the "Big Four" and the "Daily Dozen." Which skills do you want to develop?

GRIPPING	THROWING	STROKING or HITTING	JUMPING
Wrestling	Baseball	Tennis	Basketball
Weightlifting	Softball	Racquetball	Volleyball
Hockey	Football	Badminton	High Jump
Baseball	Wrestling	Golf	Long Jump
Football		Baseball hitting	Triple Jump
		Softball hitting	
		Swimming	

KICKING	SPRINTING	SKIING, SKATING	BALANCE-CO-ORDINATION
Soccer	40-100 yd. dash	Ice Skating	Gymnastics
Football	Most Sports	Roller Skating	Diving
Martial Arts	Football	Snow Skiing	Wrestling
Swimming	Baseball	Water Skiing	Basketball
	Basketball		
	Soccer		

FLEXIBILITY	DEPTH PERCEPTION	STAMINA ENDURANCE	BODY ALIGNMENT
All Sports	All Sports	Distance Running	Program that develops the body in total balance by systematic exercises
Very Important	Particularly	Swimming	
	Riflery	Basketball	
	Archery	All Sports	
	Pitching		
	Shooting		
	Basketball		
	Golf		
	Racquetball		

PSYCHOLOGICAL - MENTAL

Setting Goals
Breaking Personal Records
School Records
City, State
National, World Records
Needed for all Sports

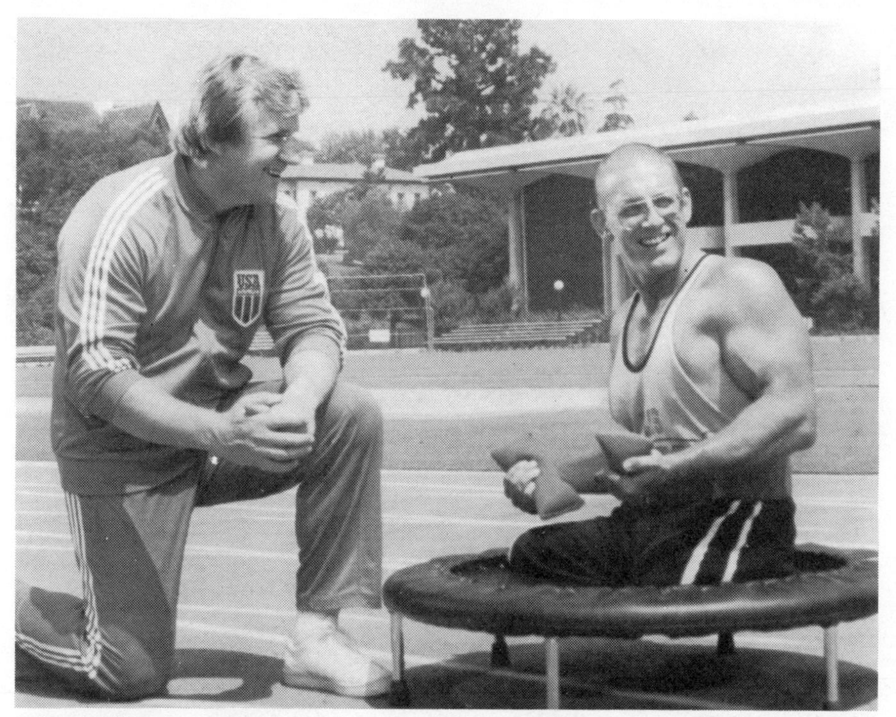

Robert J. Wieland, an incredible athlete despite losing both legs in combat in Viet Nam, works out with author. Wieland, a popular "motivator" is widely known for his "Strive for Success" lectures and frequent television appearances.

These are very important athletic skills that you can develop and will help you become a better athlete and person. Take a look at the list again. The whole program can be done with Sanbags on your rebound unit.

Using your rebound unit and your Sanbags follow this program and reap that athletic success.

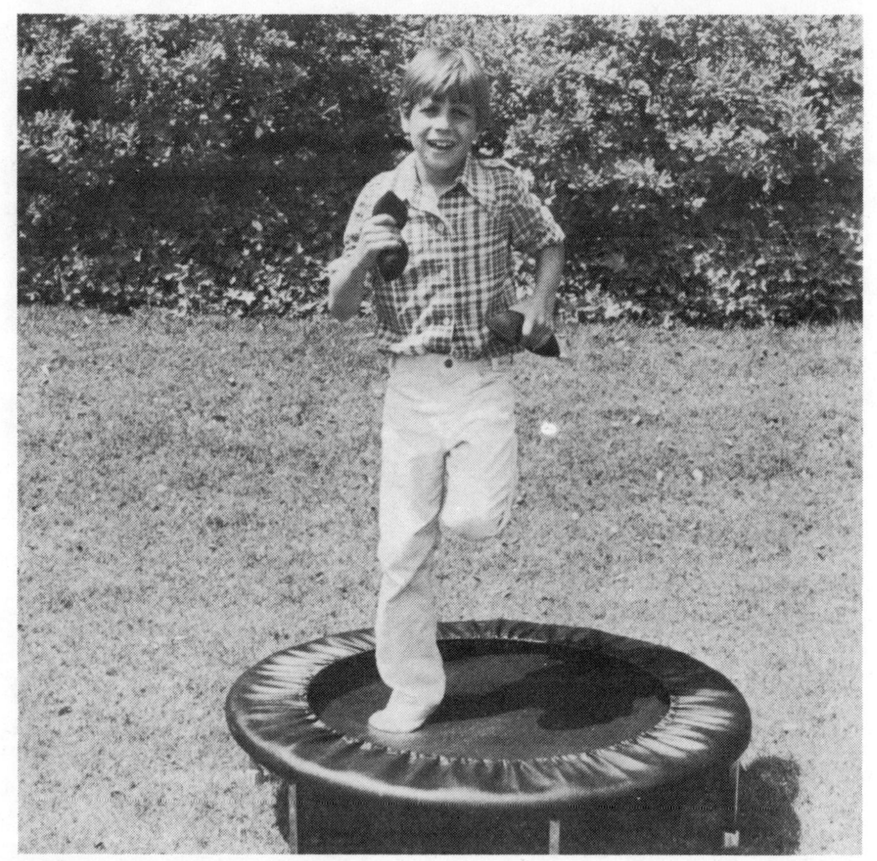
Robert Sneider demonstrates the jog easy.

If you have been running 1-5 miles per day, swimming 1000 yards or more, or in season in any sport, your program should be as follows:

Start with 2 minutes in each position and add 1 minute each week till you reach 3 minutes total for all four exercises (12 minutes for all). You should use this program every day. If you feel this is not adequate, increase each exercise till you can do each exercise with 1.36 kilo Sanbags in each position 10 minutes or 40 minutes total.

Several Olympic athletes that I am training are up to forty minutes a day with 5 pound Sanbags. They are in terrific shape, resting pulse 42, and body fat content 5%. (See section Sanbagging Principles, Chapter 14.)

If you are a younger athlete, six years of age or so, start with only 30 seconds in each position with .45 kilo Sanbags, work up to 5 minutes in each exercise by adding 15 seconds a week. Then add Sanbag weight later. It is important here that you take your time developing.

These basic exercises will improve all athletic skills from coordination to muscular strength. When you are consistent, doing these exercises every day, you will really improve. The first three months of this program can make a tremendous difference to your entire health and sports program.

THE BIG FOUR

Exercise	
1. Lymphatic Bounce	Excellent for all athletes whether 3 years old or a major leaguer in any pro sport; cleanses the lymphatic system, develops balance.
2. Shuffle	Important for balance skills, coordination, strength to leap, lower back, great for all athletes in season or getting in shape pre-season.
3. Jog	Excellent for toning body for every sport, particularly football, basketball, volleyball, etc.
4. Sprint High Knee	Excellent for track & field, tennis, racquetball, soccer, and more.

An Important Point To Remember

In order for you to really benefit from the Sanbagging routines, it is important that you do **all exercises in order** (unless otherwise prescribed). Start with exercise #1 and work to whatever the last number is in your particular sports program.

Working from exercise #1 to the last exercise would be one set. Set two would start from exercise #1 to the end of your program. You do as many sets as indicated in your routine, always starting from the beginning and going to the end.

A More Personalized Approach

THE BIG FOUR — BASIC GUIDELINES BY AGE GROUP

For the Lymphatic Bounce, Shuffle, Jog, and Sprint High Knee*

Age	Beginner Program	Intermediate Program	Advanced Program	Sanbag Weight
1½ - 6 years	30 sec.	40 sec.	1 min.	.45 kilo
6 - 12 years	30 sec.	40 sec.	1 min.	.45 kilo
Junior High Athlete	30 sec.	1 min.	1½ min.	.45 kilo
High School Athlete	45 sec.	1 min.	2 min.	.45 kilo
College Athlete	45 sec.	1½ min.	2½ min.	.45 kilo
Age Group Athlete	30 sec.	1½ min.	2½ min.	.45 kilo
Masters Athlete	30 sec.	1½ min.	2½ min.	.45 kilo

*Do suggested time in **each** exercise. Ex: 30 sec. bounce, 30 sec. shuffle, 30 sec. jog, 30 sec. sprint.

Do this program every day with .45 kilo Sanbags. Every month, add more weight if possible. Remember, take time to build up to your goal of 1.36 kilo Sanbags for 20 min. — Add 1 set per week of the four exercises till you reach your goal.

The younger the child, the more moderate the program. For the more advanced (12-20 years old) who are competitive in organized sports, then of course more activity will be required. This is what we will call the **Training Base Program** for all sports conditioning, flexibility, and strength. With this valuable training base, you will be able to learn your sports techniques that much better.

It is interesting to note that a Houston Astros pitcher, while doing this program of these basic exercises with 1.36 kilo Sanbags, discovered a new pitch. He hopes to make it the greatest year ever. He improved his pitching technique noticeably and his conditioning is at an all time high (resting pulse 42).

INTERVAL PROGRAM WITH THE BIG FOUR AND SANBAGS

For Men and Women

Beginner	**Intermediate**	**Advanced**
(New to "Sanbag" rebounding, young child)	(1-3 mos. rebounding Young Athlete 7-13 years old)	(15-20 min. rebounding 1-5 miles jogging runner, swimmer, or in top shape)
15 sec. Jog	25 sec. Jog	45 sec. Jog
5 sec. Lymphatic Bounce	5 sec. Lymphatic Bounce	5 sec. Lymphatic Bounce
15 sec. Shuffle	25 sec. Shuffle	45 sec. Shuffle
5 sec. Lymphatic Bounce	5 sec. Lymphatic Bounce	5 sec. Lymphatic Bounce
15 sec. Sprint	25 sec. Sprint	45 sec. Sprint
5 sec. Lymphatic Bounce	5 sec. Lymphatic Bounce	5 sec. Lymphatic Bounce
60 seconds Total	90 seconds Total	150 seconds Total
Repeat this set three times in row, and end your program with an easy 2 min. jog. Use .45 kilo Sanbags.	Repeat this set three times in a row and end your program with an easy 1 min. jog. Use .91 kilo Sanbags.	Repeat 3 times in a row. Slow jog 2 min. after each set. Use 1.36 kilo Sanbags.
Increase 1 set a week till you can do up to eight minutes, increase easy jog 1 min. per week till you jog 8 min. Leave Sanbag weight the same.	Increase 1 set per week till you reach 8 sets or 12 min. Increase slow jog 1 min. after each week till you reach 8 min.	Increase 1 set each week till you reach 8 sets or 20 min., slow jog after each till you reach 16 min.
TOTAL: 12 Minutes	TOTAL: 17 Minutes	TOTAL: 36 Minutes

The Interval Program with your Sanbags using the "Big Four" is a real tool to athletic conditioning and strength building for all sports. The beginner can move into the moderate program by completing his 12 minutes total. The moderate can move to the advanced. Have a wristwatch or a small clock nearby so you can see where you are.

For you beginners, if you exceed more than double resting pulse rate (Example: Resting Pulse Rate 70, 70 x 2 equals 140) or if you feel continually fatigued, it is time to cut back on the sprint segment of your program. This program of interval rebound Sanbagging is for you if you want to be really in shape. You will enjoy it.

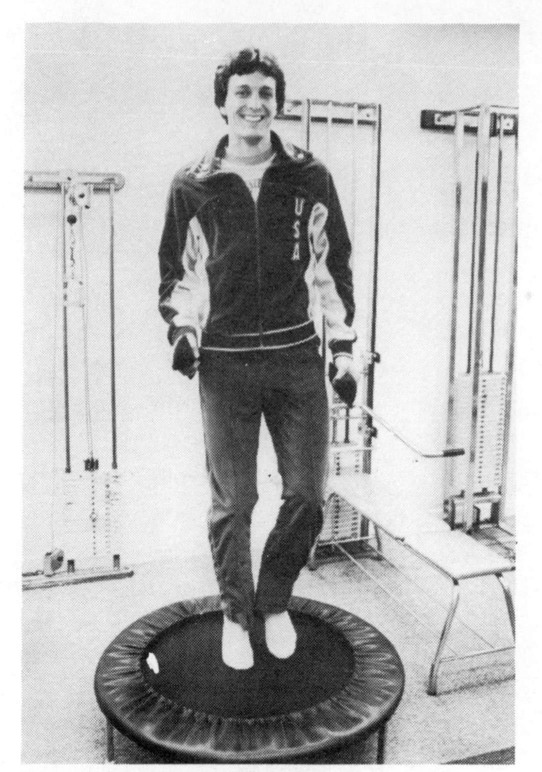

Kenny Sutton, doing the jog easy.

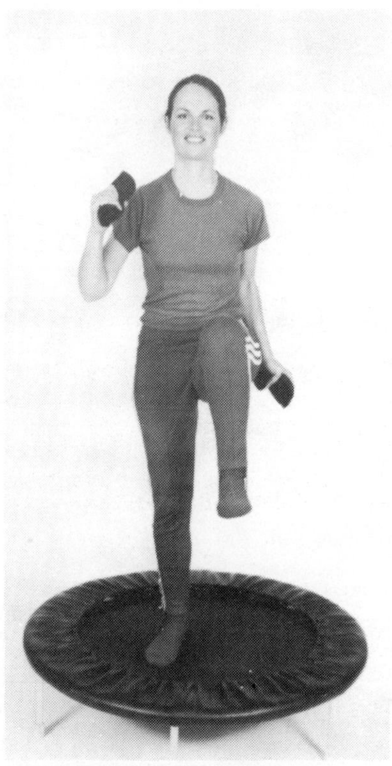

Lynn Grimditch, sprint high knee.

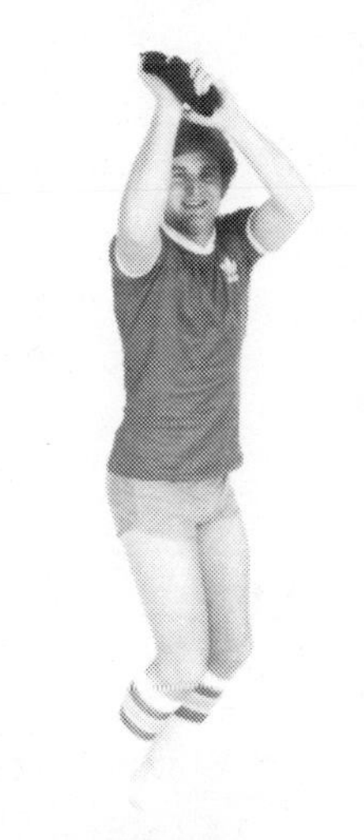

SANBAGGING EXERCISES FOR YOUR FAVORITE SPORT

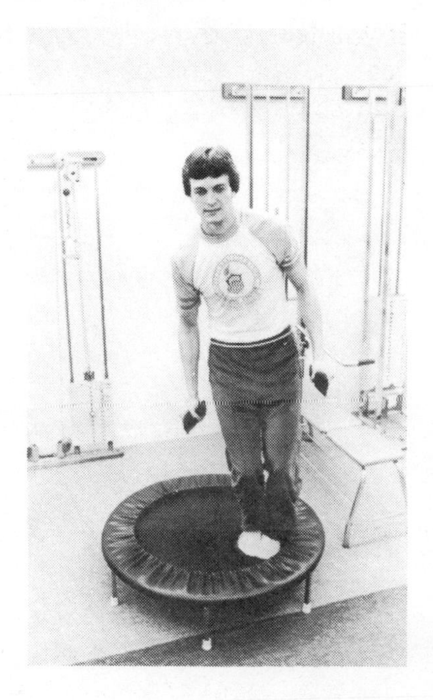

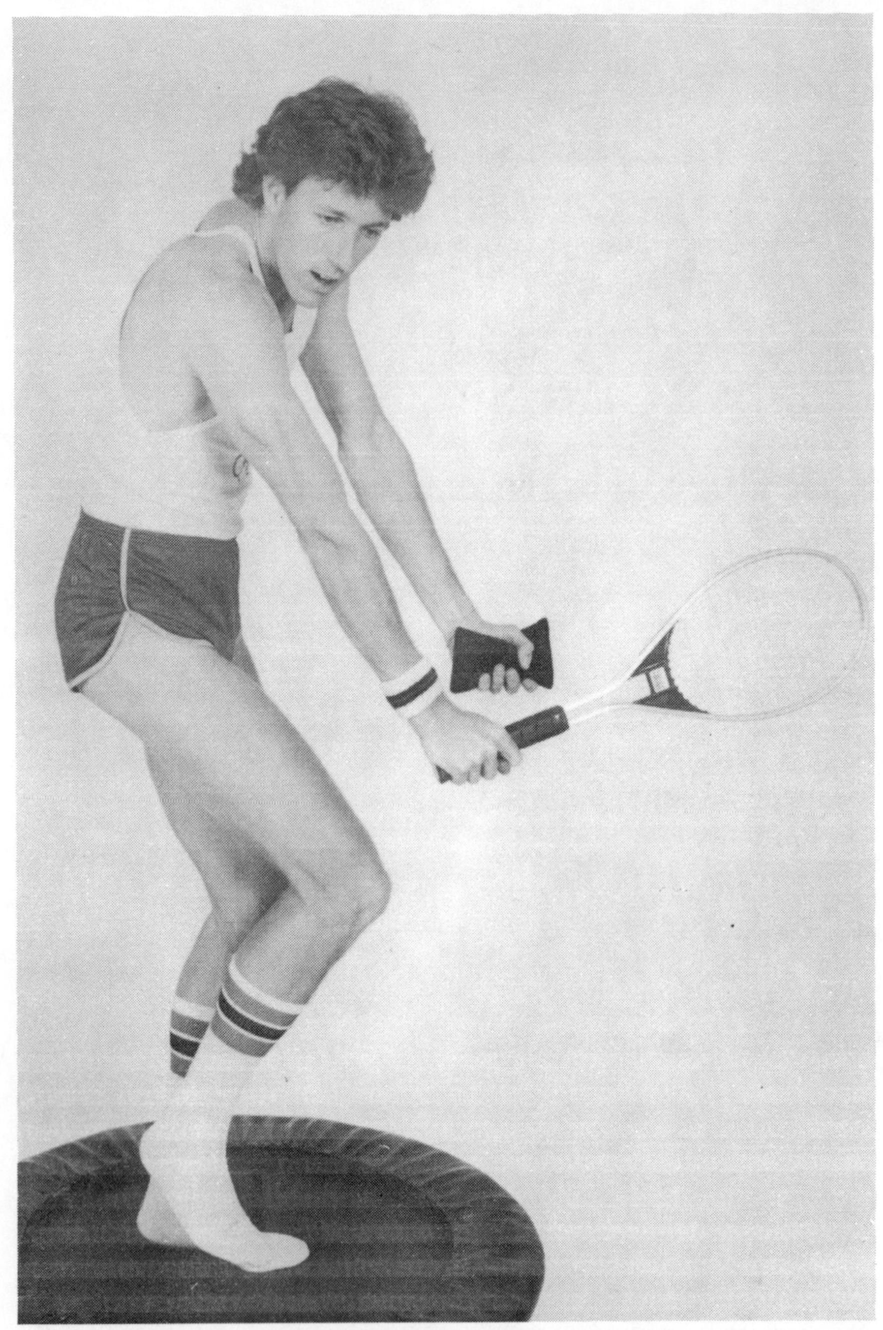

Dwight Stones shows how doing backhand stroke with Sanbag develops motor skills. (See chapter on "Sanbagging Principles", Point 6, Page 124.)

Tennis

The 'Big Four' is a must as a warmup

THE BASIC FOUR

Exercise	Wt.	Time	Sets	Goal
Lymphatic Bounce	.45 kilo Sanbags	30 sec.	3	3 sets of 2½ min.
Shuffle	.45 kilo Sanbags	30 sec.	3	3 sets of 2½ min.
Jog Easy	.45 kilo Sanbags	30 sec.	3	3 sets of 2½ min.
Sprint High Knees	.45 kilo Sanbags	30 sec.	3	3 sets of 2½ min.

Start your program with .45 kilo Sanbags by alternating between Lymphatic Bounce, Shuffle, Jog Easy, and Sprint High Knee at 30 seconds each. Repeat this three times in your warmup program. Add 15 seconds every week on each set till you reach 2½ min. in each exercise three times. Total time, 30 min.

It would be very desirable that you increase Sanbag dosages every month by .45 kilos. Eventually using 1.36 kilo Sanbags in your tennis warmup. This activity is excellent warmup before you play your match. Put this program on your tennis court today. All you need is some light Sanbags and a rebound unit and watch your game improve.

Working with many tennis professionals, teachers, players, and students of the game, there are several major keys to your sport. They are:

1. Cardio-Respiratory Fitness — you can't play if you are overweight or have an injury.
2. Flexibility — tight joint, muscular imbalance leads to many injuries.
3. Strength — if you are not explosive, you can't reach those hard shots, your body will be injured easier, too.
4. Technique — your technique will improve with fitness.
5. Will or Desire — you may have desire, but if you are not fit, you will only end up injured or frustrated.

For over two years, I have been coaching and training one of California's finest age group tennis players. He was always complaining of little injuries, particularly knees, ankles, etc. We started to develop a program of flexibility, strength training including our Sanbagging program on the rebound unit. Within weeks, this fine player went from being one of the best players in the state to beating the No. 1 player at the end of the tennis season. What was most incredible, his injury problem virtually disappeared.

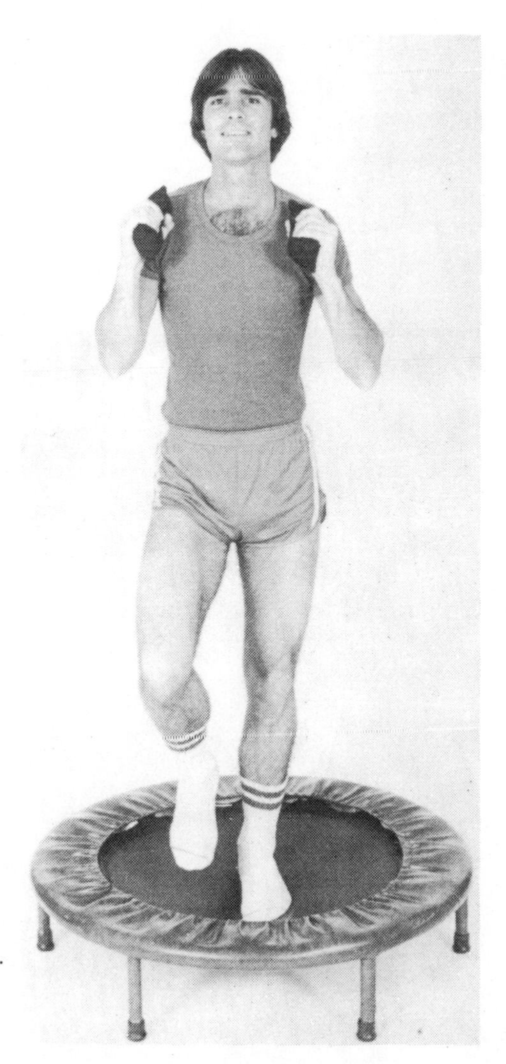

T.J. McCavitt, beginning of press.

THE DAILY DOZEN

Sanbagging will improve your tennis, too!

Exercise	Wt.	Reps/Time	Sets	Goals
1. Curl	.45 kilo	10	2	5 sets of 20 reps. with 1.36 kilo Sanbags
2. Press	.45 kilo	10	2	
3. Upright Row	.45 kilo	10	2	
4. Tricep Press	.45 kilo	10	2	
5. Squeeze	.45 kilo	10	2	
6. Curl & Press	45 kilo	10	2	
7. Side Raise	.45 kilo	10	2	
8. Crossover	.45 kilo	10	2	
9. Sprint High Knee	.45 kilo	45 sec.	2	3½ minutes
10. Press Up & Out	.45 kilo	10	2	5 sets, 20 reps, 1.36 kilo bags
11. Pullover	.45 kilo	10	2	
12. Jog Easy	.45 kilo	1 min.	2	7 minutes

Add 1 rep. each day till you reach 20 reps. Start with 2 sets and one set after you reach 20 reps. Remember, TRAIN, DON'T STRAIN. If you see this is too much, don't push. This program is best done by jogging easy and then doing your exercises on your rebound unit.

Using these exercises with beginning players in our fitness centers, I have seen great improvement in stamina, flexibility, and ability to improve technique. This program is very effective if it is done consistently.

Other drills that you can do on your rebound unit with your versatile Sanbags:

Exercise	Wt.	Reps/Time	Sets	Goals
1. Forehand Stroke	.45 kilo	12	2	5 x 25 with 1.36 kilo Sanbags
2. Backhand Stroke	.45 kilo	12	2	5 x 25 with 1.36 kilo Sanbags
3. Serve	.45 kilo	12	2	5 x 25 with 1.36 kilo Sanbags
4. Side to Side Movement	.45 kilo	12	2	5 x 25 with 1.36 kilo Sanbags

Add one rep. per day till you reach twenty-five repetitions, add .45 kilo every month to your Sanbags. These exercises will emulate your tennis game. These drills are excellent in improving your game. May I suggest that you do these exercises in front of a mirror so you can actually see your stroking technique.

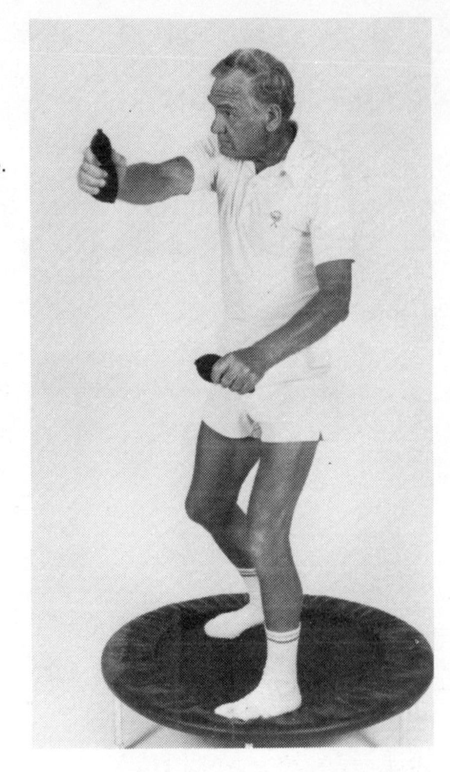

Forehand stroke.

Don Allen, 67, top-ranked tennis player in age group, attorney by profession, has been Sanbagging for about eight months.

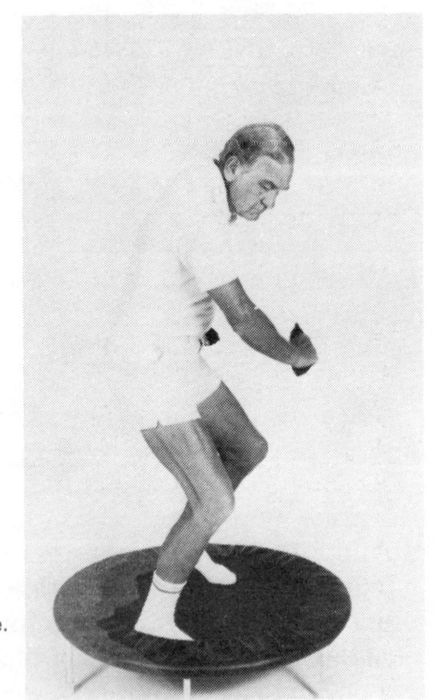

Backhand stroke.

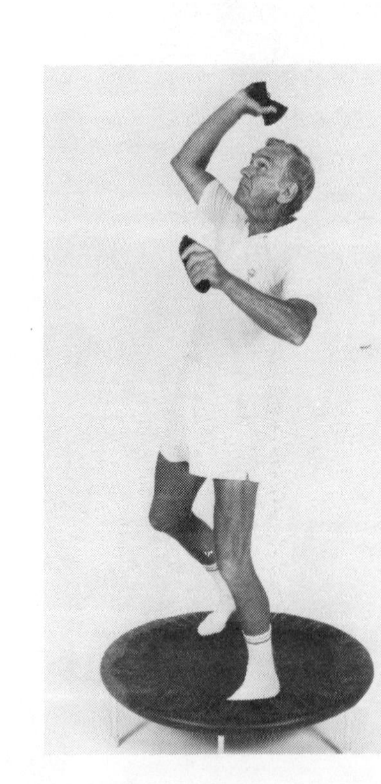

Serve.

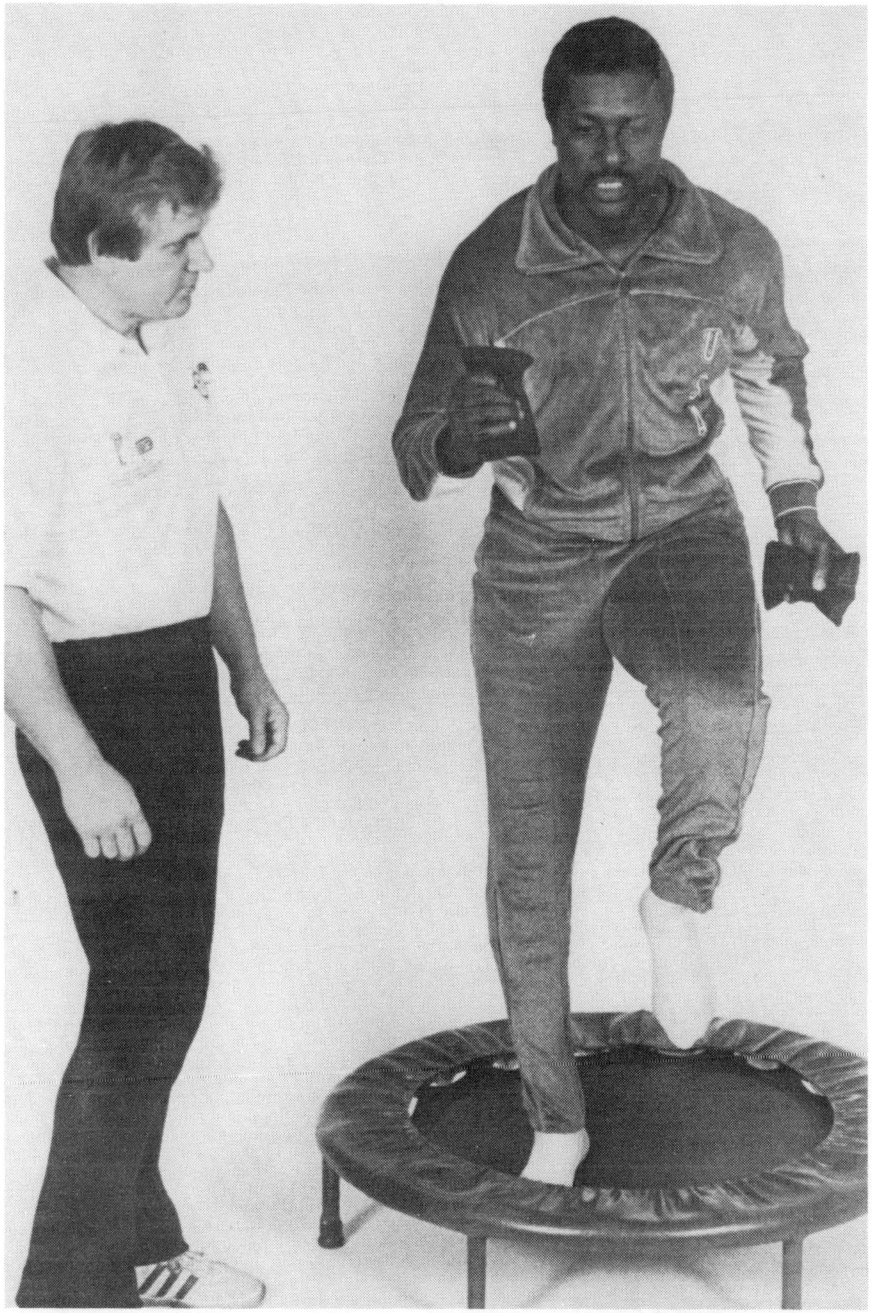

Football

Pre-season, in-season maintenance —with your Sanbagging program

Harry instructs James C. Butts, 1976 Olympics triple jump silver medalist (56′¾″) in the sprint high knee.

Football players are told by their coaches to work out by lifting weights, develop their techniques for their position, do windsprints, analyze movies. I am very familiar with football training as I have worked with some of the biggest names in this sport.

Sanbagging on a rebounding unit has many of the necessary components in developing the all around football player in more than just running and weight training. Most of your top football players develop the major prime movers for the sport (like chest, shoulders, quadriceps). Many times a program that develops the total body is neglected. Results are injuries and inefficient productivity in the sport. Coaches love to see a well-conditioned athlete, fully developed (muscular conditioning). This is your program for pre-season conditioning and maintenance even during the season.

THE BASIC FOUR

Exercise	Wt.	Reps/Time	Sets	Goals
1. Lymphatic Bounce	.45 kilo	30 sec.	2	6 sets of each exercise with 1.36 kilo Sanbags
2. Shuffle	.45 kilo	1 min.	2	
3. Jog	.45 kilo	1½ min.	2	
4. Bounce	.45 kilo	1 min.	2	

Add 1 set each till you reach 6 sets of each exercise using the 1.36 kilo Sanbags. Add .45 kilo to your Sanbag every month. Work out daily. Those who find this program easy can add one set each week till you reach 10 sets in all with 1.36 kilo Sanbags. TOTAL TIME: 40 minutes with 1.36 kilo Sanbags.

The football player who is in shape will feel confident, will not be injured as easy, and will respond more readily in the classroom, too. The above "Basic Four" program is excellent for someone coming off a knee injury or surgery. Check with your doctor for his approval. This program is very kind to your joints.

THE DAILY DOZEN

Sanbagging Your Way to Excellence on the Gridiron

Exercise	Wt.	Reps/Time	Sets	Goals
1. Curl	.45 kilo	12	3	8 sets of 20 reps with 1.36 kilo Sanbags.
2. Press	.45 kilo	2	3	
3. Upright Row	.45 kilo	12	3	
4. Tricep Press	.45 kilo	12	3	
5. Squeeze	.45 kilo	12	3	
6. Curl & Press	.45 kilo	12	3	
7. Side Raise	.45 kilo	12	3	
8. Crossovers	.45 kilo	12	3	
9. Sprint High Knee	.45 kilo	½ min.	3	4 minutes
10. Press Up & Out	.45 kilo	12	3	8 sets of 20 reps with 1.36 kilo Sanbags.
11. Pullovers	.45 kilo	12	3	
12. Jog Easy	.45 kilo	1½ min.	3	12 minutes

Your goal as a football player is to increase a set a week till you reach 8 sets, add .45 kilo Sanbags a month, till you reach 1.36 kilo. Your total goal is 8 sets of 12 reps. in all exercises: 4 minute Sprint High Knee, 12 minutes Jog Easy. This program will really make you a solid performer in the football program.

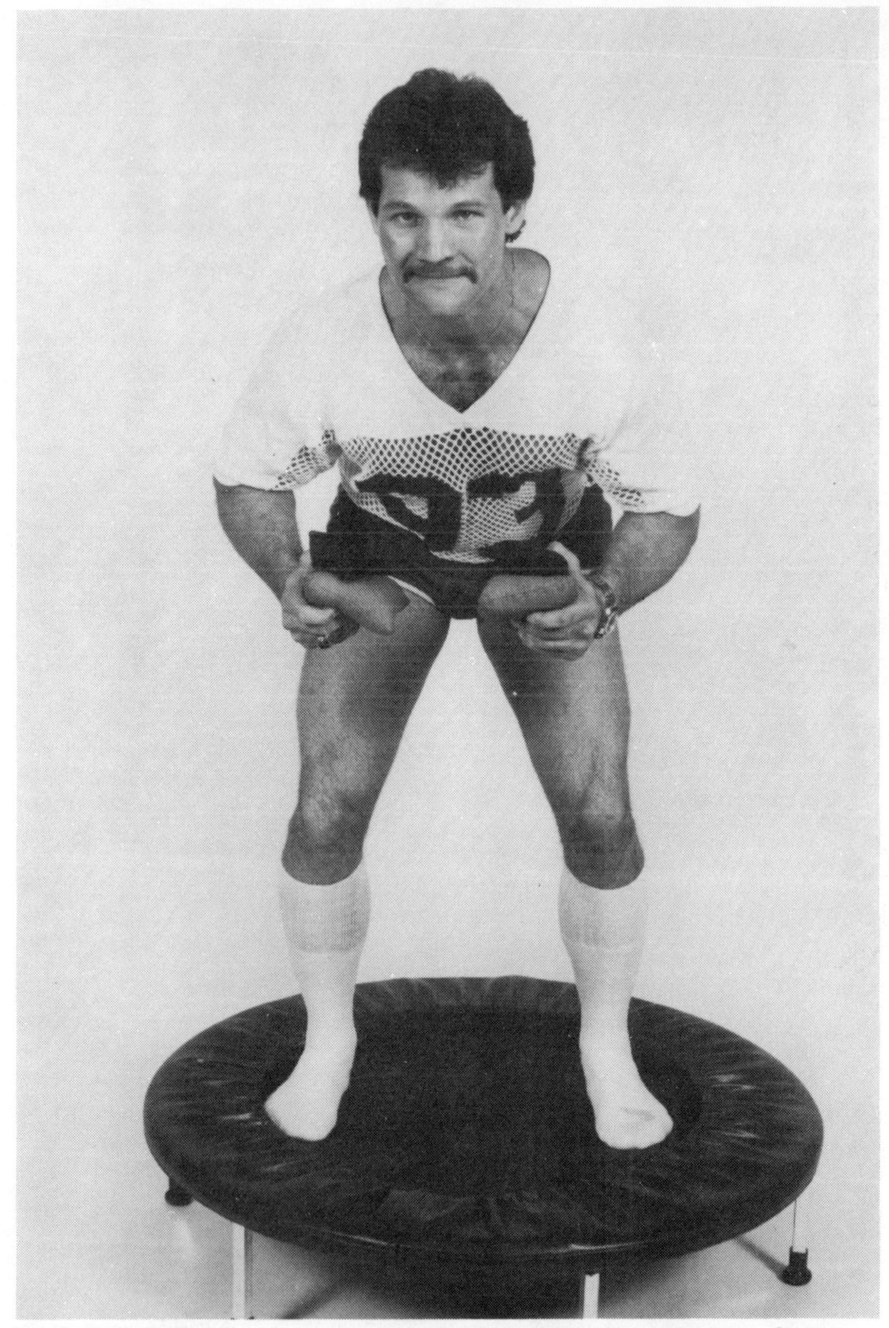

Bob Orosz, linebacker, Ohio State, demonstrates the blocking position, using heavy Sanbags, two in each hand.

FOOTBALL
HEAVY BODY BUILDING PROGRAM WITH SANBAGS

After you have been running 1-5 miles per day, and lifting weights 3 times per week. Try this and really get into shape.

Exercise	Wt.	Reps/Time	Sets	Goals
1. Curl	1.36 kilo	25	3	10 sets of 25 reps using 1.36 kilo Sanbags
2. Press	1.36 kilo	25	3	
3. Upright Row	1.36 kilo	25	3	
4. Tricep Press	1.36 kilo	25	3	
5. Squeeze	1.36 kilo	25	3	
6. Curl & Press	1.36 kilo	25	3	
7. Side Raise	1.36 kilo	25	3	
8. Crossover	1.36 kilo	25	3	
9. Sprint High Knee	1.36 kilo	½ min.	3	5 min.
10. Press Up & Out	1.36 kilo	25	3	10 sets of 25 reps with 1.36 kilo Sanbags
11. Pullover	1.36 kilo	25	3	
12. Jog Easy	1.36 kilo	2½ min.	3	25 min.

Set a goal of adding one set per week, until you reach 10 sets of 25 reps. with 1.36 kilo Sanbags, add 15 seconds to sprint each week in the ten weeks until you are sprinting 5 minutes. Jog up to 25 minutes by adding one set of 2½ minutes per week. This program is for the advanced football player. Remember, if you feel sore or tired, take it easy until you build up. This program will definitely get you ready for a gruelling schedule from high school to pro football.

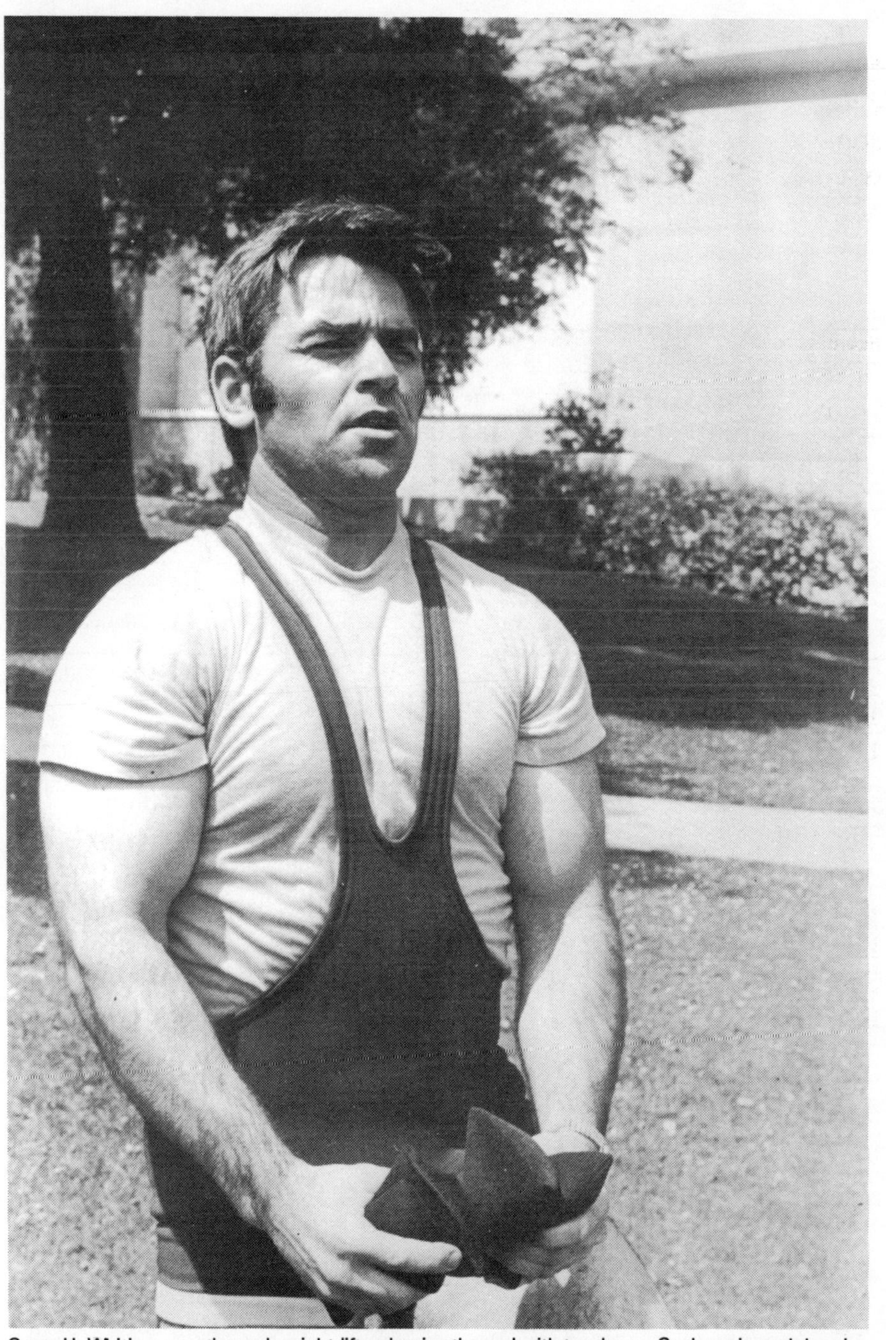

Geary H. Whiting, wrestler and weight lifter, begins the curl with two heavy Sanbags in each hand.

Basketball

Sanbagging is your key to a great season

After coaching college basketball for three years, I can tell you that a player in today's sports arena needs to be fit. Much depends on your attitude, but more depends on your ability to move, shoot, play defense and stay in school academically. Try this program.

THE BASIC FOUR — SANBAGGING ROUTINE

Exercise	Wt.	Reps/Time	Sets	Goals
Lymphatic Bounce	.45 kilo	30 sec.	2	8 sets of each exercise with 1.36 kilo Sanbags
Shuffle	.45 kilo	1½ min.	2	
Jog	.45 kilo	1½ min.	2	
Bounce	.45 kilo	1 min.	2	

Add 1 set each week till you reach 8 sets of each exercise. The total is 32 minutes. Pre-season you can go to as much as 12 sets with 1.36 kilo Sanbags. In season, cut it back to six sets. Add .45 kilo Sanbags each month till you reach 1.36 kilo bags. Conditioning can be a real key to a great defense. Hustle can mean the difference between making a team or not. You will be amazed at your ability to stay injury free by following this program.

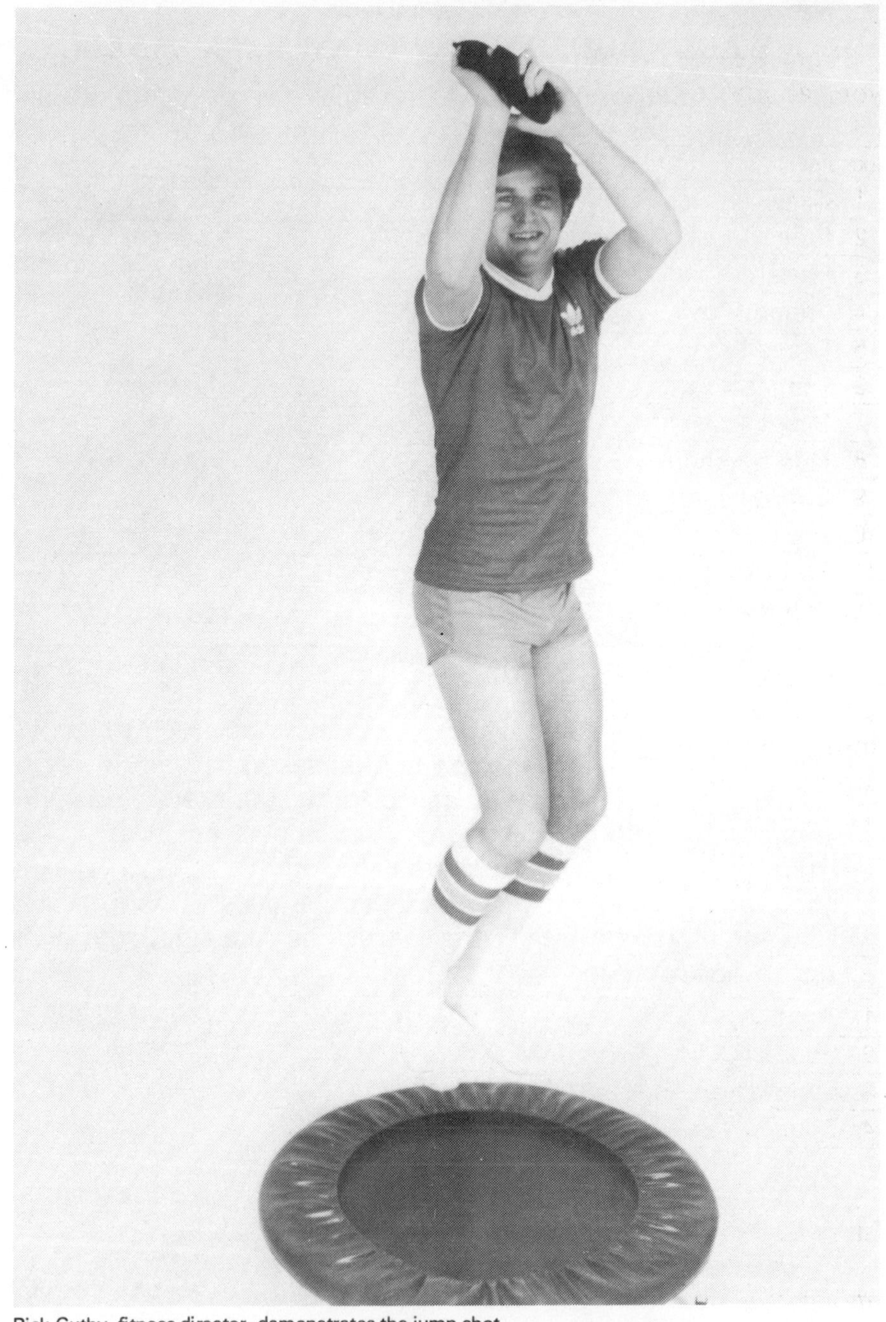

Rick Guthy, fitness director, demonstrates the jump shot.

THE DAILY DOZEN

From PeeWee to the NBA, you will see a total difference in your ability to play the game of basketball.

Exercise	Wt.	Reps/Time	Sets	Goals
1. Curl	.45 kilo	14	3	8 sets of 14 with 1.36 kilo Sanbags
2. Press	.45 kilo	14	3	
3. Upright Row	.45 kilo	14	3	
4. Tricep Press	.45 kilo	14	3	
5. Squeeze	.45 kilo	14	3	
6. Curl & Press	.45 kilo	14	3	
7. Side Raise	.45 kilo	14	3	
8. Crossovers	.45 kilo	14	3	
9. Sprint High Knee	.45 kilo	½ min.	3	4½ min.
10. Press Up & Out	.45 kilo	14	3	8 sets of 14 with 1.36 kilo Sanbags.
11. Pullover	.45 kilo	14	3	
12. Jog Easy	.45 kilo	1½ min.	3	10 min.

Add one set a week, till you reach 8 sets of 14 reps. Add .45 kilo of Sanbag weight till you reach 1.36 kilo bags. Add ½ minute on each sprint till you reach 4½ minute in the sprint. Add 1 minute Jog Easy till you reach 9½ to 10 minute in the jog easy. Total time spent is around 32 minutes.

VERTICAL JUMP PROGRAM WITH SANBAGS

(For Basketball, Volleyball)

Exercise	Wt.	Reps/Time	Sets	Goals
1. Jog Easy	.45 kilo	1 min.	2	5 sets of each exercise with 1.36 kilo Sanbags
2. Bounce	.45 kilo	1 min.	2	
3. Sprint High Knee	.45 kilo	1 min.	2	
4. Bounce	.45 kilo	1 min.	2	

GOAL — add set of each activity until you reach five sets, total time of 20 minutes. Add .45 kilo a month until you reach 1.36 kilo Sanbags. This program will increase your vertical jump as much as 3 inches in six weeks.

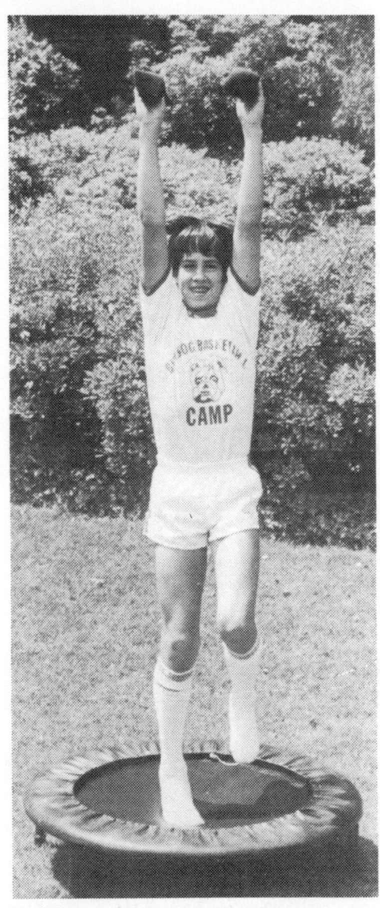

Todd Grinolds, completion of press.

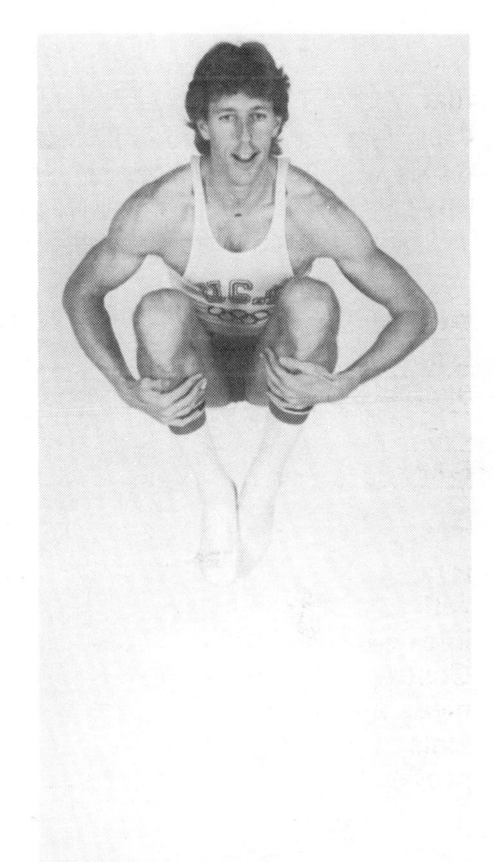

Dwight Stones develops tremendous vertical jumping ability through rebounding program.

Baseball

Sanbagging — your answer to improving your talent

Having played baseball myself (trying out with the Minnesota Twins and the Chicago White Sox), I can appreciate what it takes to play this wonderful sport. Presently, I am preparing several pro baseball players with Sanbagging on our rebound units with dramatic results. You, as a baseball player, will improve if you follow these basic guidelines every day.

THE BIG FOUR

Pre-season — every day training

Exercise	Wt.	Reps/Time	Sets	Goals
1. Lymphatic bounce	.45 kilo	½ min.	2	6 sets with 1.36 kilo Sanbags
2. Shuffle	.45 kilo	1 min.	2	6 sets with 1.36 kilo Sanbags
3. Jog	.45 kilo	1 min.	2	6 sets with 1.36 kilo Sanbags
4. Bounce	.45 kilo	1 min.	2	6 sets with 1.36 kilo Sanbags

Add 1 set a week until you reach six sets. Add .45 kilo Sanbag per month until you reach 21 minutes with 1.36 kilo Sanbags. If you find this easy, go to 10 sets.

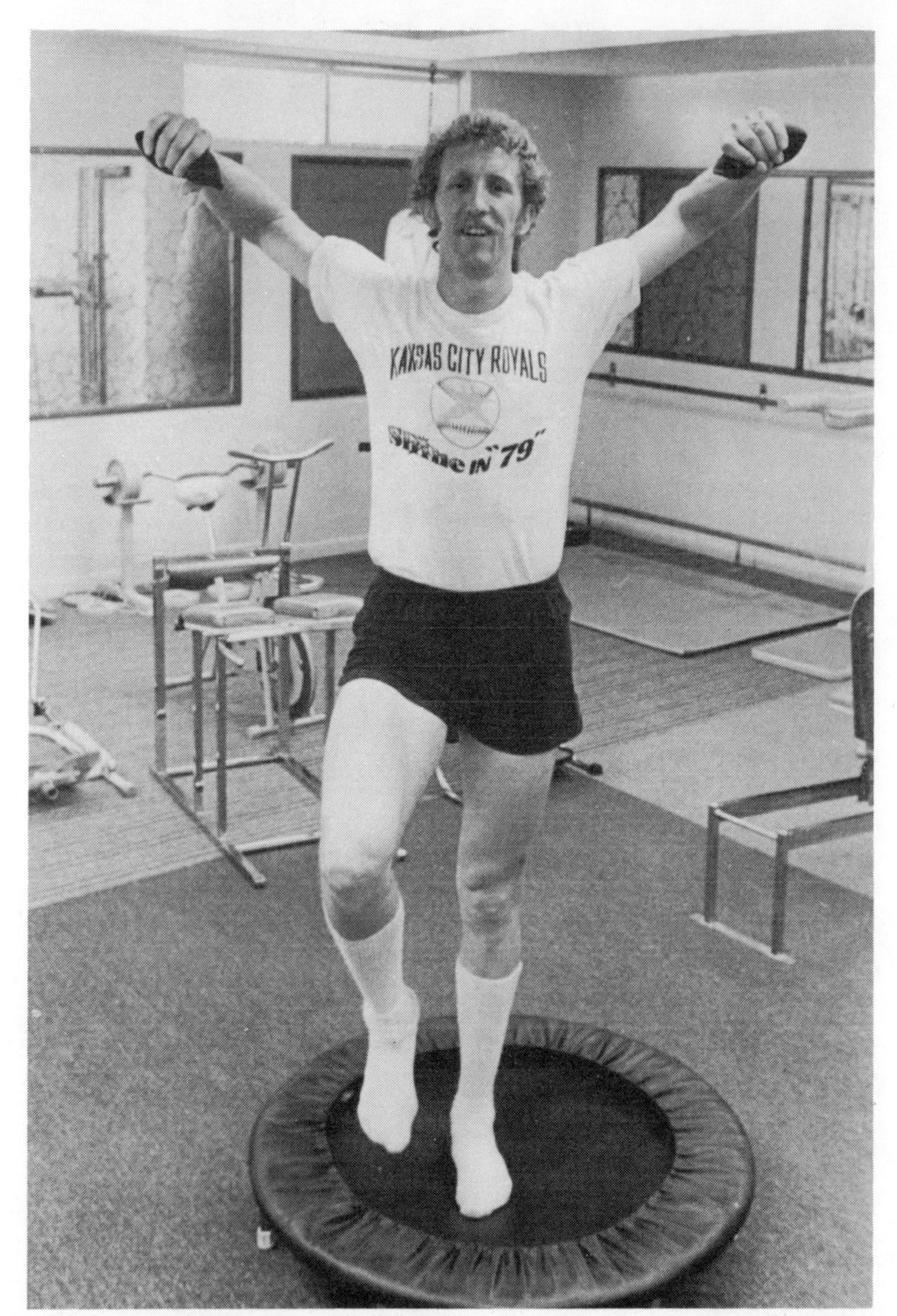

George L. Throop III, pitcher (Kansas City Royals, Houston Astros), doing side raises — excellent for shoulders and upper back (see "Daily Dozen").

THE DAILY DOZEN

Sanbagging increases endurance, develops muscles, and helps in all phases of your game.

Exercise	Wt.	Reps/Time	Sets	Goals
1. Curl	.45 kilo	12	2	6 sets with 1.36 kilo Sanbags
2. Press	.45 kilo	12	2	
3. Upright Row	.45 kilo	12	2	
4. Tricep Press	.45 kilo	12	2	
5. Squeeze	.45 kilo	12	2	
6. Curl & Press	.45 kilo	12	2	
7. Side Raise	.45 kilo	12	2	
8. Crossover	.45 kilo	12	2	
9. Sprint High Knee	.45 kilo	½ min.	2	4 min.
10. Press Up & Out	.45 kilo	12	2	6 sets with 1.36 kilo Sanbags
11. Pullover	.45 kilo	12	2	
12. Jog Easy	.45 kilo	1 min.	2	8 min.

Add 1 set per week, till you reach six sets, add .45 kilo Sanbags per month till you reach 1.36 kilo bags. Add ½ min. each week until you reach 4 minutes. On Jog Easy, add 1 minute each week. Approximate total time, 22 minutes. This program is very good in season, too. Be consistent, use it every day.

PITCHING

Sanbagging will improve your throwing. Try this program and see for yourself.

Exercise	Wt.	Reps/Time	Sets	Goals
Jog Easy (warmup)	.45 kilo	1 min.	3	8 sets of each exercise
Throwing Motion	.45 kilo	20	3	8 min. in easy jog
Squeeze (Forearms, wrist)	.45 kilo	20	3	8 sets of each exercise
Curl Press (Biceps, forearms)	.45 kilo	20	3	
Sprint High Knee (Total Body)	.45 kilo	½ min.	3	4 min.

Add 1 set a week until you reach 8 sets. Jog easy 8 minute total. Sprint High Knee 4 minutes. Add .45 kilo Sanbag every month until you reach 1.36 kilo bags. Total time for routine is approximately 20 minutes.

Besides doing these excellent conditioning routines, try to get enough sleep, study the game, keep your head full of positive thoughts about your future. Many times the athlete that does the little things will get the job. I know you can improve; give this routine a try.

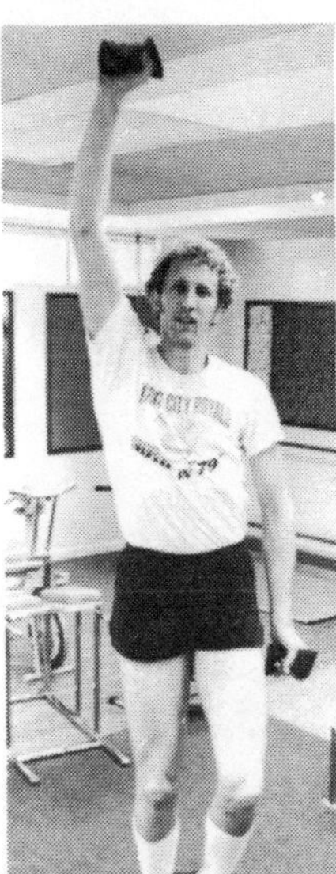

George Throop

Mid-point, throwing motion.

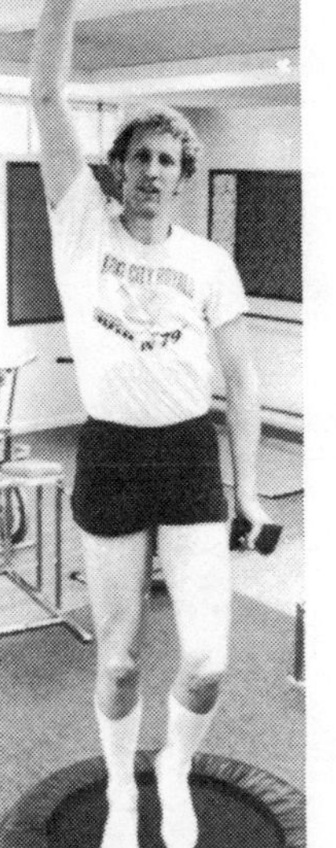

Completion, throwing motion.

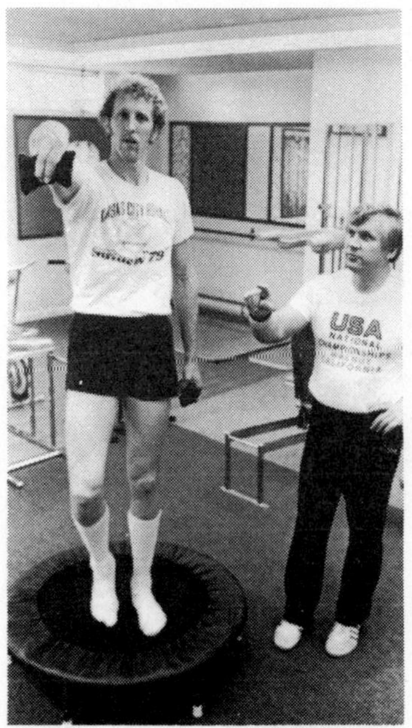

Harry explaining pitching technique.

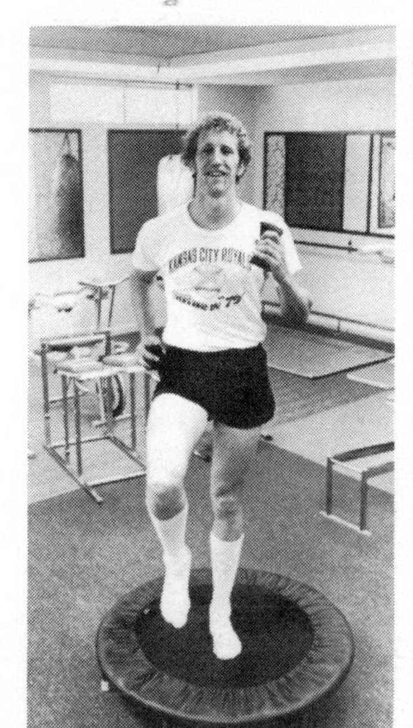

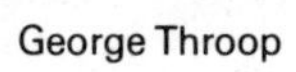

George Throop

Sprint High Knee.

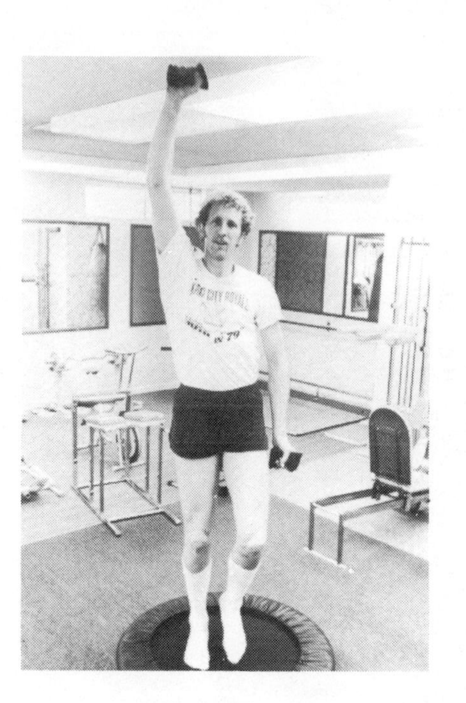

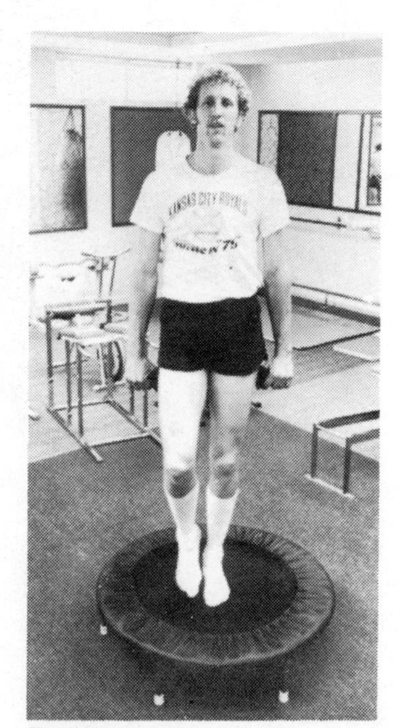

The squeeze.

Track & Field

Stay in shape year-round

You, as a track athlete, need to stay in shape year around. There is much good that you can do on your world class training center, the consistency of Sanbags and a small rebound unit. Presently, I am coaching and training these athletes with some of the programs mentioned below: Dwight Stones, 10 time world record holder in the high jump; Dan Ripley, former world record

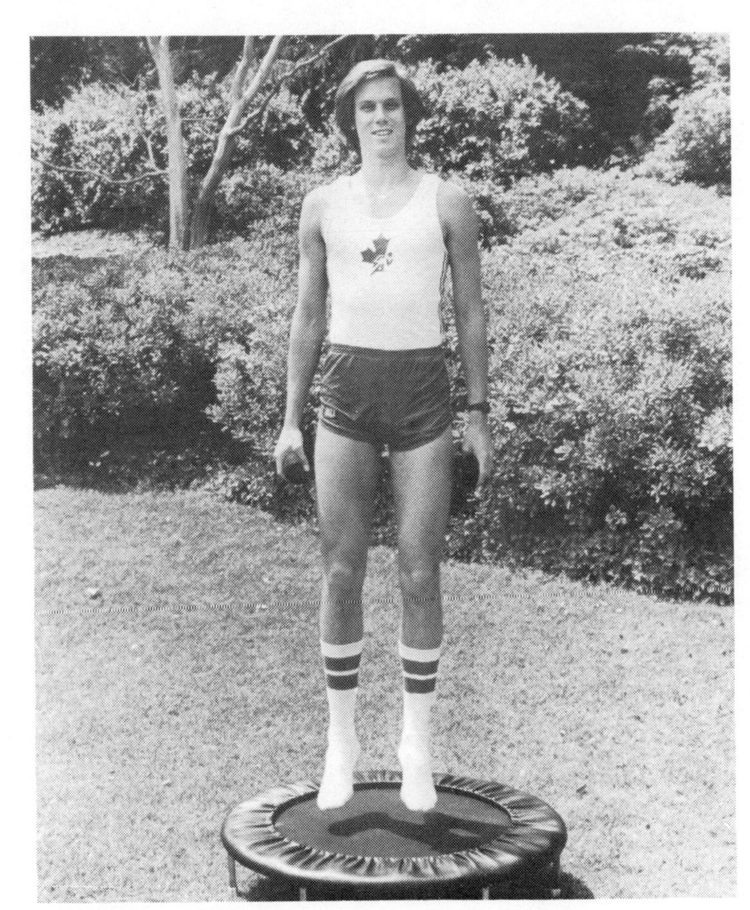

Greg Joy, the bounce.

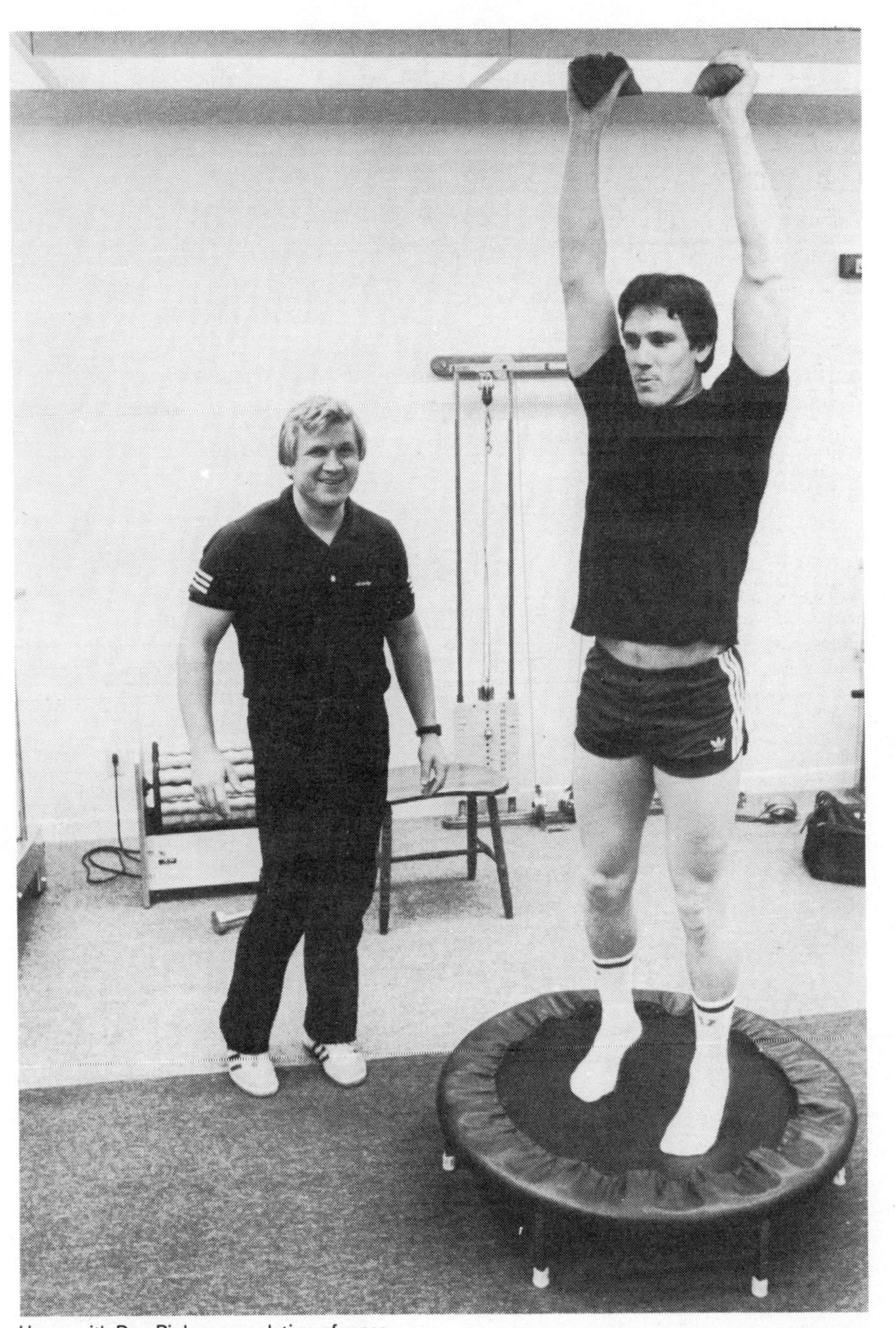

Harry, with Dan Ripley; completion of press.

holder, 18′ 5¾″ pole vault; Greg Joy, silver medalist, high jump, 1976 Olympic Games; James Butts, silver medalist, triple jump, 1976 Olympics. There are many other athletes from all age groups who are benefitting with this tremendous strength and conditioning tool.

RUNNING PROGRAM

Three programs for . . .

Sprinters	**Middle Distance**	**Distance**
(40-440 yard dash)	(400-1500 meters)	(1 mile to marathon)

BIG FOUR

Training for the Sprinter to stay in shape year round

Exercise	Wt.	Time	Sets	Goals
1. Lymphatic Bounce	.45 kilo	15 sec.	1-3	8 sets, add 5 sec. per week. 2½ min. total
2. Shuffle	.45 kilo	30 sec.	1-3	8 sets, add 15 sec. per week until you can do 3 min.
3. Jog Easy	.45 kilo	30 sec.	1-3	8 sets, add 30 sec. per week until you can do 4½ min.
4. Sprint High Knee	.45 kilo	30 sec.	1-3	8 sets, add 30 sec. per week until you can do 4½ min.
		Total: 1¾ min.		Total: 15½ min.

Add 5 seconds on the Lymphatic Bounce each week. Add 15 seconds on the Sprint every week. Add 30 seconds a week on the shuffle and jog easy. Increase Sanbag weight every month until you are using 1.36 kilo Sanbags. Younger athletes are encouraged to add weight and sets at a slower pace.

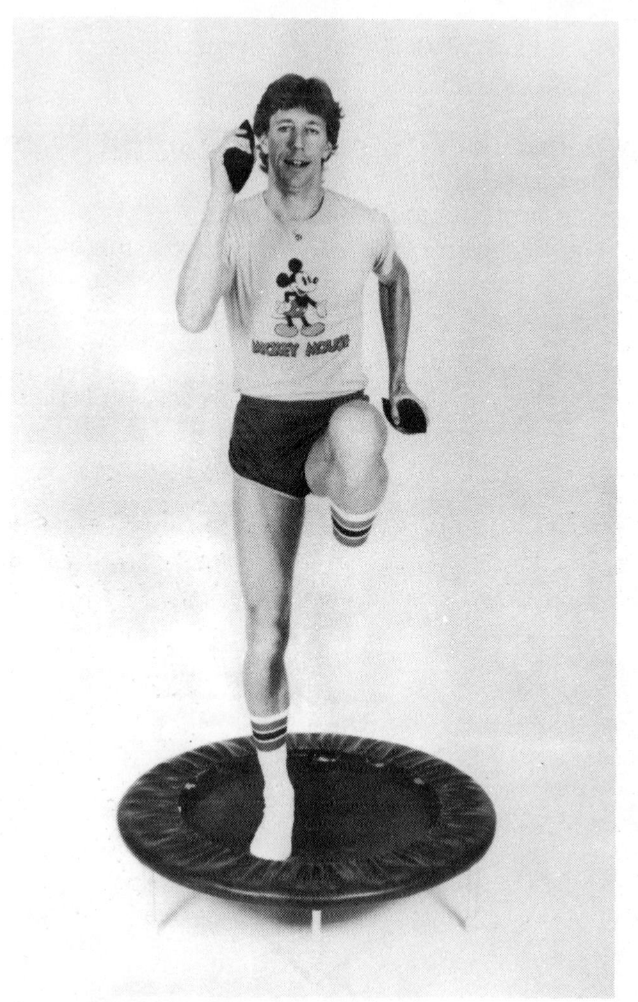

Dwight Stones, sprint high knee.

BIG FOUR

Middle Distance (400 meters - 1500 meters)

Warm-up

Exercise	Wt.	Time	Sets	Goals
1. Lymphatic Bounce	.45 kilo	1 min.	2	8 sets, add 15 seconds a week, total time, 3 min.
2. Shuffle	.45 kilo	1½ min.	2	8 sets, add 30 sec. per week, total 7½ min.
3. Jog Easy	.45 kilo	2 min.	2	8 sets, add 30 sec. per week total 8 min.
4. Sprint High Knee	.45 kilo	1½ min.	2	8 sets, add 15 sec. per week total time 3½ min.
		Total: 6 min.		

Add 15 seconds per week on Lymphatic Bounce and Sprint, add 30 seconds per week on the Shuffle and Jog Easy. Add Sanbag weight every 15 days, goal: 1.36 kilo bags in 1½ months.

BIG FOUR

Distance 1500 meters to the Marathon

Exercise	Wt.	Time	Sets	Goals
1. Lymphatic Bounce	.45 kilo	1 min.	3	10 sets, all 15 sec. per week 3½ min. total
2. Shuffle	.45 kilo	2 min.	3	10 sets, add 1 min. per week until you reach 12 min.
3. Jog Easy	.45 kilo	2 min.	3	10 sets, add 1 min. per week until you reach 12 min.
4. Sprint High Knee	.45 kilo	1 min.	3	10 sets, add 15 sec. per week until you reach 3½ min.

Add 15 sec. per week on Lymphatic Bounce and Sprint High Knee. Add 1 minute a week on Jog Easy and Shuffle. Sanbag weights should be added every 15 days until you reach 1.36 kilo bags. TOTAL TIME: 30 minutes.

JUMPING PROGRAM

High Jump, Long Jump, Triple Jump, Pole Vault, etc.

Exercise	Wt.	Time	Sets	Goals
1. Jog Easy	.45 kilo	2 min.	1	3 sets of 6 minutes with 1.36 kilo Sanbags
2. Bounce	.45 kilo	1 min.	1	
3. Sprint High Knee	.45 kilo	1 min.	1	
4. Shuffle	.45 kilo	1 min.	1	
5. Lymphatic Bounce (Warm-Down)	.45 kilo	1 min.	1	
		Total: 6 min.		

Add 1 set per week until you can do 3 sets of six minutes. Add .45 kilo Sanbag weight every two weeks until you reach 1.36 kilo. You can add more sets in the bounce if you wish. This is a warmup for the "Daily Dozen."

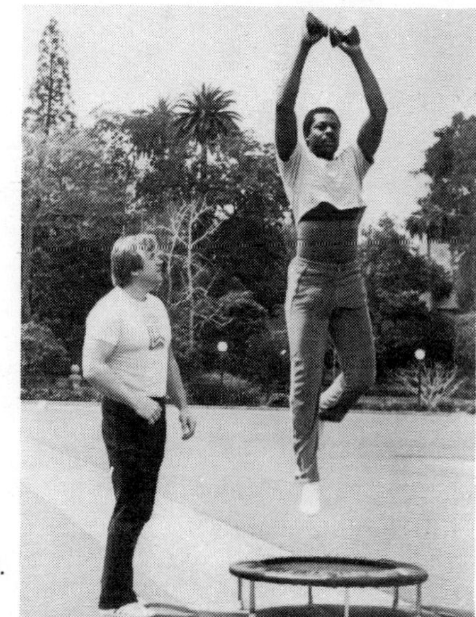

James Butts, the bounce.

THROWING PROGRAM

Shot Put, Discus, Javelin, Hammer, etc.

Exercise	Wt.	Time	Sets	Goals
1. Jog Easy	.45 kilo	1 min.	1	Add 1 min. on each exercise every week, goal: 3 sets of each exercise with 1.36 kilo bags
2. Bounce	.45 kilo	1 min.	1	
3. Shuffle	.45 kilo	1 min.	1	
4. Sprint High Knee	.45 kilo	1 min.	1	
5. Lymphatic Bounce	.45 kilo	1 min.	1	

Add 1 set every week until you reach 3 sets in each exercise. Add .45 kilo Sanbag weight every two weeks until you reach 1.36 kilo bags.

SANBAG RESISTANCE PROGRAM FOR THROWERS

(Bodybuilding) Warm-up Using Chart at Left

Exercise	Wt.	Time	Sets	Goals
1. Curl & Press	.45 kilo	20	2	Work up to 5 x 20 with 1.36 kilo Sanbags
2. Tricep Press	.45 kilo	20	2	
3. Pullover	.45 kilo	20	2	
4. Press Up & Out	.45 kilo	20	2	
5. Squeeze	.45 kilo	20	2	

Add 1 set a week until you can do 5 x 20, add .45 kilo Sanbag weight every two weeks until you can do 1.36 kilo bags; younger athletes go slower.

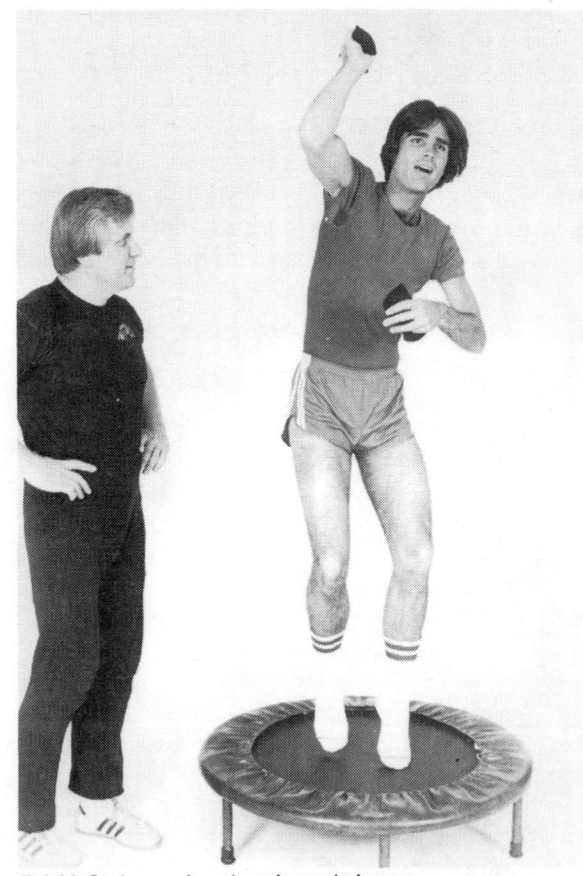

T.J. McCavitt practices throwing technique.

Lynn Grimditch

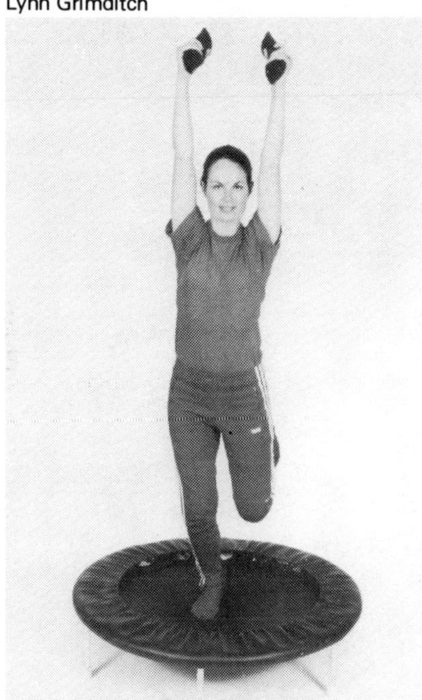

Press.

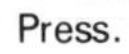

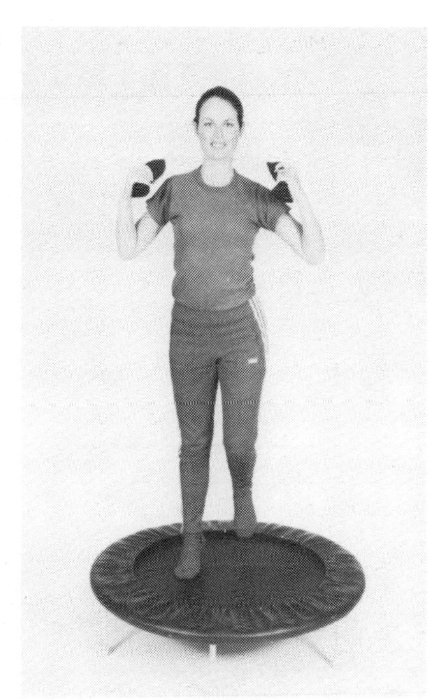

Return to starting position.

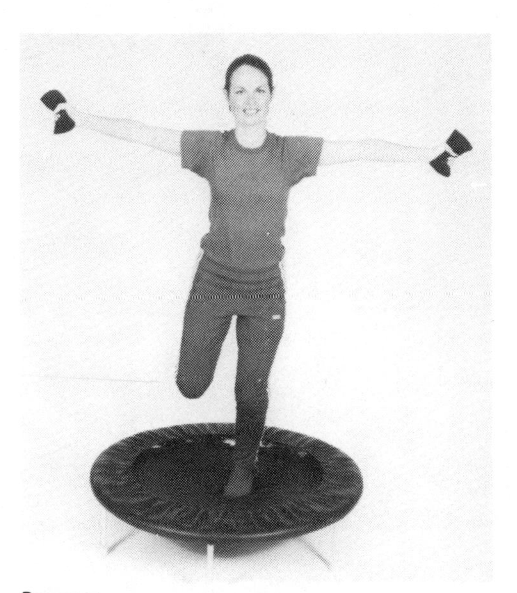

Press out.

SANBAGGING WITH THE DAILY DOZEN

Your Strength and conditioning Package that will improve any track & field activity.

Exercise	Wt.	Time	Sets	Goals
1. Curl	.45 kilo	12	2	8 sets of 12 with .45 kilo Sanbags Add .45 kilo every 15 days until you reach the 1.36 kilo Sanbags
2. Press	.45 kilo	12	2	
3. Upright Row	.45 kilo	12	2	
4. Tricep Press	.45 kilo	12	2	
5. Squeeze	.45 kilo	12	2	
6. Curl & Press	.45 kilo	12	2	
7. Side Raise	.45 kilo	12	2	
8. Crossover	.45 kilo	12	2	
9. Sprint High Knee	.45 kilo		2	3½ min. in 8 weeks
10. Press Up & Out	.45 kilo	12	2	
11. Pullover	.45 kilo	12	2	
12. Jog Easy		1 min.		9 min. in 8 weeks

Add 1 set every week until you reach 8 sets. Do these exercises while you jog, bounce, or shuffle. Add 15 seconds on Sprint High Knee, 30 seconds on Jog Easy every week. Add .45 kilo Sanbag weight every two weeks, until you reach 1.36 kilo Sanbags.

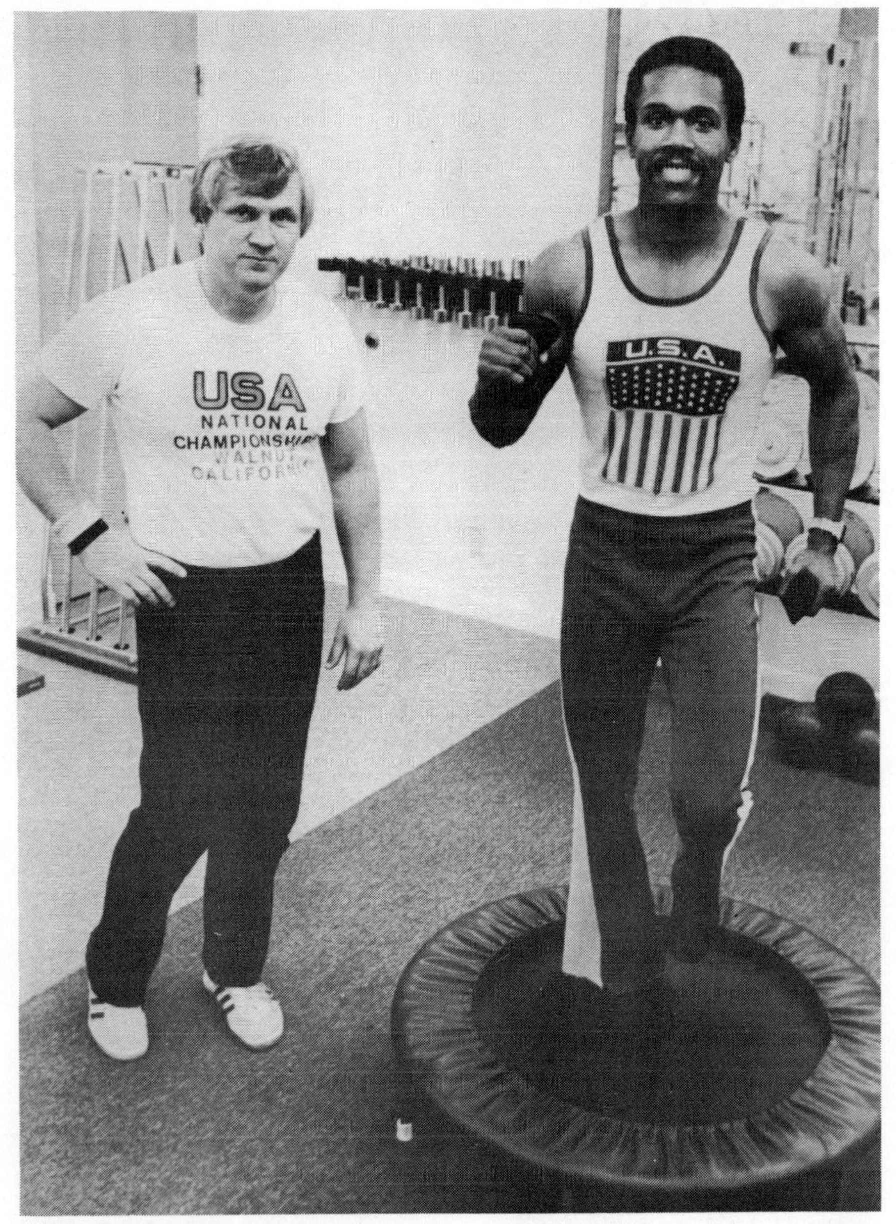

Hainsley Best, jog easy.

EXCELLENT RESULT WITH THIS BODY BUILDING SPECIAL! TRY THIS TODAY!

For the Advanced Athlete in-season

Exercise	Wt.	Reps/Time	Sets	Goals
1. Jog Easy	.45 kilo	2 min.	2	6 sets total
2. Curl & Press	.45 kilo	20	2	Add 1 set per week until you reach 6 sets.
3. Sprint	.45 kilo	1 min.	2	Add .45 kilo Sanbags every two weeks.
4. Curl & Press	.45 kilo	20	2	6 x 20 each Sanbag
5. Sprint	.45 kilo	1 min.	2	Weight Training Exercise with 1.36 kilo Sanbags
6. Curl & Press	.45 kilo	20	2	
7. Sprint	.45 kilo	1 min.	2	
8. Lymphatic Bounce (Warm-Down)	.45 kilo	2		

Add 1 set per week until you reach 6 sets. Add .45 kilo to your Sanbags weight every two weeks. This is an excellent conditioner. Do these at least five times a week.

Golf

Lower your heart rate, stay in shape — improve your game

Warm-Up: "Big Four"

Exercise	Wt.	Reps/Time	Sets	Goals
1. Jog Easy	.45 kilo	1 min.		8 sets of 1 min. each Total: 8 min. Easy Jog
2. Curl & Press	.45 kilo	10	2	8 x 10 with 1.36 kilo bags
3. Squeeze	.45 kilo	10	2	8 x 10 with 1.36 kilo bags
4. Bounce	.45 kilo	1 min.		8 sets of 1 min. each Total: 8 min.
5. Upright Row	.45 kilo	10	2	8 x 10 with 1.36 kilo bags
6. Shuffle	.45 kilo	1 min.		8 sets of 1 min. each Total: 8 min.
7. Pullover	.45 kilo	10	2	8 x 10 with 1.36 kilo bags
8. Sprint High Knee	.45 kilo	30 sec.		8 sets of 30 sec. each Total: 4 min.
9. Lymphatic Bounce	.45 kilo	1 min.		8 sets of 1 min. each Total: 8 min.

Add one set per week until you reach 8 sets. Add .45 kilo Sanbag weight every two weeks, until you reach 1.36 kilo bags. On jog, shuffle, bounce, and Lymphatic Bounce, add 15 seconds per week. Add ½ minutes on Jog Easy. Leave reps the same. Those of you who are not in good condition, go up to 3 sets only.

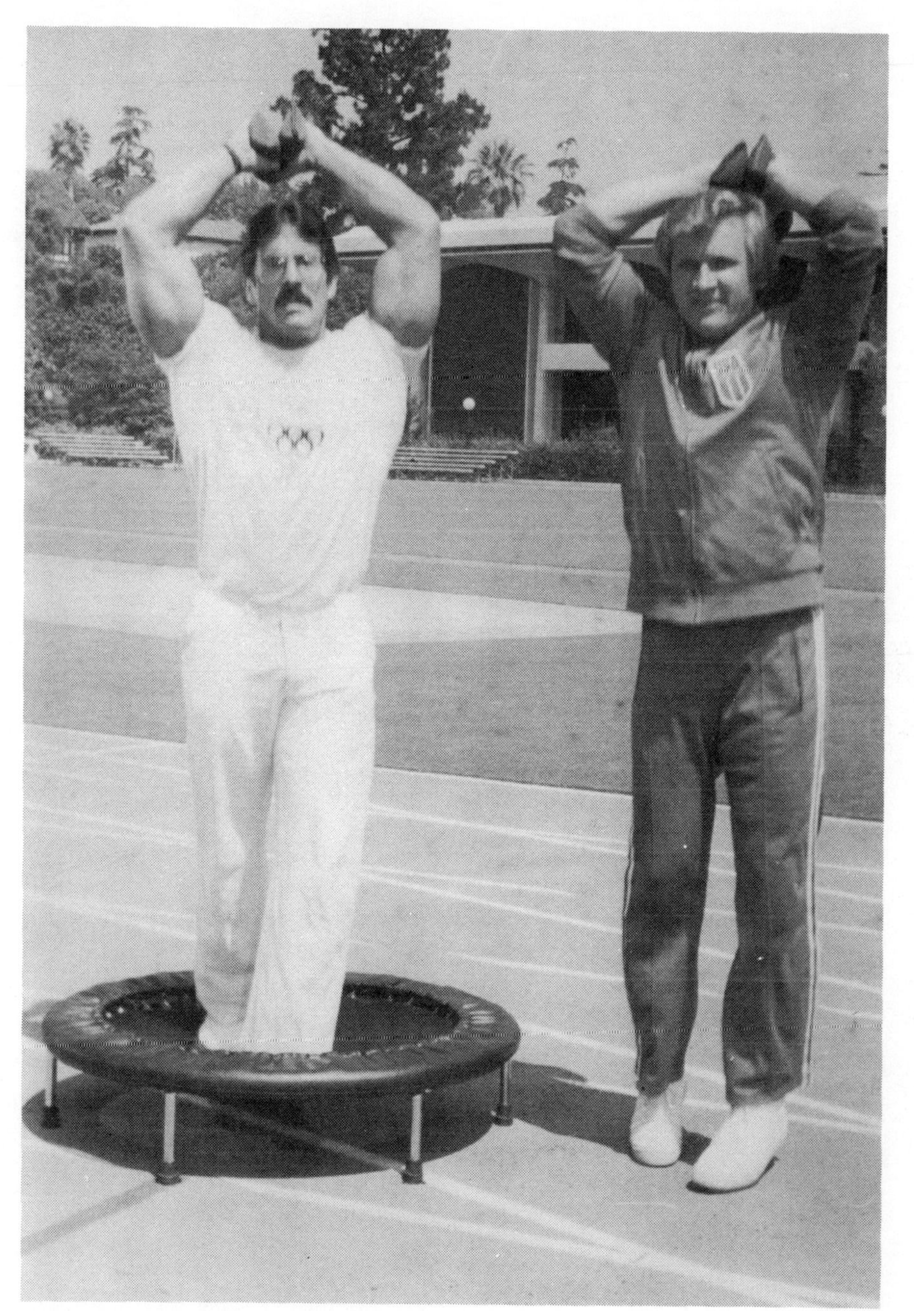

Mr. Universe, Mike Mentzer, doing the pullover.

Racquetball

Get in shape first

WARM-UP WITH BIG FOUR

Exercise	Wt.	Reps/Time	Sets	Goals
1. Jog Easy	.45 kilo	1 min.	2	6 sets of 1 min. with 1.36 kilo
2. Curl & Press	.45 kilo	20	2	6 x 20 with 1.36 kilo bags
3. Bounce	.45 kilo	1 min.	2	6 sets of 1 min. with 1.36 kilo bags
4. Squeeze	.45 kilo		2	6 x 20 with 1.36 kilo bags
5. Sprint High Knee	.45 kilo	30 sec.	2	Add 15 sec. per week Total: 2 min.
6. Pullover	.45 kilo	20	2	6 x 20 with 1.36 kilo bags
7. Lymphatic Bounce	.45 kilo	1 min.	2	6 sets of 1 min. each

Add 1 set every week until you reach 6 sets of 20 in Sanbag weight training exercises. Add .45 kilo every 2 weeks, until you reach 6 x 20 with 1.36 kilo Sanbags. Increase 15 seconds a week in the Sprint, 1 minute a week on Jog Easy, Bounce, Lymphatic Bounce (6 x 1 minute sets with 1.36 kilo Sanbags). This is a great supplement to your game, it works. I know, I use this every day.

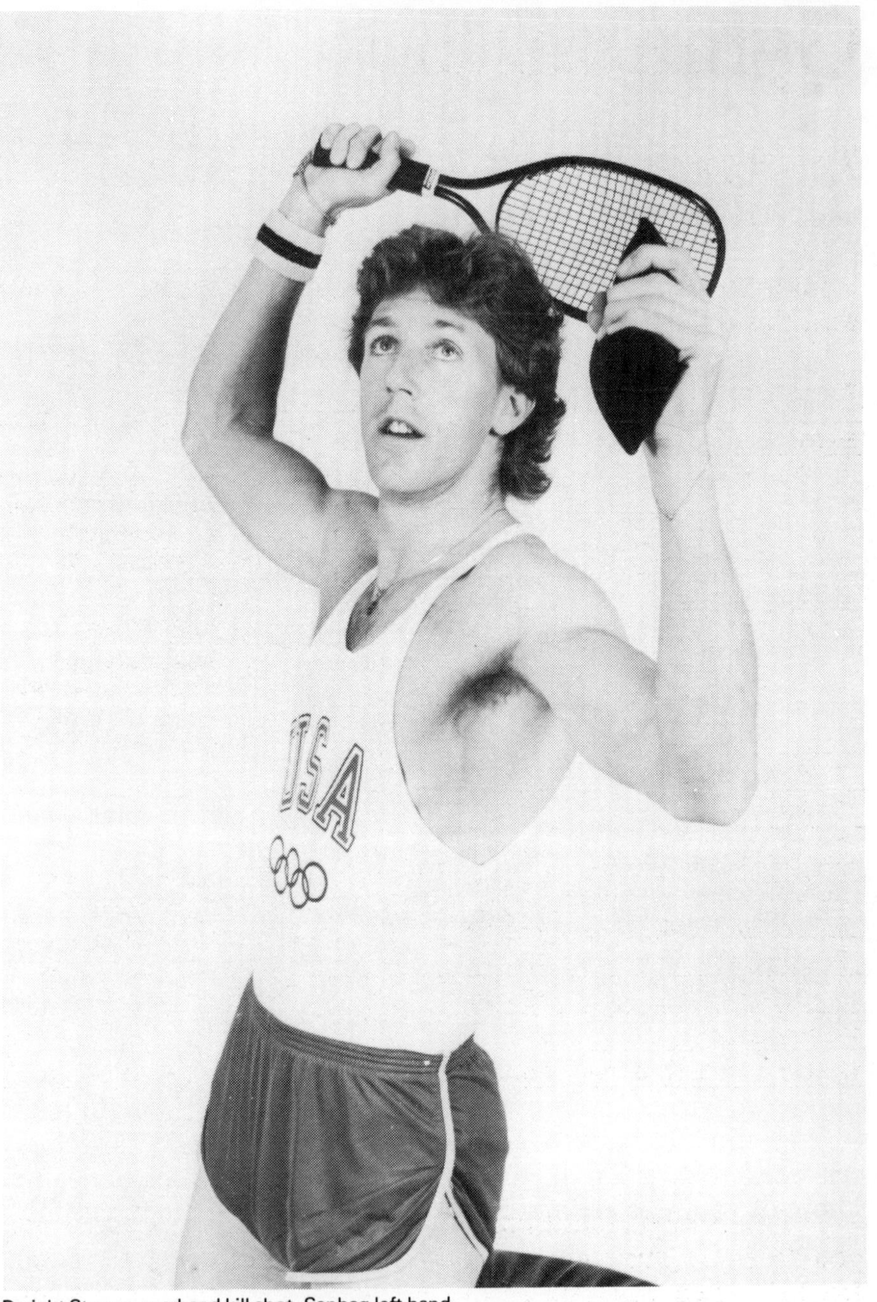

Dwight Stones, overhand kill shot, Sanbag left hand.

Gymnastics

Tumbling, apparatus work, floor exercise

Improve your techniques, develop strong joints and ligaments with this quick Sanbag routine.

Warm-up: Do the Big Four

Exercise	Wt.	Reps/Time	Sets	Goals
1. Bounce	.45 kilo	30 sec.	1	Add 1 set every week in each exercise until you reach 8 sets.
2. Sprint High Knee	.45 kilo	30 sec.	1	
3. Curl & Press	.45 kilo	20	1	Add .45 kilo on your Sanbags every two weeks until you reach 1.36 kilo Sanbags
4. Side Raise	.45 kilo	10	1	
5. Pullover	.45 kilo	20	1	
6. Shuffle	.45 kilo	1 min.	1	
7. Press	.45 kilo	20	1	
8. Tricep Press	.45 kilo	20	1	
9. Jog Easy	.45 kilo	1 min.	1	
10. Upright Row	.45 kilo	20	1	
11. Squeeze	.45 kilo	20	1	
12. Lymphatic Bounce	.45 kilo	1 min.	1	

The most important thing, if you are a young gymnast, is that you do enjoy this routine. Add other exercises from the "Daily Dozen" when you can do this easily. If you are a very strong gymnast, you can add more sets. This is an excellent warm-up before practice, too.

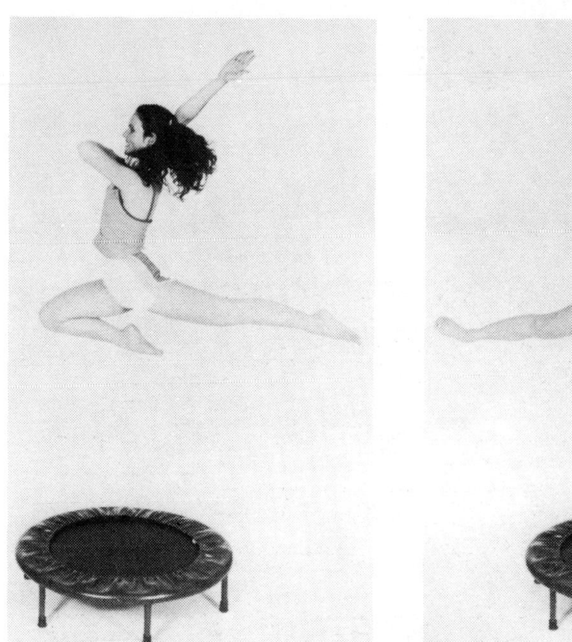
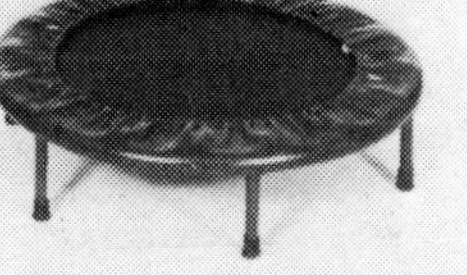
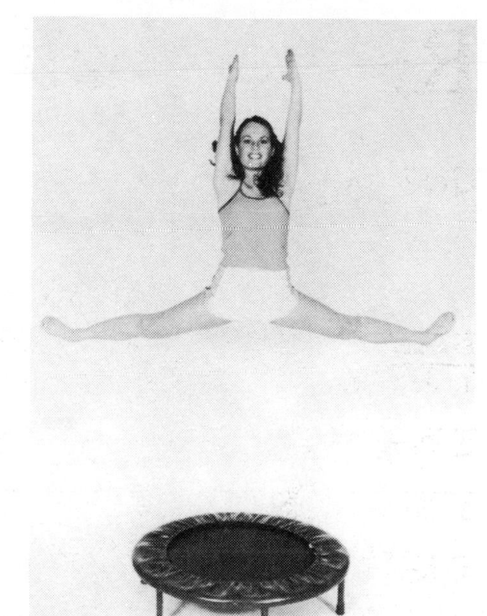
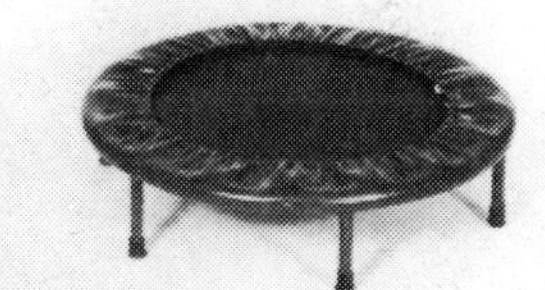

Lynn Grimditch demonstrates stag leap (left) and split with arms up.

UPPER BODY PROGRAM FOR THE GYMNAST

Exercise	Wt.	Reps	Sets	Goals
1. Curl	.45 kilo	20	2	Add 1 set a week until you reach 8 sets. Add .45 kilo Sanbag weight every two weeks until you reach 1.36 kilo Sanbags
2. Curl & Press	.45 kilo	20	2	
3. Upright Row	.45 kilo	20	2	
4. Lateral Raise	.45 kilo	12	2	
5. Pullover	.45 kilo	20	2	
6. Tricep Press	.45 kilo	20	2	
7. Press Up & Out	.45 kilo	20	2	
8. Curl & Press	.45 kilo	20	2	
9. Crossover	.45 kilo	20	2	

Young gymnasts can increase a little slower. Remember that the important thing here is developing the muscle through the full range. Older, stronger gymnasts can increase weight right on schedule. This program will definitely develop a powerful upper body. Try it!

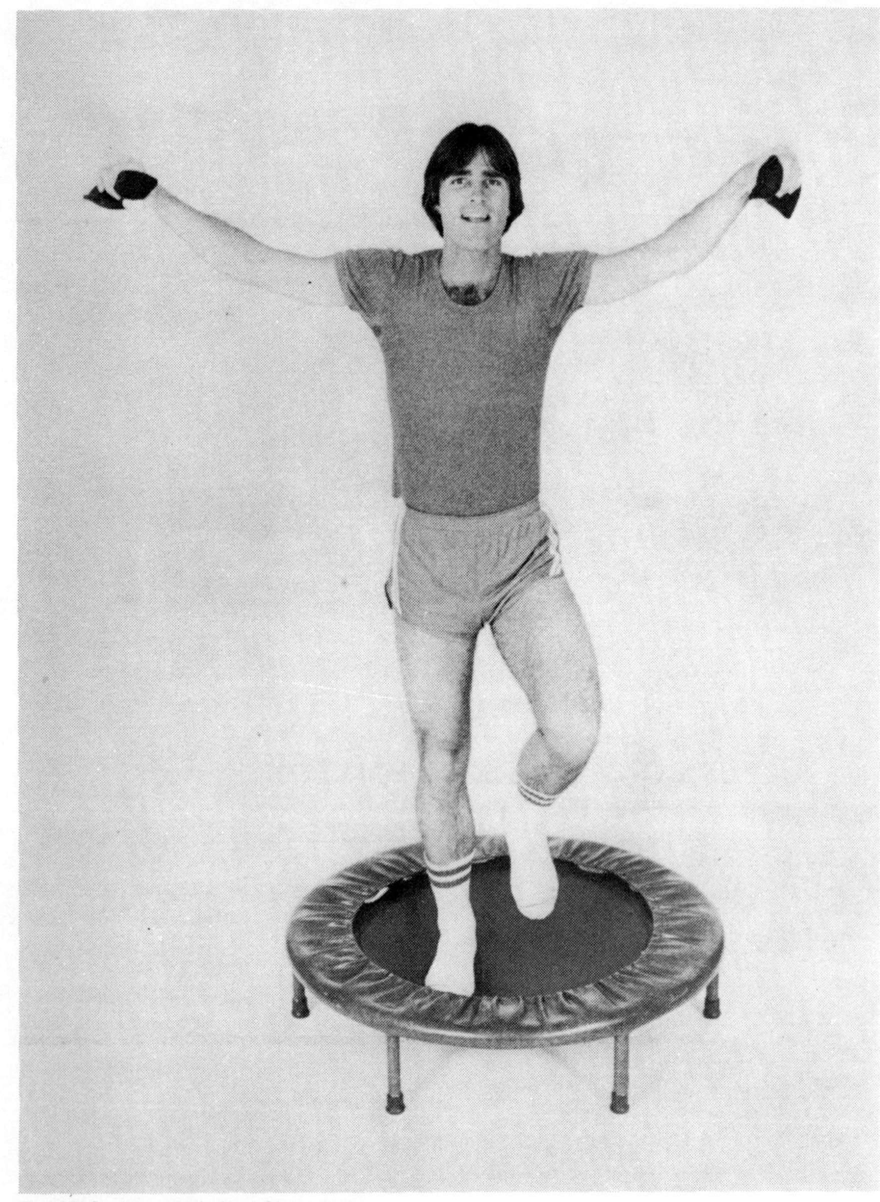

T.J. McCavitt, completion of lateral raise.

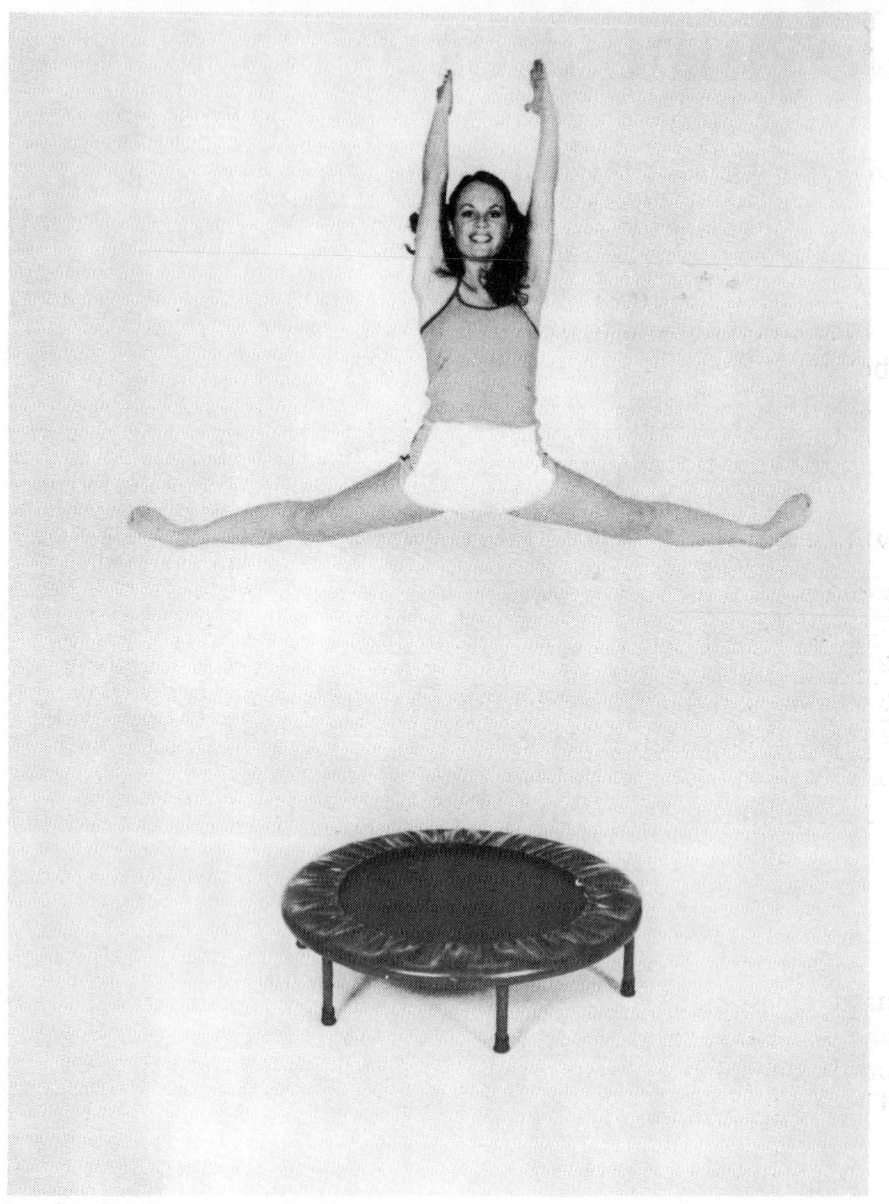

Lynn Grimditch demonstrates split with arms up.

Jogging

Amaze yourself with your progress

Try running on the rebound unit with your Sanbags. You will be amazed at your progress. it is so **easy on your joints.**

Warm-Up: Big Four

Exercise	Wt.	Reps/Time	Sets	Goals
1. Jog Easy	.45 kilo	3 min.	2	Add 1 set per week until you reach 8 sets with 1.36 kilo Sanbags
2. Bounce	.45 kilo	1 min.	2	
3. Sprint High Knee	.45 kilo	1 min.	2	
4. Jog Easy	.45 kilo	2 min.	2	
5. Lymphatic Bounce	.45 kilo		2	Total Time: 48 min.

Your goal is to condition. Add 1 set every week in each exercise until you reach 8 sets. This is terrific for those rainy days or if you are in a hotel room. Add .45 kilo Sanbag weight every month until you reach 1.36 kilo. Those overweight, keep it at 3 sets. Those who jog already, go for the 8 sets.

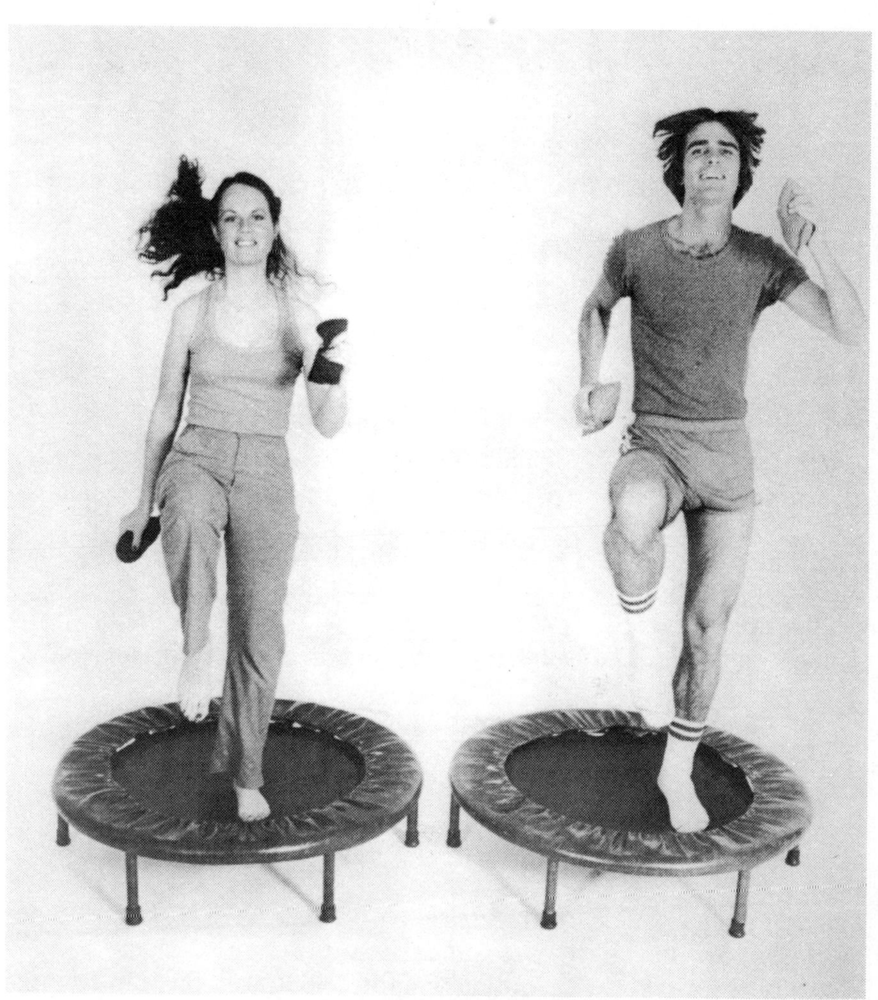

Lynn Grimditch, T.J. McCavitt demonstrate sprint high knee.

Soccer

Build stamina to play the whole game

Here's a program that will keep you going strong, and increase that stamina you need to play the whole game.

Warm-up: The Big Four

Exercise	Wt.	Time	Sets	Goals
1. Jog Easy	.45 kilo	2 min.	2	8 sets total
2. Bounce	.45 kilo	1 min.	2	Add 1 set per week on all activities
3. Sprint High Knee	.45 kilo	30 sec.	2	
4. Slalom	.45 kilo	30 sec.	2	
5. Lymphatic Bounce	.45 kilo	1 min.	2	Total Time: 48 min.
6. Jog Easy	.45 kilo	2 min.	2	

Add 1 set a week until you reach 8 sets. Add 15 seconds per week on Sprint High Knee and Slalom; on all others add 30 seconds per week. Add Sanbag weight, .45 kilo every month until you reach 1.36 kilo Sanbags. This is an excellent program for pre-season conditioning.

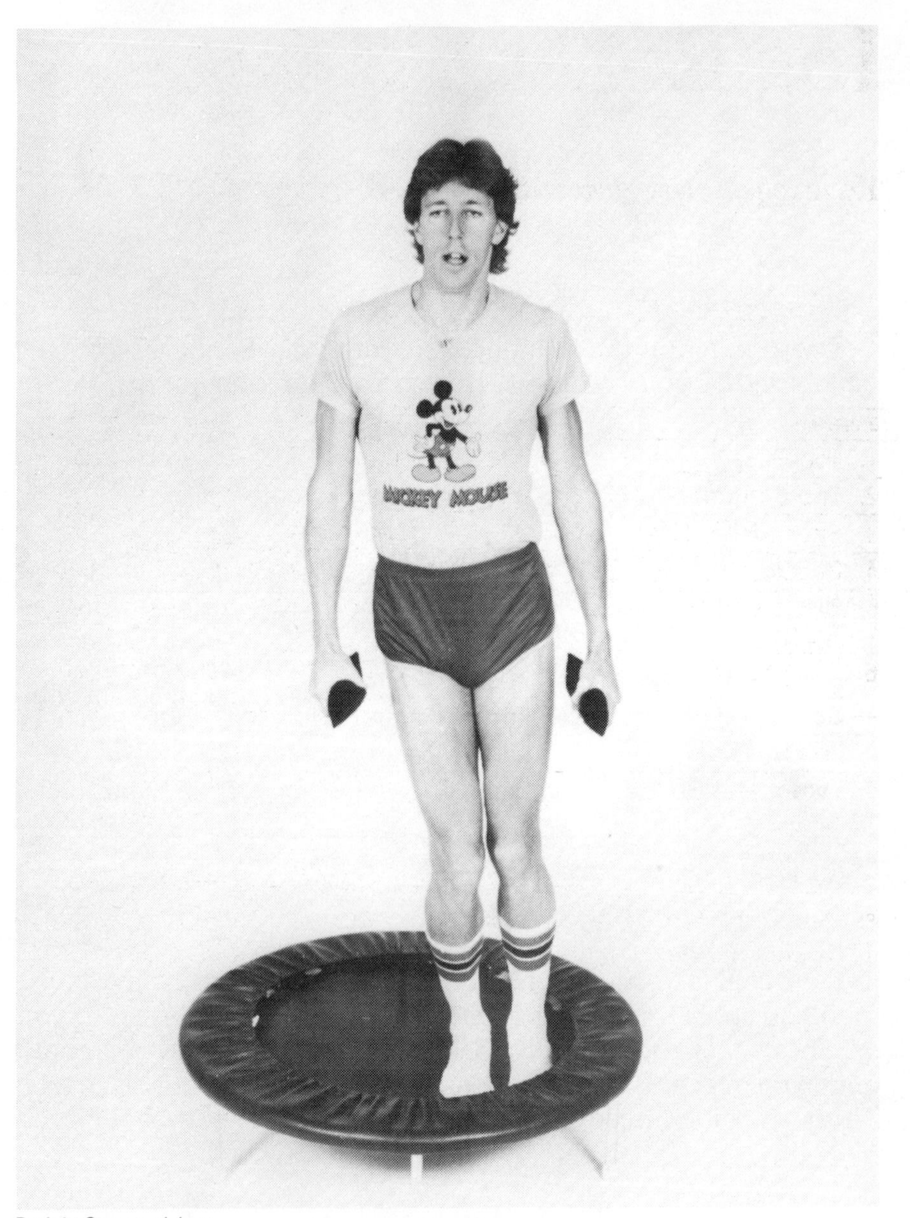

Dwight Stones, slalom.

Ice/Roller Skating

Your legs, important to success

Exercise	Wt.	Time	Sets	Goals
1. Jog Easy	.45 kilo	1 min.	2	8 sets in each exercise until you reach 1.36 kilo Sanbags
2. The Slalom	.45 kilo	1 min.	2	
3. Sprint High Knee	.45 kilo	30 sec.	2	
4. Shuffle	.45 kilo	1 min.	2	
5. Bounce Side to Side	.45 kilo	1 min.	2	
6. Lymphatic Bounce	.45 kilo	1 min.	2	Total Time: 48 min.

Add 30 seconds per week in all exercises except Sprint, add 15 seconds per week. Add resistance every month until you reach 1.36 kilo Sanbags. Add 1 set every week until you reach 8 sets.

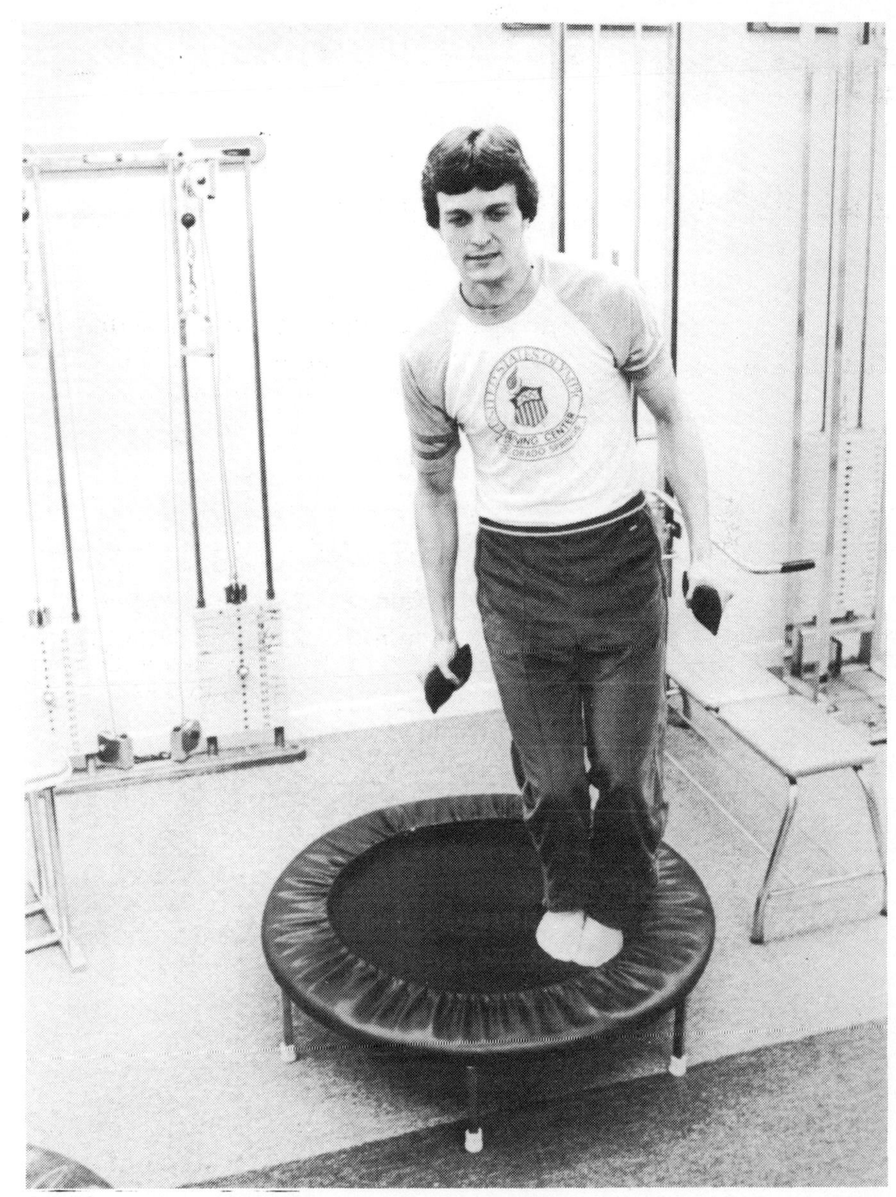

Kenny Sutton, bounce side to side.

Skiing — Water/Snow

Enjoy your sport and prevent injury

Try these simple and fun exercises.
Warm-up: The Big Four

Exercise	Wt.	Time	Sets	Goals
1. Jog Easy	.45 kilo	2 min.	2	Add one set per week until you reach 8 sets with 1.36 kilo Sanbags
2. Slalom Exercise	.45 kilo	1 min.	2	
3. Bounce	.45 kilo	1 min.	2	
4. Sprint High Knee	.45 kilo	30 sec.	2	
5. Lymphatic Bounce	.45 kilo	1 min.	2	
6. Jog Easy	.45 kilo	2 min.	2	

Add 15 seconds a week on Sprint High Knee. All the rest add 30 seconds. Add one set every week until you reach 8 sets. Add .45 kilo Sanbags every month until you reach 1.36 kilo bags doing eight sets. This program is designed for your personal level of fitness. You may find 2-3 sets plenty for you rather than working up to 8 sets. Those suffering any joint damage, overweight, etc., keep it to 3 sets total.

Wayne Grimditch

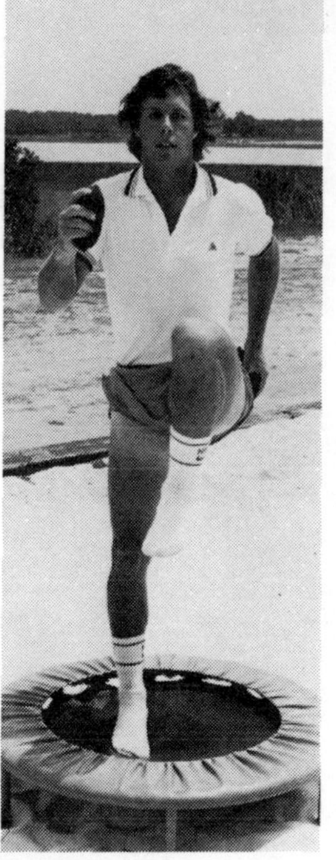

Sprint high knee.

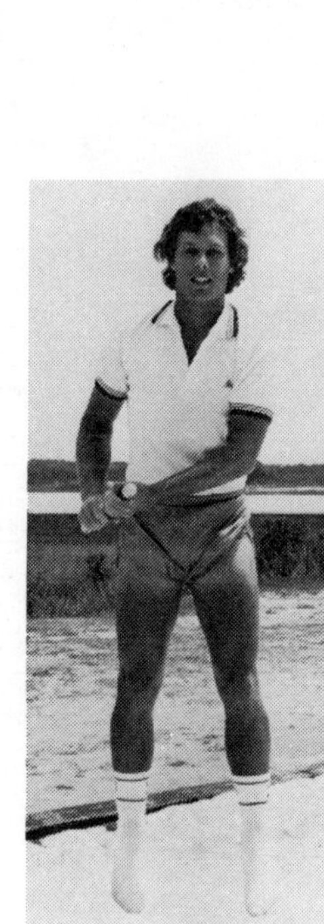

Primary technique drill for water ski jumping.

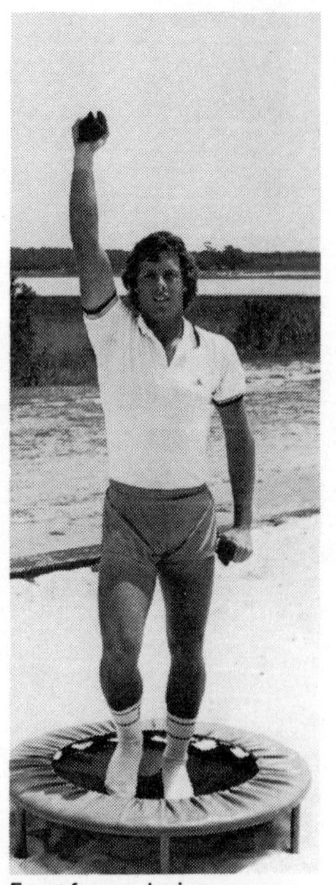

Front forward raise.

Swimming

Conditioning, strength, through Sanbagging

This is a great program for you who have a desire to improve your swimming fitness levels.

Warm-up: The Big Four

Exercise	Wt.	Reps/Time	Sets	Goals
1. Jog Easy	.45 kilo	1 min.	2	Add 30 sec. per week on Jog Easy, Shuffle, Bounce, and Lymphatic Bounce until you reach 8 sets by adding 1 set a week
2. Shuffle	.45 kilo	1 min.	2	
3. Pullover	.45 kilo	20	2	
4. Tricep Press	.45 kilo	20	2	
5. Side Raise	.45 kilo	15	2	
6. Curl & Press	.45 kilo	20	2	
7. Bounce	.45 kilo	1 min.	2	Add 1 set of 20 a week until you reach 8 x 20
8. Sprint High Knee	.45 kilo	1 min.	2	
9. Lymphatic Bounce	.45 kilo	1 min.	2	On Sprint add 15 sec.
				Total Time: 58 min.

Continue to improve your strength by adding resistance every month. Start with .45 kilo Sanbags, add .45 kilo every month until you reach 1.36 kilo Sanbags. You can do this program as a pre-season resistance program for swimming. Once again, be careful not to over train. Keep to 3 sets if you are a beginner, eventually building up to 8 sets.

Dwight Stones

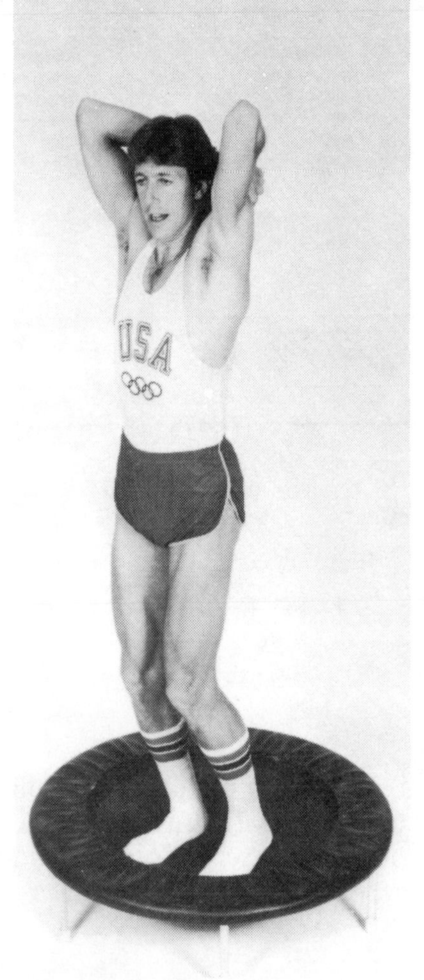

Beginning, tricep press.

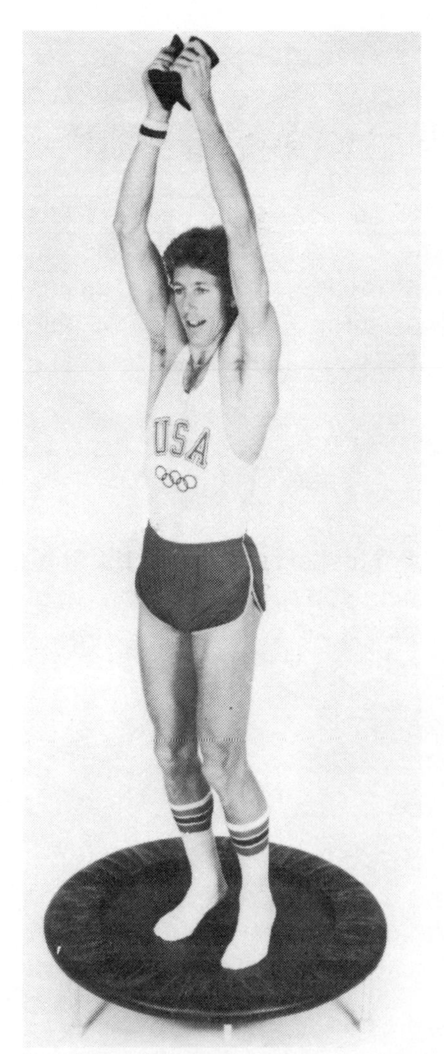

Completion, tricep press.

Hockey

Off-the-ice aid to better performance

Warm-up: The Big Four

Exercise	Wt.	Reps/Time	Sets	Goals
1. Jog Easy	.45 kilo	1 min.	1	Add 1 set of each exercise per week until you reach 8 sets.
2. Shuffle	.45 kilo	1 min.	1	
3. Squeeze	.45 kilo	25	1	
4. Curl & Press	.45 kilo	20	1	Add .45 kilo Sanbag weight per month until you reach 1.36 kilo Sanbags
5. Bounce	.45 kilo	1 min.	1	
6. Sprint High Knee	.45 kilo	30 sec.	1	
7. Lymphatic Bounce	.45 kilo	1 min.	1	

This excellent conditioning and bodybuilding program will help you to maintain excellent hockey stamina. If you are a young player or out of condition, start with only 3 sets. You can add other exercises from the "Daily Dozen" as you get stronger.

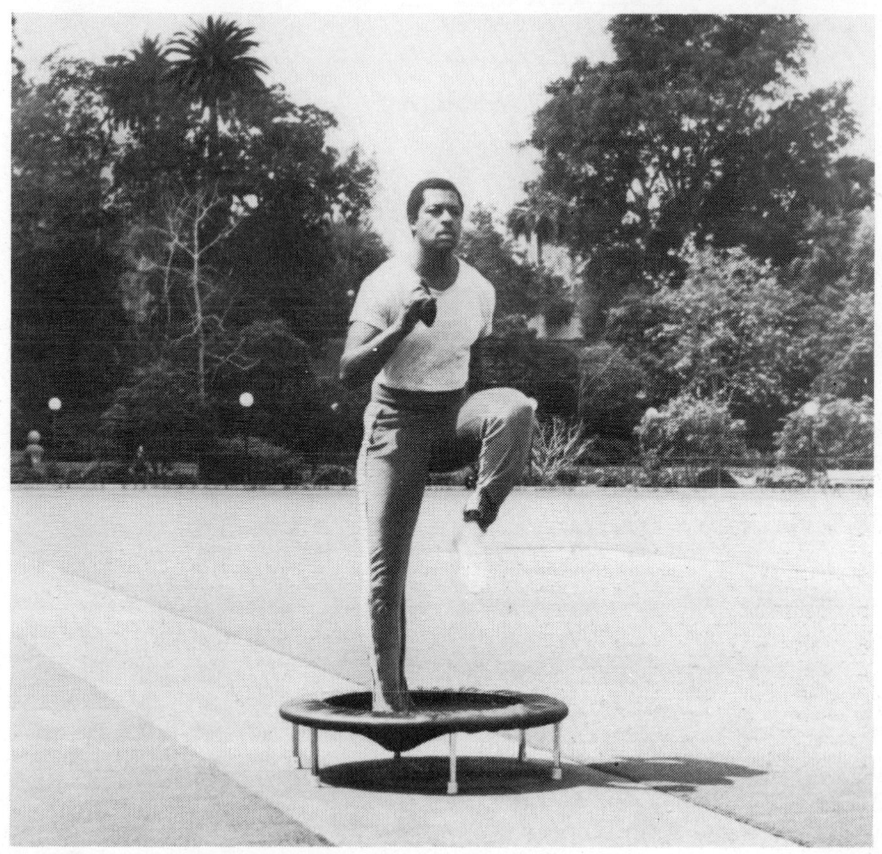

James Butts, sprint high knee, on track.

Martial Arts

Improve balance, condition, coordination

Excellent program for balance, conditioning, coordination. Move up your belt ranking with this super program.

Warm-up: The Big Four

Exercise	Wt.	Reps/Time	Sets	Goals
1. Shuffle	.45 kilo	1 min.	1	Add 1 set of each exercise until you reach 8 total sets. Add 1 set a week. Add .45 kilo every month until you reach 1.36 kilo Sanbags.
2. Curl & Press	.45 kilo	20	1	
3. Sprint High Knee	.45 kilo	30s ec.	1	
4. Pullover	.45 kilo	20	1	
5. Bounce	.45 kilo	1 min.	1	
6. Side Raise	.45 kilo	20	1	
7. Press Up & Out	.45 kilo	20	1	
8. Jog Easy	.45 kilo	1 min.	1	
9. Lymphatic Bounce	.45 kilo			

This excellent training is being used by Eugene Pickett (First Degree Black Belt, Captain U.S. Olympic Martial Arts team). You can improve if you do this at least 4 times a week.

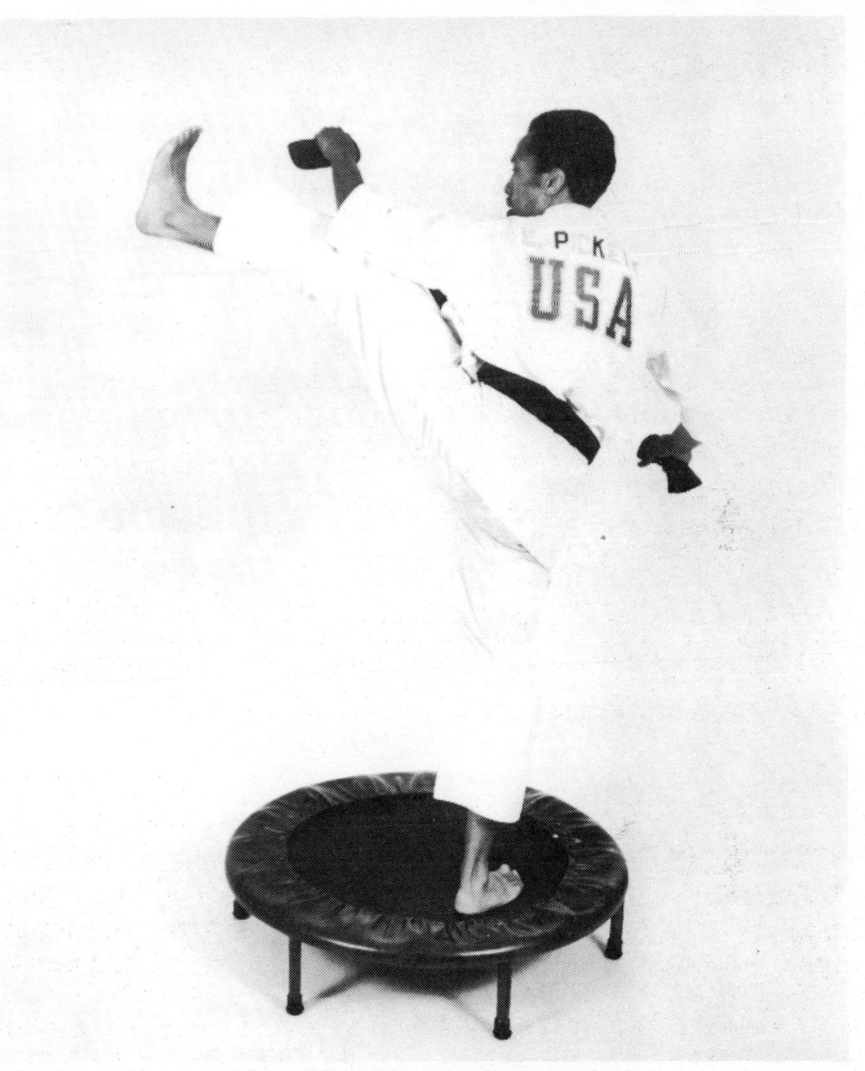

Eugene Pickett Jr., captain, U.S. martial arts team, demonstrates the high kick.

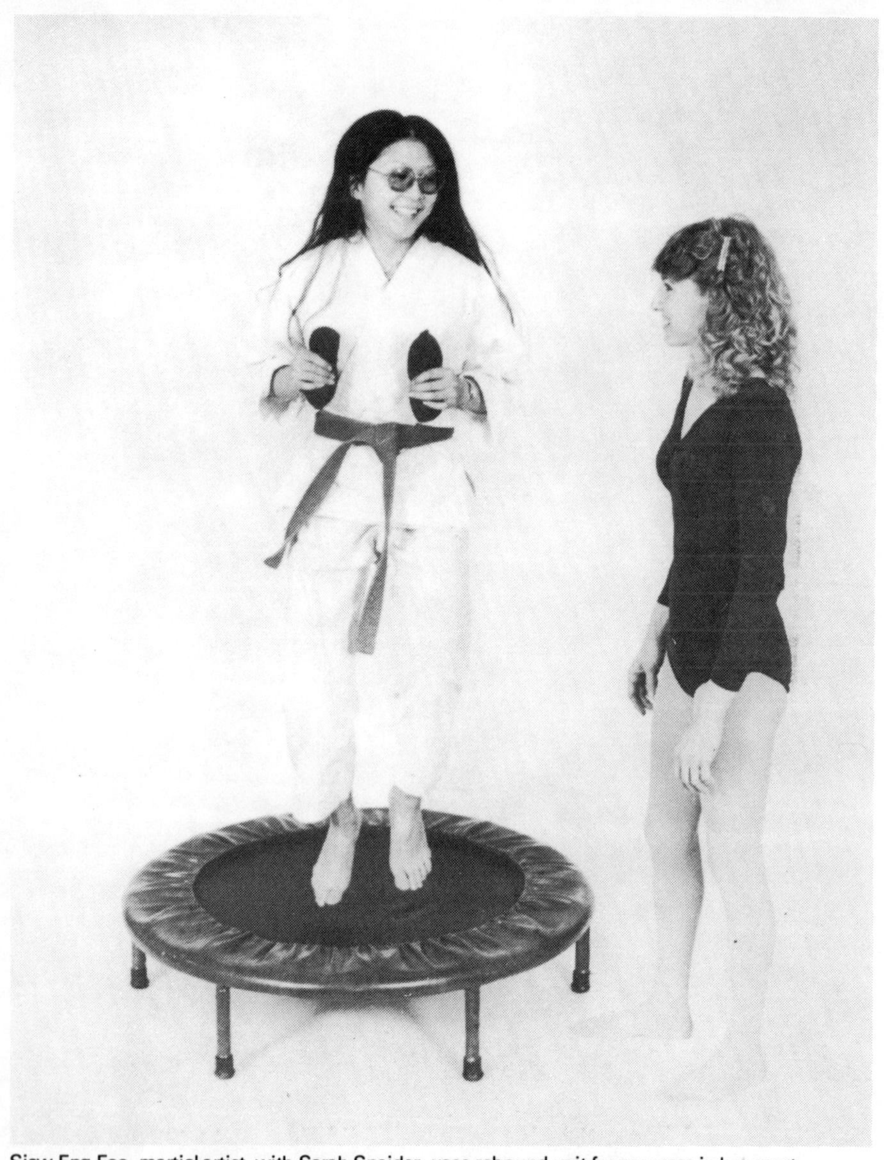

Siew Eng Foo, martial artist, with Sarah Sneider, uses rebound unit for progress in her sport.

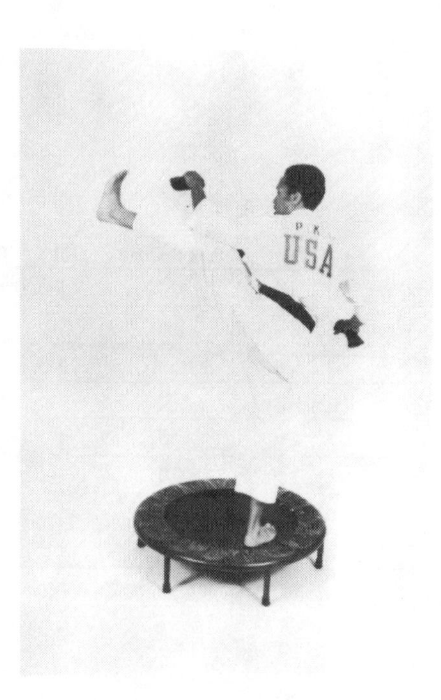

Bowling

Pick up those spares, using Sanbags

Warm-up: The Big Four

Exercise	Wt.	Reps/Time	Sets	Goals
1. Jog Easy	.45 kilo	1 min.	1	Add 1 set each week until you reach 8 sets. Add .45 kilo every month
2. Shuffle	.45 kilo	1 min.	1	
3. Curl	.45 kilo	15	1	
4. Pullover	.45 kilo	15	1	
5. Bounce	.45 kilo	1 min.	1	
6. Curl & Press	.45 kilo	15	1	
7. Sprint High Knee	.45 kilo	30 sec.	1	
8. Lymphatic Bounce	.45 kilo	1 min.	1	

Bowling is a sport of high levels of concentration, leg strength, and, above all, control. Surprise yourself and improve your score by trying this excellent conditioner. Those a little overweight and out of shape, stay with 3 sets for a while.

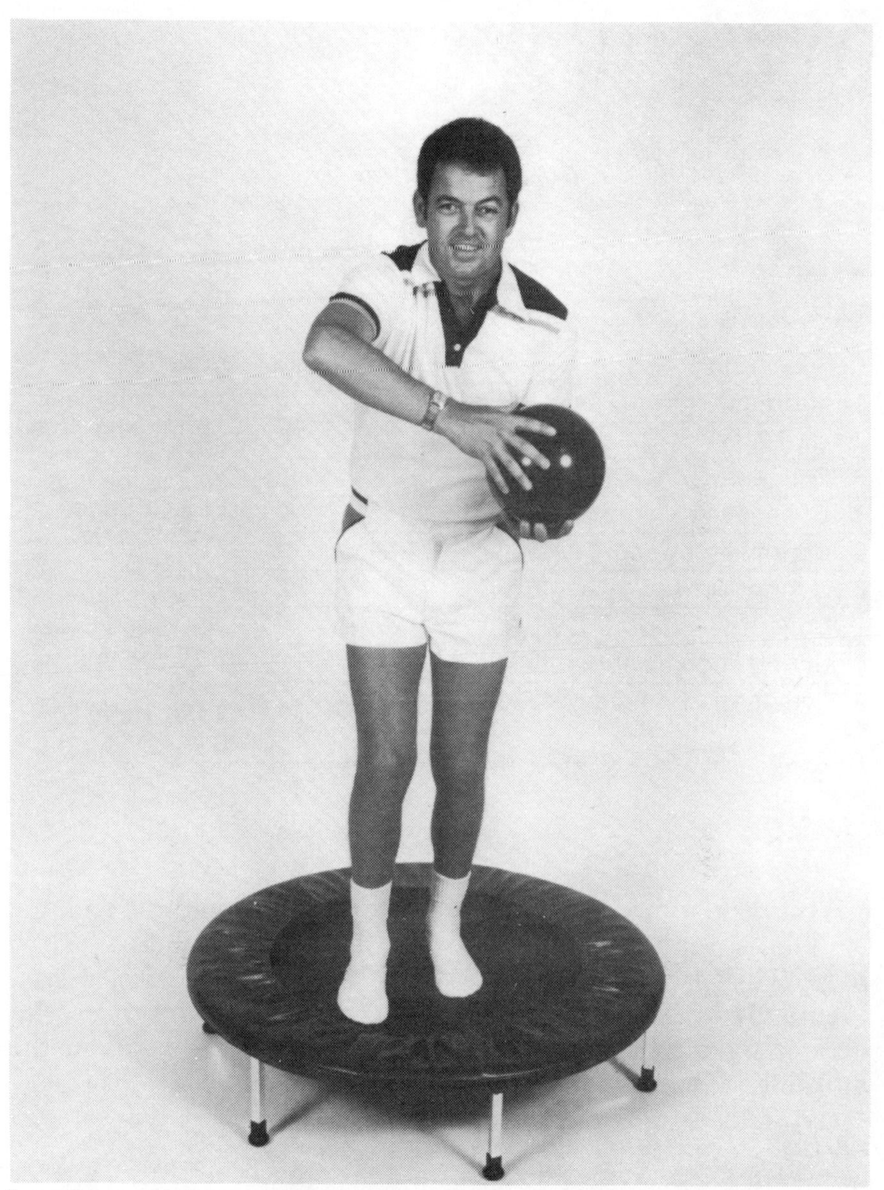

Roger Chaney, athletic coach, rebound exercise trainer, demonstrates bowling technique.

Wrestling

Win with super condition, stamina

Warm-up: The Big Four

Exercise	Wt.	Reps/Time	Sets	Goals
1. Jog Easy	.45 kilo	1 min.	2	Add 15 sec. on Sprint High Knee every week. Add 30 sec. on Jog Easy, Bounce. Goal: 8 sets.
2. Curl & Press	.45 kilo	20	2	
3. Squeeze	.45 kilo	20	2	
4. Bounce	.45 kilo	1 min.	2	
5. Sprint High Knee	.45 kilo	30 sec.	2	
6. Upright Row	.45 kilo	20	2	Add 1 set of 20 each week until you reach 8 x 20 with 1.36 kilo Sanbags.
7. Squeeze	.45 kilo	20	2	
8. Spring High Knee	.45 kilo	30 sec.	2	
9. Lymphatic Bounce	.45 kilo	1 min.	2	Total Time: 50 min.

Your goal as a wrestler is to be in top shape. Do this by adding .45 kilo of Sanbag weight every month until you can do 1.36 kilo bags. This program should be done every day at least 3 sets, eventually working up to 8 sets. May I recommend for those who do not have time that you split this program: 2-3 sets in the morning, 2-3 sets in the evening.

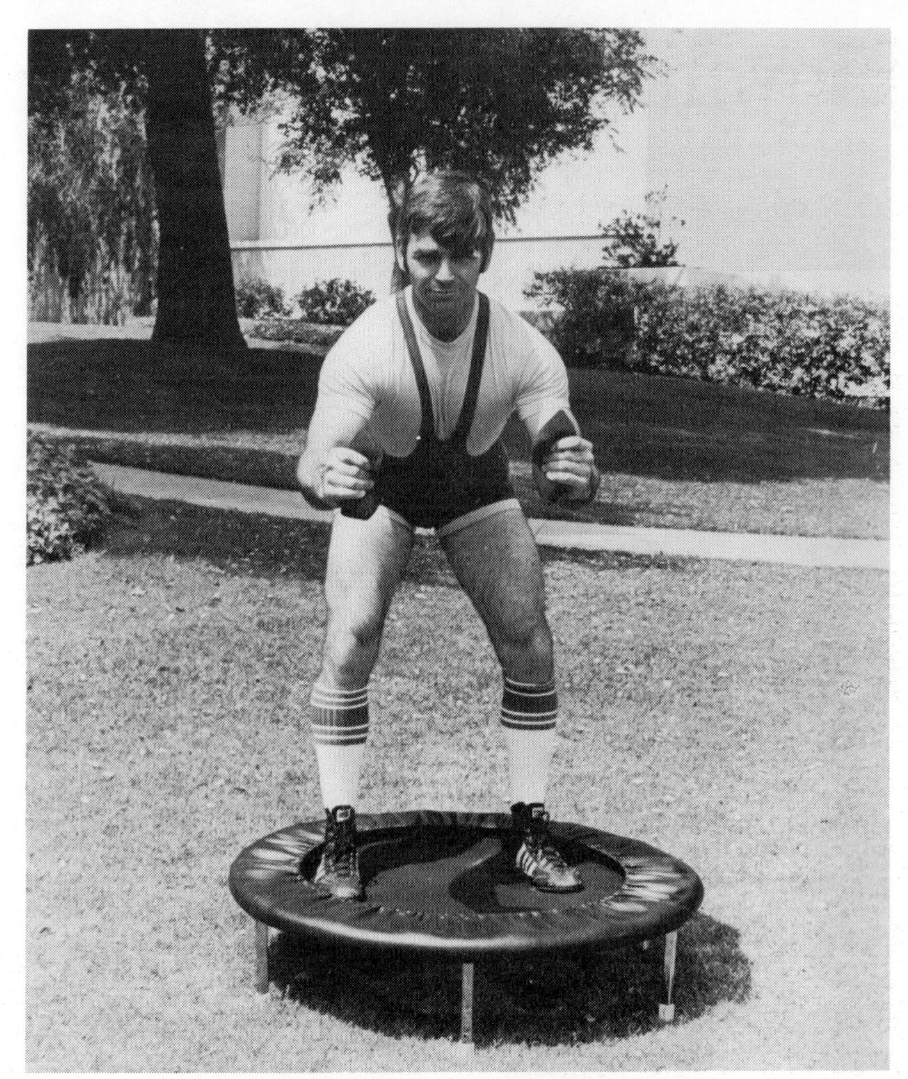

Geary Whiting, doing the squeeze.

Bicycling

Stay fit, give your joints a break

Warm-up: The Big Four

Exercise	Wt.	Reps/Time	Sets	Goals
1. Jog Easy	.45 kilo	2 min.	2	Add 1 min. on each exercise each week till you do 8 sets
2. Bounce	.45 kilo	1 min.	2	
3. Squeeze	.45 kilo	25	2	
4. Pullover	.45 kilo	20	2	
5. Curl & Press	.45 kilo	20	2	Do 8 sets total
6. Shuffle	.45 kilo	2 min.	2	Add 1 set a week till you do 8 x 25 or 8 x 20 with 1.36 kilo Sanbags.
7. Lymphatic Bounce	.45 kilo	1 min.	2	
				Total Time: 48 min.

This is an excellent program to help your bicycling fitness, plus it works your grip. Go slowly if you are a sporadic rider. This is sure to help you in your activity and sure will give you variety in your training.

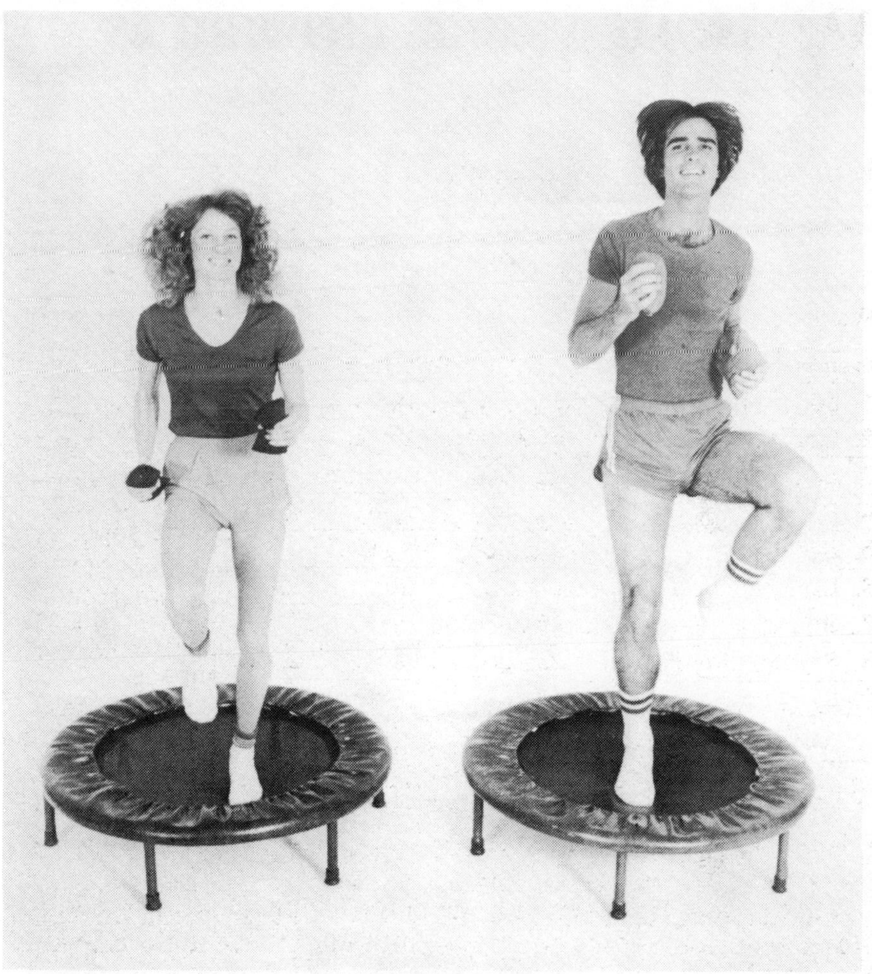

Sarah Sneider and T.J. McCavitt demonstrate jogging.

SOME EXCELLENT DRILLS TO IMPROVE YOUR ATHLETIC SKILLS

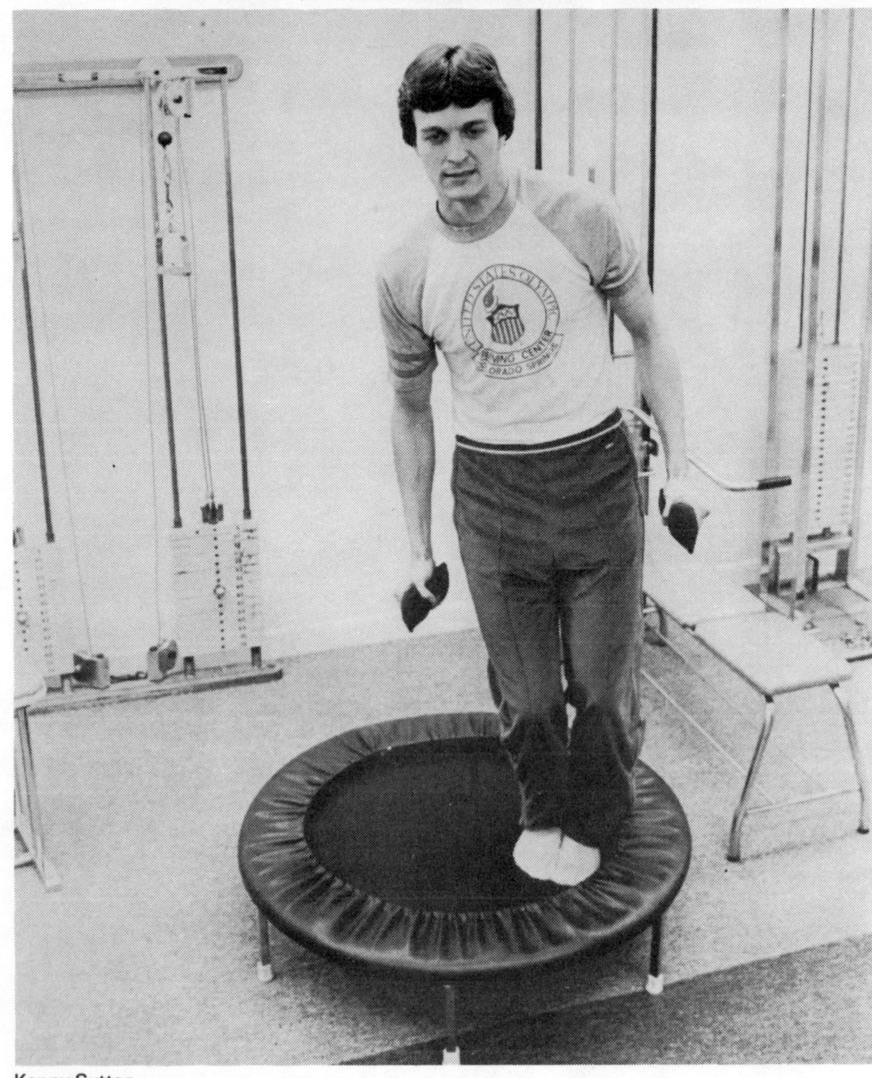

Kenny Sutton

SLALOM

Purpose: Excellent for skiing, baseball, joint conditioning for all sports.

Place .45 kilo Sanbags in hands, put both feet together and bounce side to side on your rebound unit bending the knees.

Program: Start with 20 bounces, add one set a week till you reach 5-6 sets, add .45 kilo Sanbag weight every two weeks.

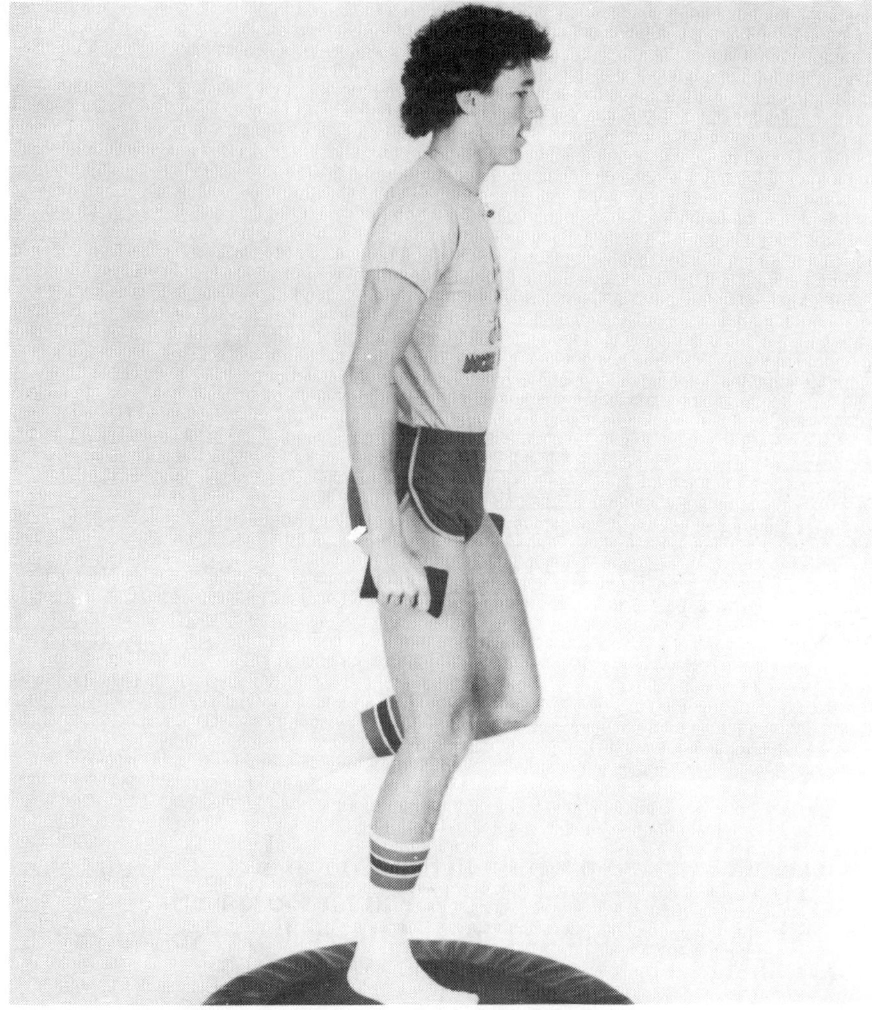

Dwight Stones, one-legged turns.

ONE-LEGGED TURNS

Purpose: Excellent for balance in all sports; balance helps all athletes to control their bodies in outstretched or awkward positions.

Place .45 kilo Sanbags in hand, center yourself in center of mat on one foot, jump and turn to your right, and then turn to your left.

Program: Start with 10 turns to the left, 10 turns to the right, add one set a week till you reach 5-6 sets, add .45 kilo Sanbag weight every two weeks.

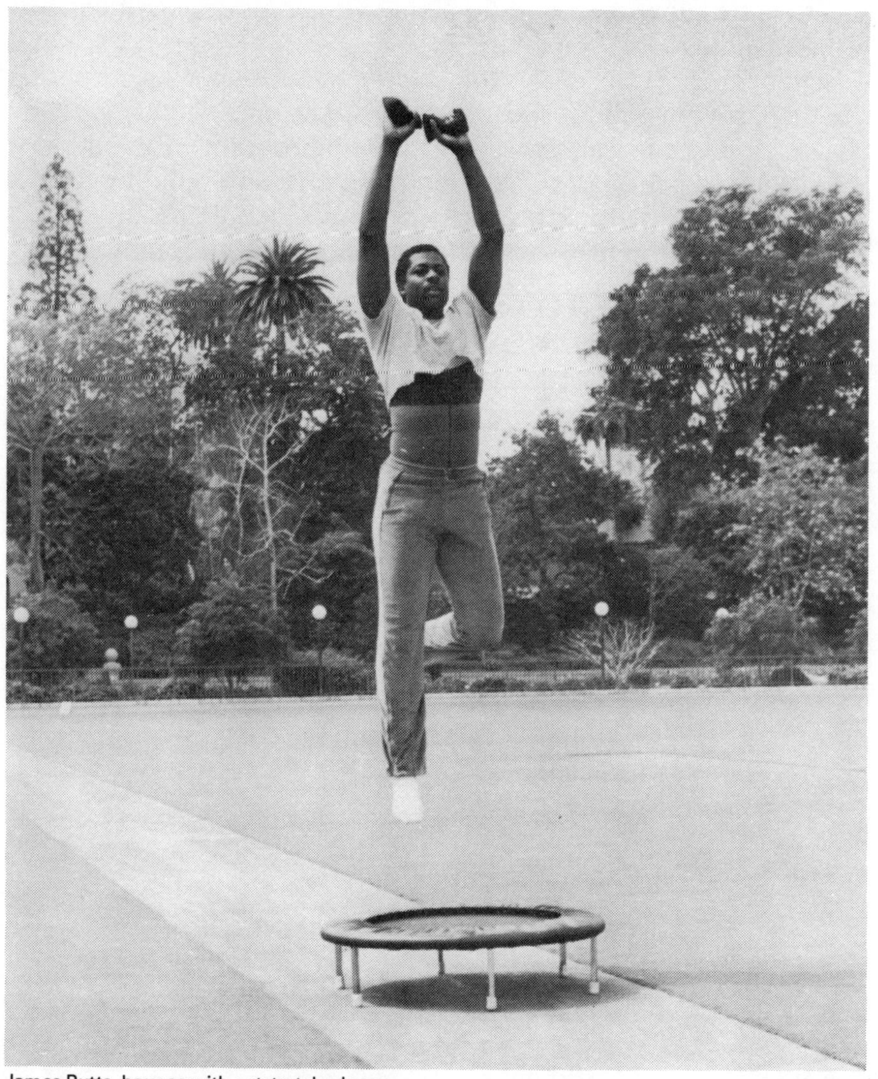
James Butts, bounce with outstretched arms.

HIGH LEAP WITH OUTSTRETCHED HANDS

Purpose: Excellent drill for defensive skills (volleyball, football, basketball), vertical jump improvement.

Place .45 kilo Sanbags in hands, stand in center of mat, then jump with outstretched hands as high as possible.

Program: Start with 10 repetitions, add 1 set every week till you reach 5-6 sets, add .45 kilo Sanbags weight every two weeks.

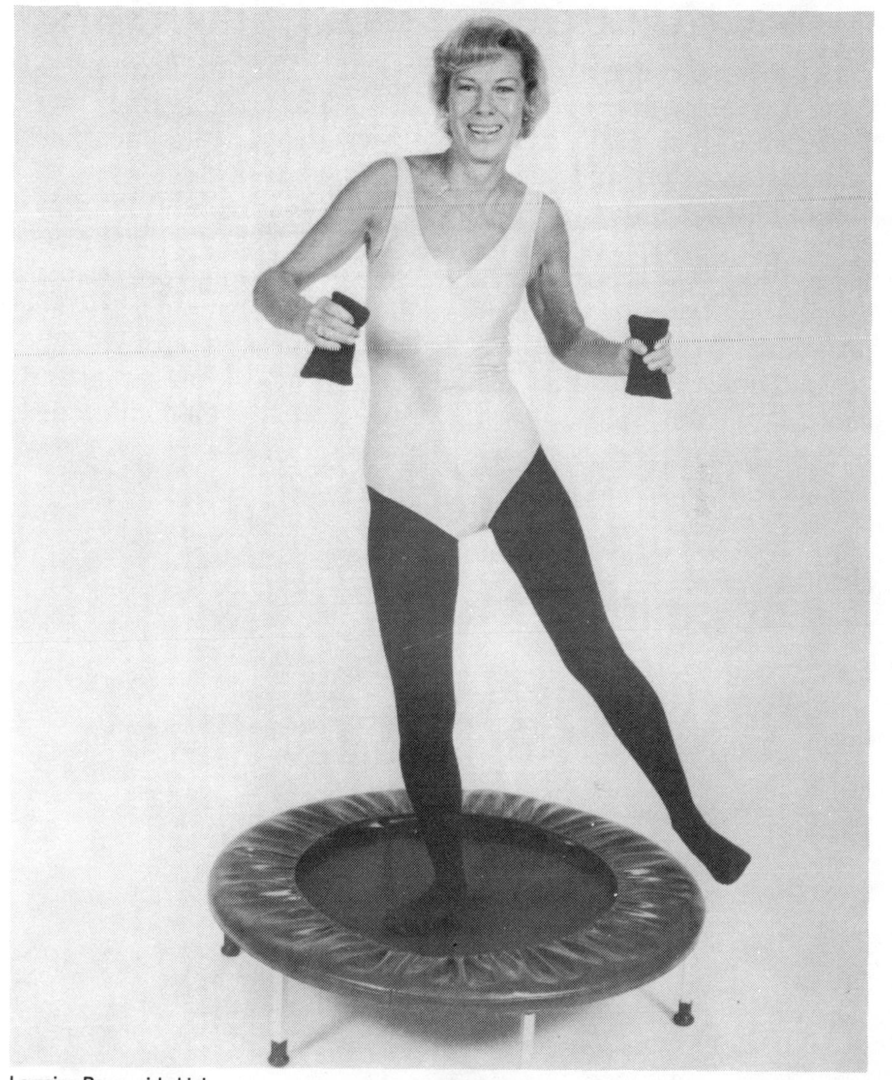
Lorraine Rapp, side kicks.

SIDE KICKS

Purpose: Tremendous exercise for ankles and lower legs, excellent for skating, skiing, good conditioner for hips and thighs, too.

Place .45 kilo Sanbags in hands, start in center of mat, kick leg to side alternating right and left legs.

Program: Start with 10 repetitions, add 1 set every week till you reach 5-6 sets, add .45 kilo Sanbags weight every two weeks.

WHAT ABOUT OTHER SPORTS?

Have we forgotten your sport? Don't become discouraged, there is a lot of improvement you can make by doing the "Basic Four," and the "Daily Dozen." Review the program mentioned in earlier chapters and start your workouts today.

The programs described above can be adapted and improved with just a little of your imagination. That's what makes Sanbagging the most versatile sports training program in existence today. The most important thing you can **do** is **try** these programs. You can do these in your home at a cost of time, energy, and finances that just about anyone of you can afford. Take that first step forward to being that well-conditioned, enthusiastic functional human being with the wonderful benefits of Sanbagging.

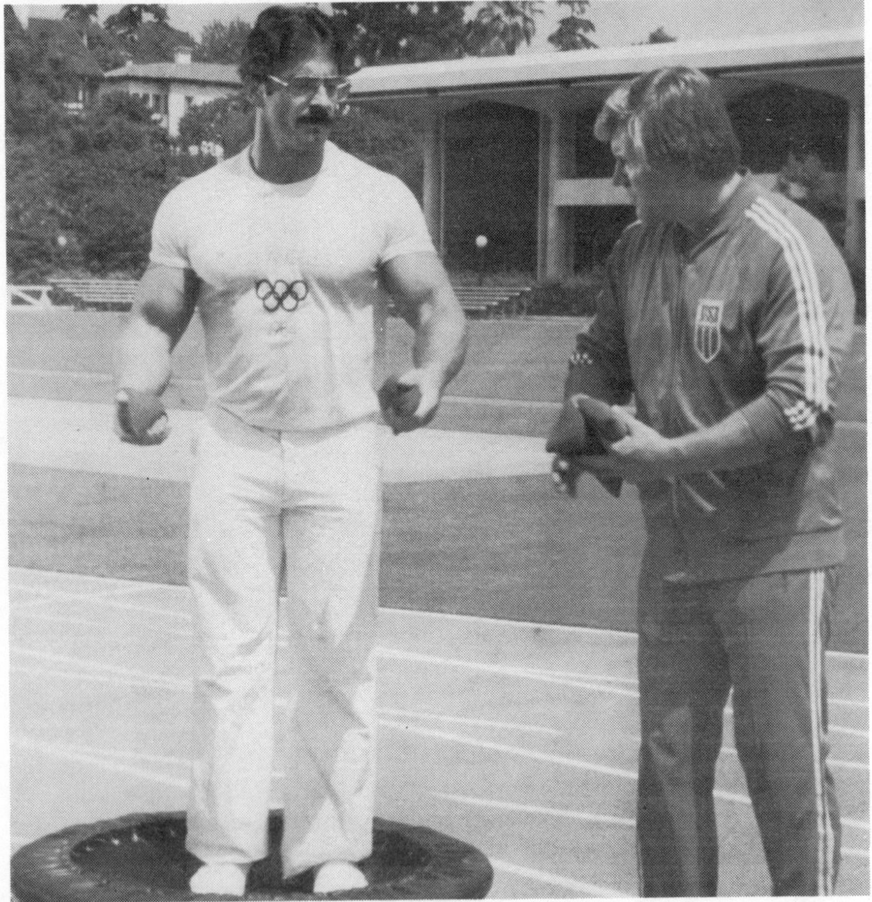

Mike Mentzer, Mr. Universe, with Harry, doing the squeeze.

Sanbagging is a must for every sports training program whether in your school, health club, or training center.

Sanbagging is a most versatile program for athletic conditioning, sports skills development, strength building, etc. It can very easily fit in any sports training schedule as an adjunct program or as **the program** for your sports conditioning needs.

HOW TO USE "SANBAGGING" IN YOUR OVERALL PROGRAM

Monday	**Tuesday**	**Wednesday**	**Thursday**
Stretching Sanbagging your sports skill — what- ever sport you play or individual Weight Training Drills, etc.	Competition Technique Development Films, etc.	Stretching Sanbagging your sports skill — with your coach or team. Weight Training Drills, etc.	Competiton Technique Development Films, etc.

Friday	**Saturday**	**Sunday**
Stretching Sanbagging your sports skill and with your team or sport Weight Training Drills, etc.	Competition in your sports	R E S T

As you can see, the possibilities of using Sanbagging as a vehicle for overall athletic development is immeasurable. You coaches who do not have budgets for the expensive weight training apparatus, this program is at a fraction of the cost.

Example: Full line of Nautilus, $12,000 - $20,000; Universal $4,000; machines, $1,000's. One rebound unit: retail price approximately $150. Sanbags and books to $60.00 — your entire fitness package for less than $210.00. Quite a bargain in these inflationary times. Check this program out and help yourself and your teams to real success.

Chapter 14

Sanbagging Principles

That will produce excellent results

1. If the Sanbags become **too light** for you, and if you are advanced, a strong athlete (lineman in football, weight lifter, etc.) then you can combine the Sanbags and make the weights **heavier.** Example: If you put a 1.36 kilo Sanbag together with a .91 kilo Sanbag, you have a 2.27 kilo Sanbag. The bags are pliable enough to combine. Many of you may be thinking that .45 kilo Sanbags are too light for the program. You can combine the bags and make heavier Sanbags.

You can combine: .91 kilo bag with .91 kilo bag, you have 1.82 kilo bag.

.91 kilo bag with 1.36 kilo bag, you have 2.27 kilo bag.

1.36 kilo bag with 1.36 kilo bag, you have 2.72 kilo bag.

My experience with this program is that anything past 2.72 kilo in the Sanbagging exercise are too much for about 95% of all people (including athletes).

2. Doing the Sanbagging exercises slowly with a **concentrated effort** will make the bags heavier. **Tense the muscles** that are being worked in the exercise positions and the **bags automatically** will become heavier. It is not necessary for you to use heavier Sanbags if you follow this principle.

3. Doing more than one exercise for each body part consecutively will produce more results than if you do only one exercise for the body part. (This is known as the overload principle.)

Example: Curl followed by Upright Row, followed by Curl Press — strong emphasis on upper arms, wrists, shoulders.

This is an **advanced training technique** I recommend attempting only after about 6-8 weeks of Sanbagging.

4. Those who are interested in real **endurance training** — emphasis on **endurance** can follow a program where any one

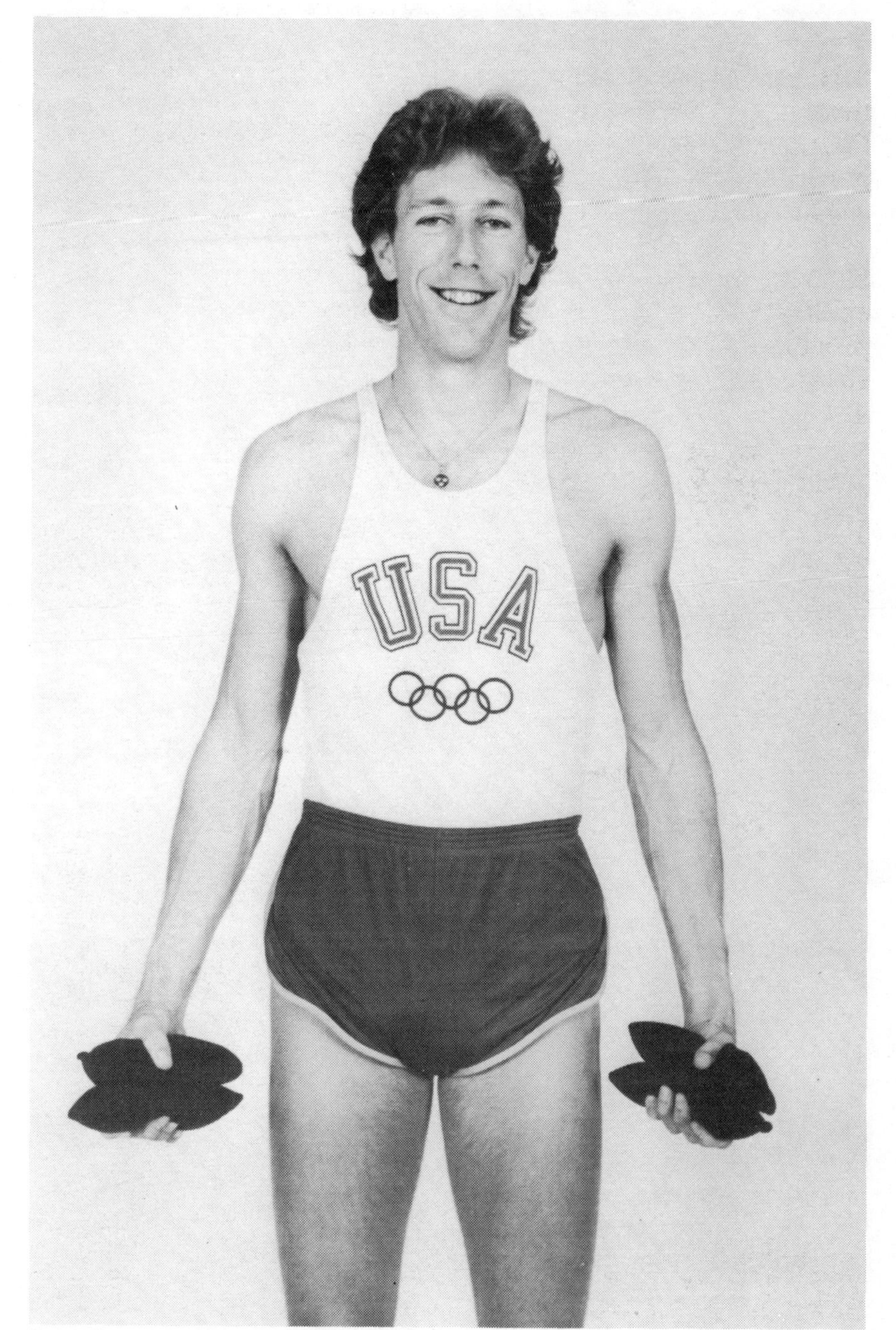

Dwight Stones shows how to combine the bags.

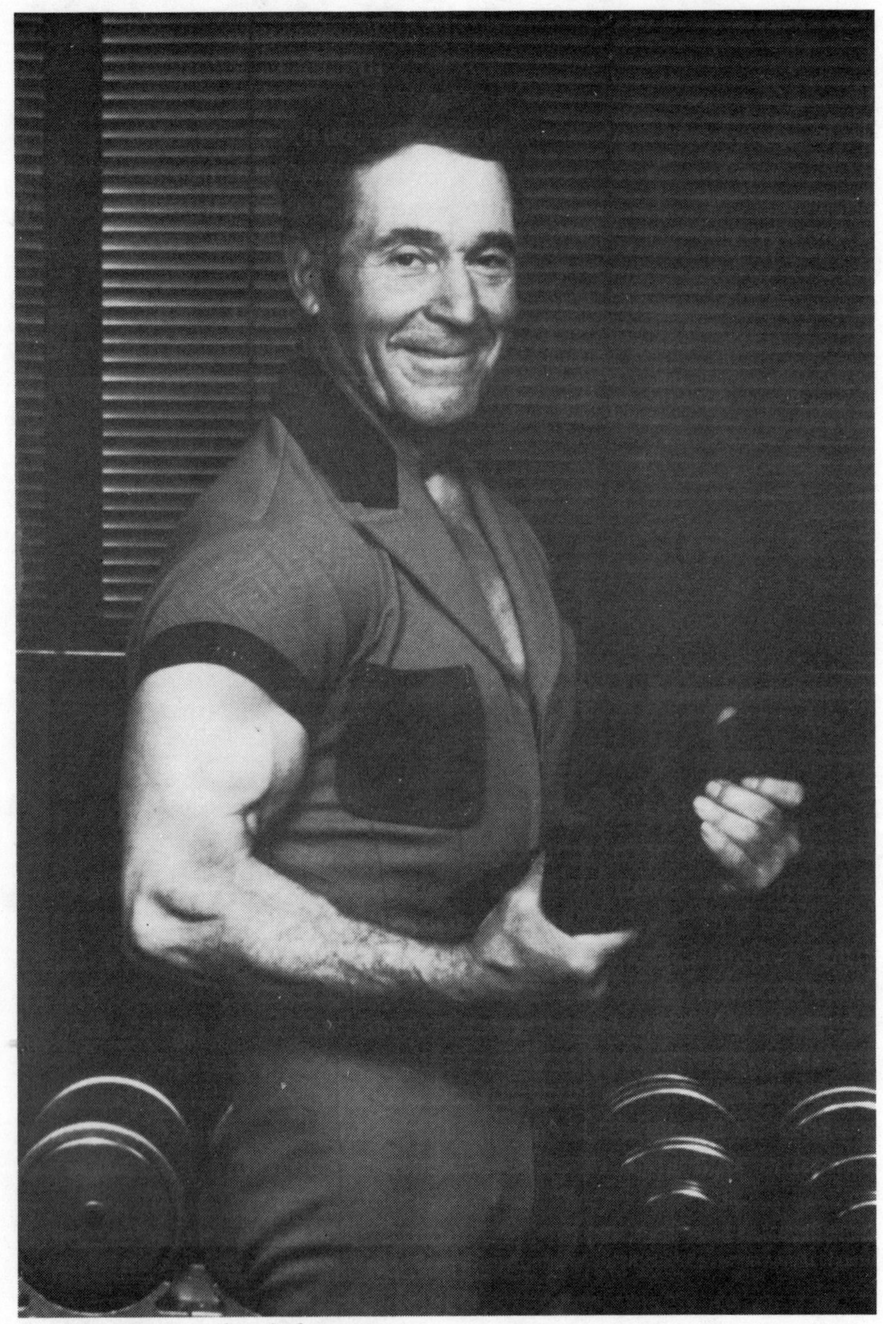

Jack LaLanne gets good results from program.

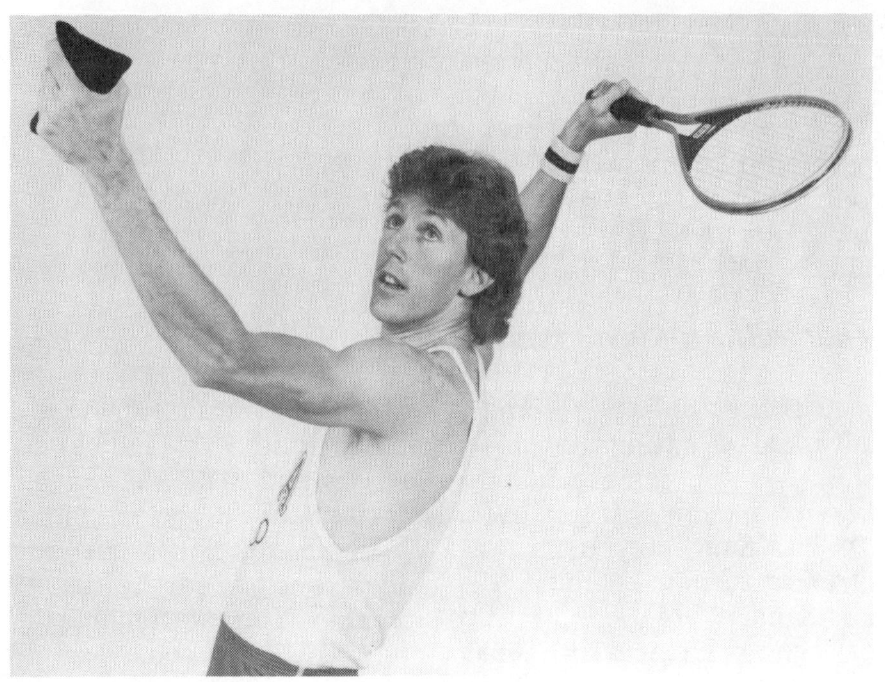

Part 5 (below) is demonstrated by Dwight Stones with racquet in one hand, Sanbag in the other, while rebounding.

exercise is done working up to 35-100 repetitions. Example: Curl & Press with .45 kilo Sanbags — start with 25 reps, add 5 reps per week till you reach 100 reps.

This type of training is excellent for the advanced pupil (6-8 weeks of Sanbagging). You can do any exercise this way. Excellent for **size reduction** and **cardio-respiratory endurance.**

5. Another excellent principle for your sports training would be to take a Sanbag in one hand and a racquet, football, baseball, etc. in the other. This really improves **technique development** for your sport and at the same time gives you strength and conditioning training.

The racquet or ball whatever becomes the resistance in one hand and Sanbag is resistance in the other.

6. Sanbagging is most effective if it is combined with your sports technique development. Example: Tennis lessons in the morning with the pro, then the Sanbagging Tennis Program at

least three times a week at home. Another example would be little league practice in the afternoon (Terrific Six at night, three times a week), etc.

The combination of Sanbagging and your favorite activity or sport can produce dozens of possibilities. This program opens the door to tremendous improvement in any sport technique skill. Use your imagination and develop your own **winning combination.**

Sanbagging is probably the most creative, enjoyable, advanced exercise program in this century. No need to strain on heavy machines, or hurt your joints jogging. This program opens all ranges of possibilities for you.

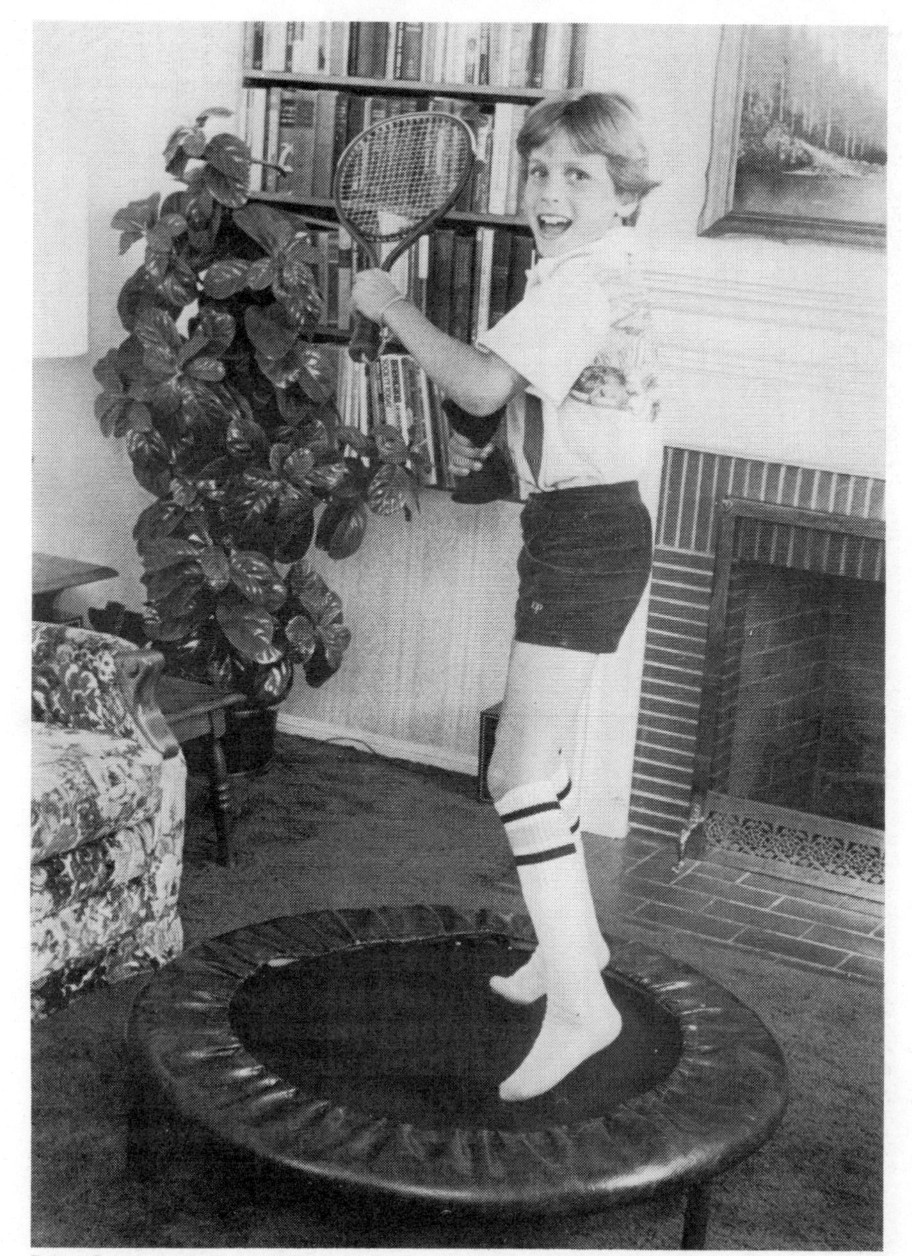

Robert Sneider improves technique using racquetball racquet while rebounding.

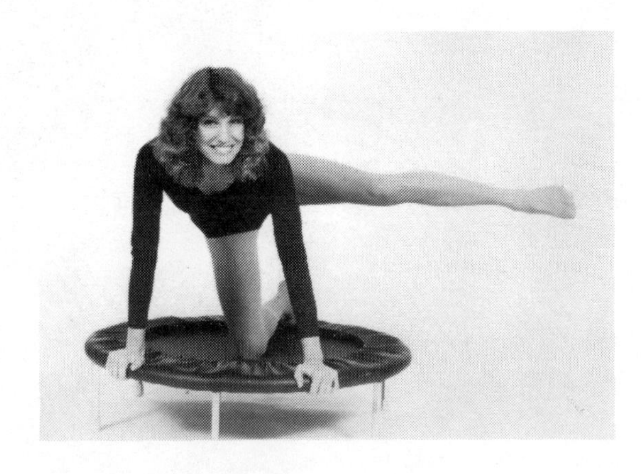

Chapter 15

Programs to Balance Your Body

The real key to injury prevention

Rebound exercise with resistance (Sanbagging) is one of the most effective programs in preventing injuries. The "Daily Dozen" program was designed to eliminate injuries. The principle of working the prime mover only (agonistic muscles) and neglecting opposite groups (antagonistic muscles) has done more to harm the athlete than help. The "Daily Dozen" was designed to be a balance between these groups. **Example:** If you are to work the bicep, one should work the tricep to balance the structure.

Many of our popular weight lifting apparatus (machines) encourage the overuse of prime movers. Unless the individual is taught the correlation between these groups and shown how to set up a sound balanced muscular program, one will, in many cases, overdo the prime mover muscular exercises on those machines. This can cause injuries and counterproductive development.

The "Daily Dozen" was designed to work both muscle groups if done in order. This will help to balance structure, improve appearance, help reduce injury, and most of all help total physical fitness. This is very different from many of your popular programs that are being done today.

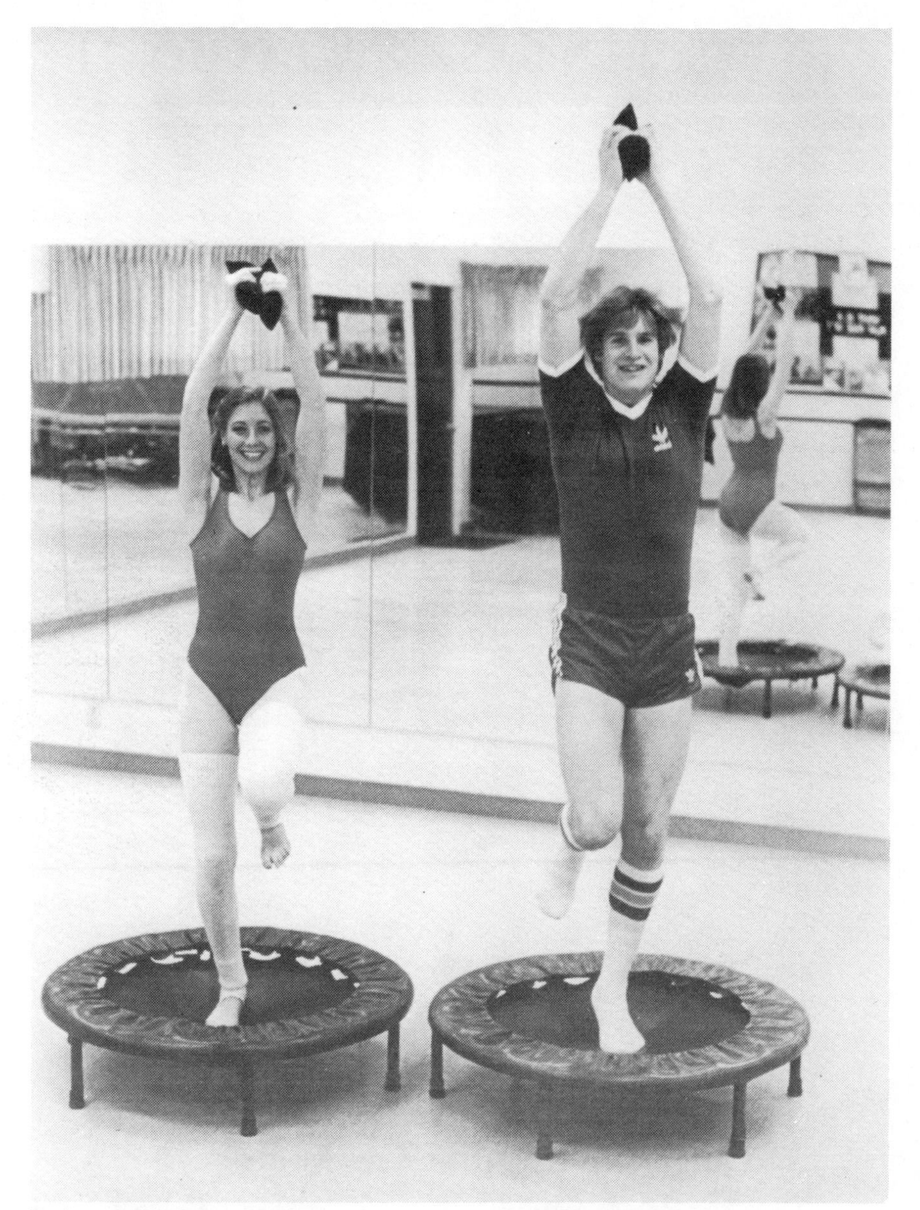

Denise and Rick Guthy.

SEVEN BASIC STRETCHING EXERCISES TO PREVENT STIFFNESS

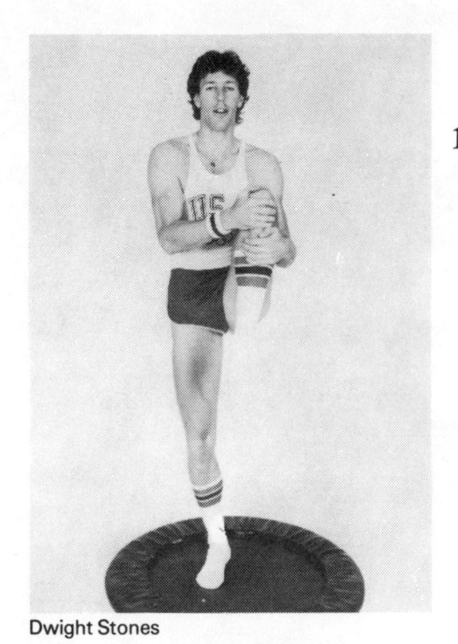

Dwight Stones

1. **Alternate Knee to Chest —** Start with left knee, draw to your chest. **Total: 20 reps**

3. **Stand & Reach — Total: 10 reps**

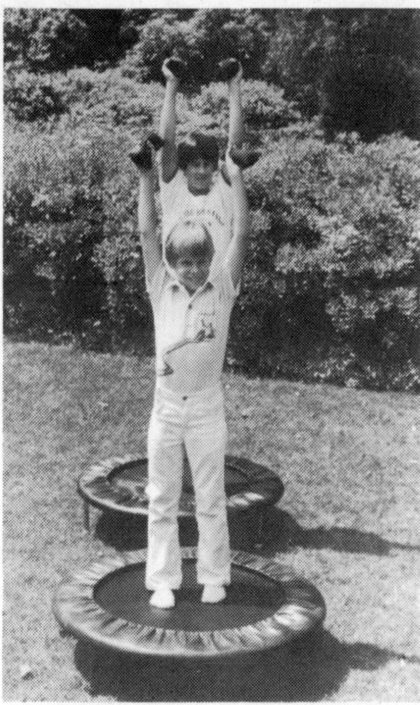

Karl Sneider and Todd Grinolds

Sarah Sneider

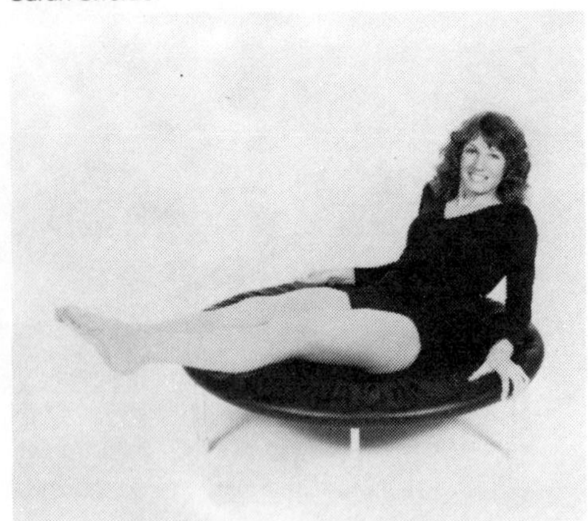

2. **Both Knees to Chest —** Bring both knees to chest while on back. **Total: 10 reps**

4. **Toe Over —** Cross feet, touch toes, alternate feet. **Total: 5 reps**

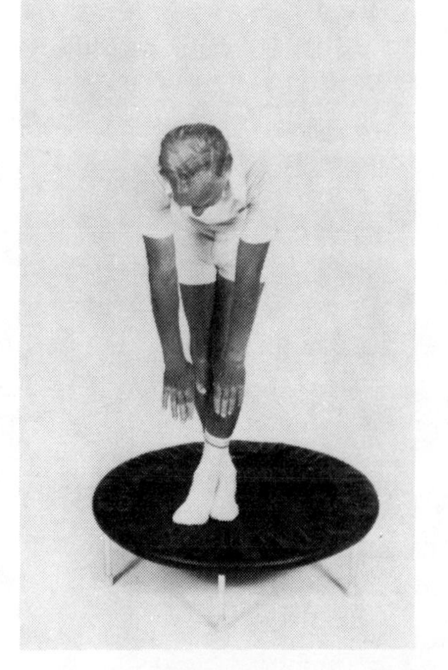

Don Allen

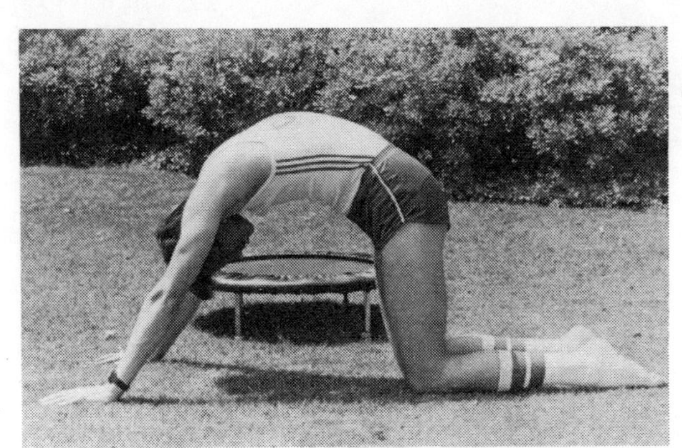

Greg Joy

7. **Partial Squat**
   Keep back straight, bend knees, squat one-fourth to one-third of the way down.
   Total: 20 reps.

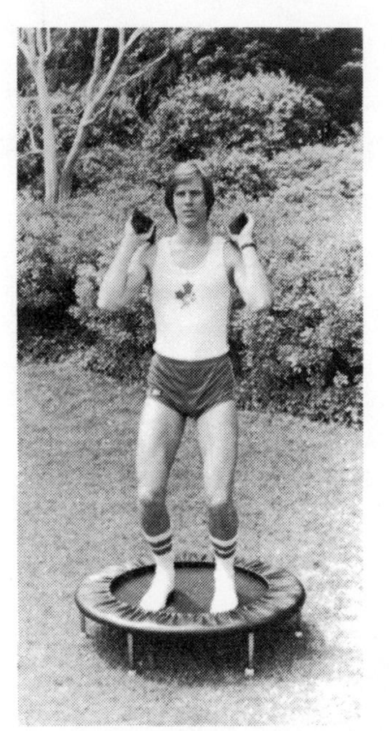

Greg Joy

5. **Back Arch:**
   Total: 8 reps

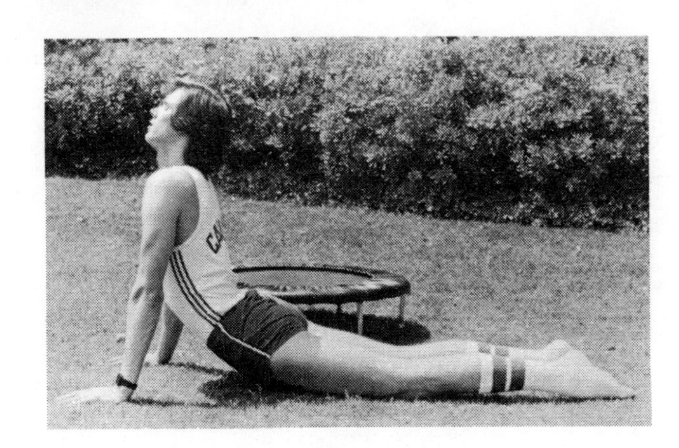

6. **Calf Raise —**
   Raise on both balls of feet.
   Total: 20 reps

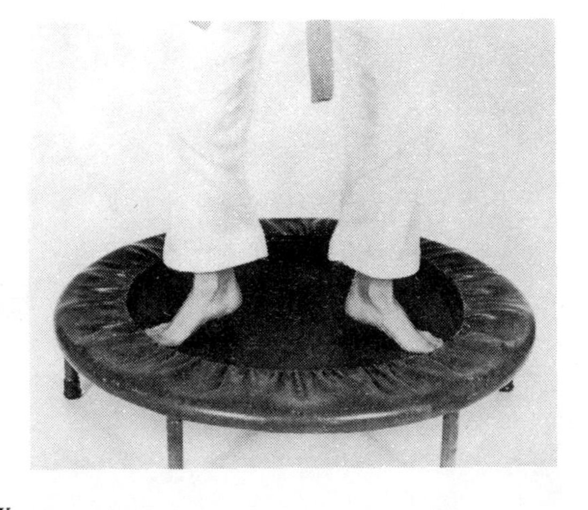

Sanbagging is an excellent form of fitness activity, but occasionally you will get stiff or tight. Try the above, before you Sanbag and after. If you are fortunate in having a swimming pool, may I encourage you to swim 2-3 times a week. This will increase flexibility and reduce injury. If you are overweight (10-100 or more pounds), or out of shape, you can overdo a Sanbag program. The stretching program above is an excellent way to reduce soreness and stiffness. Take your time. Enjoy it.

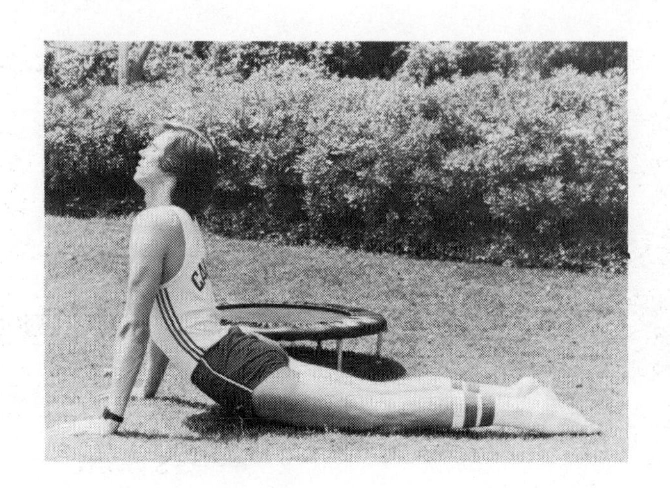

Chapter 16

Goals

Your key to making your program a success!

Much has been written and said about goals. You have heard about goals all your life, I am sure. As a fitness director and coach of world class athletes, I deal with goals every day. Just imagine if Bruce Jenner would have said: "I'd like to win the decathlon in the Olympics," without a program of **specific goals.** You and I know that it is not possible to succeed without **specific goals.**

How about the millionaire in real estate, or the housewife with a tight budget, or your child trying to make the gymnastics team? They all have something in common — that is, they have goals. Without specific well-defined goals, we don't have a destination. You are made to succeed, so outline specific goals.

BASIC FORMULA TO SUCCEED IN YOUR PROGRAM

1. I will be consistent — do the program at least three times a week.
2. I will monitor my pulse rate (keep within guidelines for my age).
3. I will take my measurements and weight weekly. I will weigh within my body weight range for my age.
4. I will not overwork on this program, but will have fun and enjoy the unique exercises program that Sanbagging develops.
5. I will encourage at least one person a week by a smile or by a card, letter or telephone call and tell several people about this program.
6. I will help keep my wonderful country strong and healthy by the example I set with the Sanbagging program.

GENERAL GOALS

These goals are too nebulous. Are you thinking this way?

1. SPORTS GOAL	I want to make my team, lose weight, reduce injuries.
2. EDUCATIONAL GOAL	I want to improve my grade point average.
3. SPIRITUAL GOAL	I want to help mankind, serve my country.
4. FINANCIAL GOAL	I want to make money.
5. LOSE WEIGHT GOAL	I want to lose weight.

Notice, the goals above are much too general. They will work much better if they are specific like:

SPECIFIC GOALS

This will help you reach your destination a lot sooner.

1. SPORTS GOAL	I want to run a 4:20 mile, lift 240 in Bench Press, hit .325, average 8 rebounds in a game, etc.
2. EDUCATIONAL GOAL	I want to improve my grade point average from 3.2 to 3.8, or I want to graduate from college in 4 yrs. etc.
3. SPIRITUAL GOAL	I want to put my faith in God into practice by helping in a nursing home twice a week, or teach church school, etc.
4. FINANCIAL GOAL	I want to improve my pay from $8,000 a year to $20,000 by giving of myself in my job.
5. LOSE WEIGHT GOAL	In six months time, I want to lose 20 pounds. I want to lose 2″ in my hips, thighs, waist, etc.

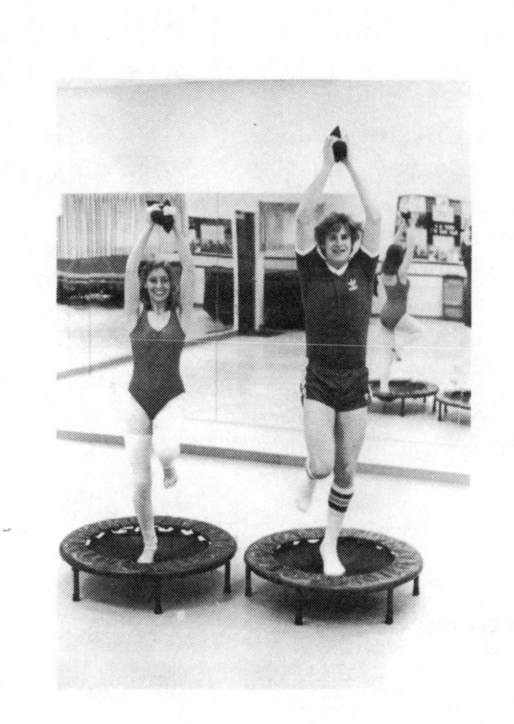

Chapter 17

In Conclusion . . .

You are truly a unique individual. There has never been another you. You are designed to succeed, to enjoy the healthy, happy life. Please take the time several minutes a day and do yourself a big favor and get in shape.

Young housewives, be courageous. You can get in shape right in your home. You don't need to leave your children two hours a day to go to the spa. Yes, all you beautiful ladies can be helped to reduce inches, improve your posture, and benefit society. This program of Sanbagging while dancing or jogging will truly make your life so much brighter.

You who are athletic and want to be top performers, the program is right here in this book for you to follow. You **can do it.** It starts with desire and goals. If you have a goal, you have a destination. Yours is the greatest time in the history of sports (salaries are escalating, it's more prestigious to be an athlete, etc.). This program could mean a college scholarship or making the local little league, FOLLOW THROUGH.

For the elderly (age is but a state of mind), with goals, with purpose; you who are 70 or 80 or better, you are needed. Keep in shape, we need your wisdom, your experience, your inspiration. This program is for you.

Those who are handicapped (special education, blind, deaf, immobilized, etc.), you are certainly going to respond to this program. You will get in shape and have fun, too.

Let's face life courageously as in the words of T. Roosevelt:

"Far better it is to dare
mighty things, to win glorious
triumphs, even though checkered
with failure, than to take rank
with those poor spirits who neither
enjoy much nor suffer much, because
they live in the grey twilight that
knows not victory nor defeat."

I challenge you to be something that you can be proud of being. I challenge you to really grow and experience the full life that is based on sound mental, spiritual, and physical habits.

You can do it! By following this amazing program of Sanbagging.©

Have fun,
Harry and Sarah Sneider

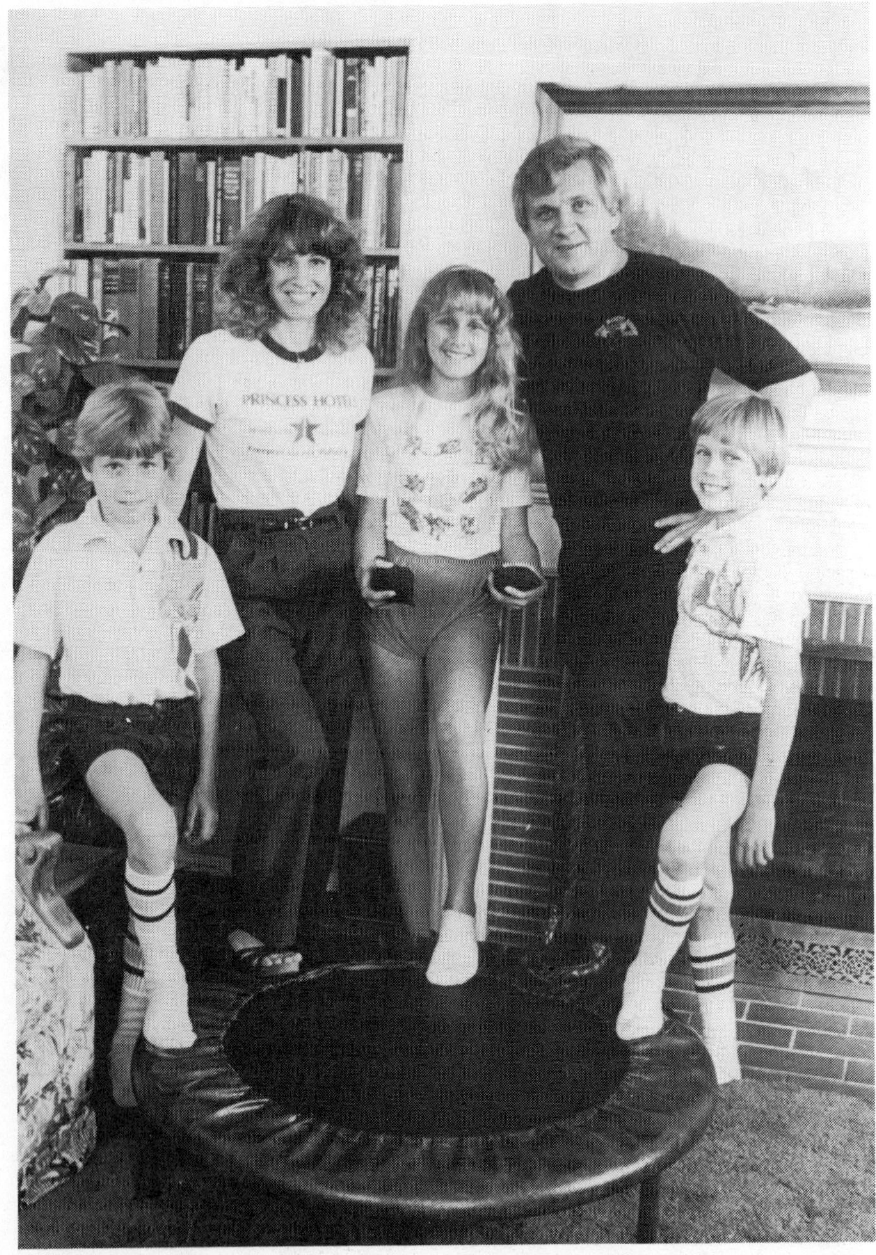

Robbie, Sarah, Debbie, Harry, Karl.

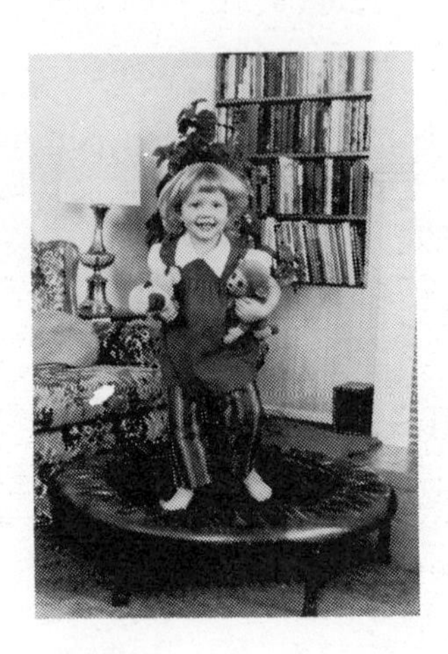

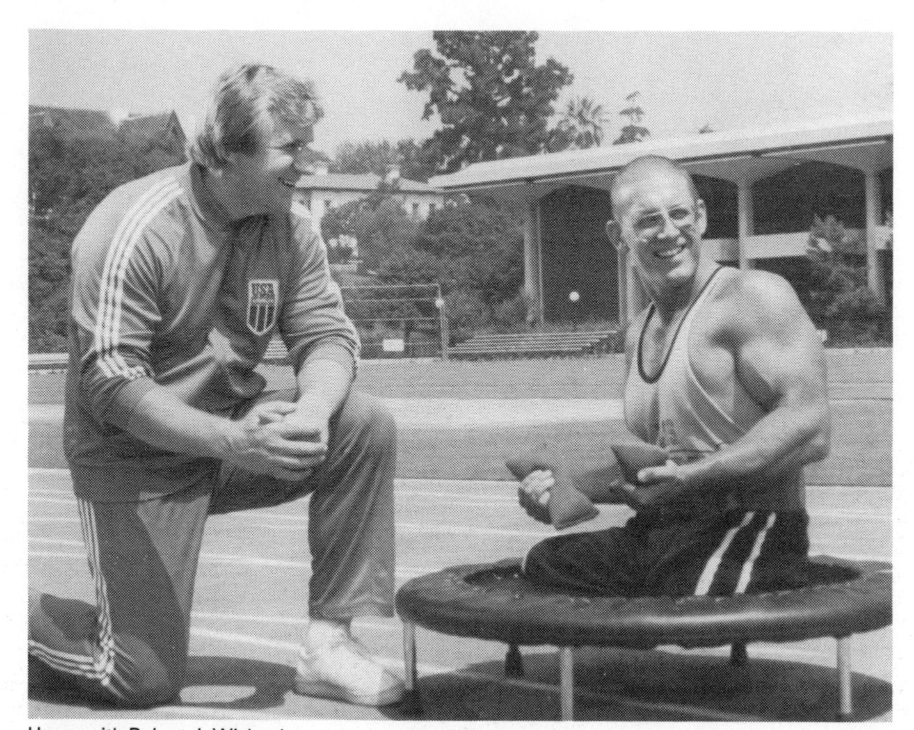

Harry, with Robert J. Wieland

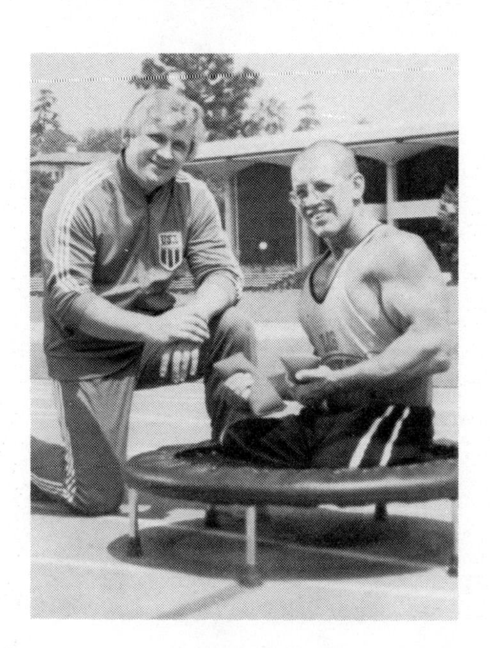

You Are What You Think

"If you think you are beaten, you are,
If you think you dare not, you don't.
If you like to win, but you think you can't
It is almost certain you won't.

"If you think you'll lose, you're lost.
For out of the world we find,
Success begins with a fellow's will —
It's all in the state of mind.

"If you think you are outclassed, you are,
You've got to think high to rise,
You've got to be sure of yourself before
You can ever win a prize.

"Life's battles don't always go
To the stronger or faster man,
But sooner or later the man who wins
Is the man WHO THINKS HE CAN!"

Anonymous

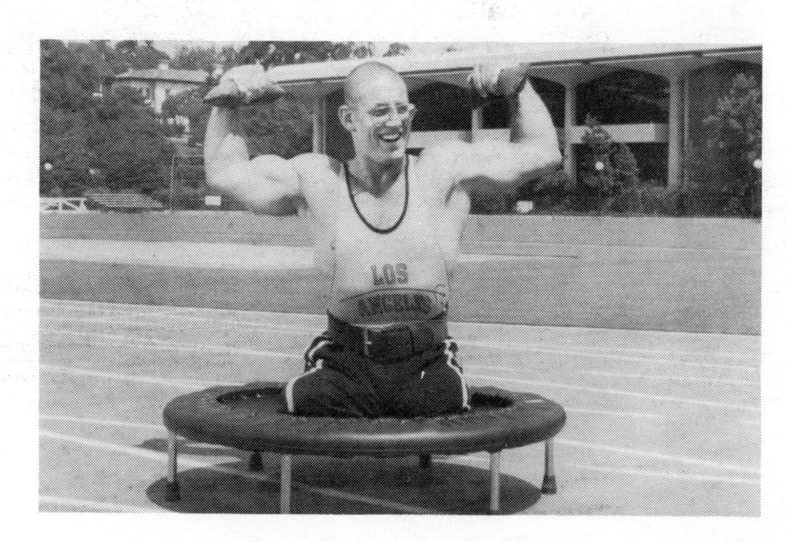

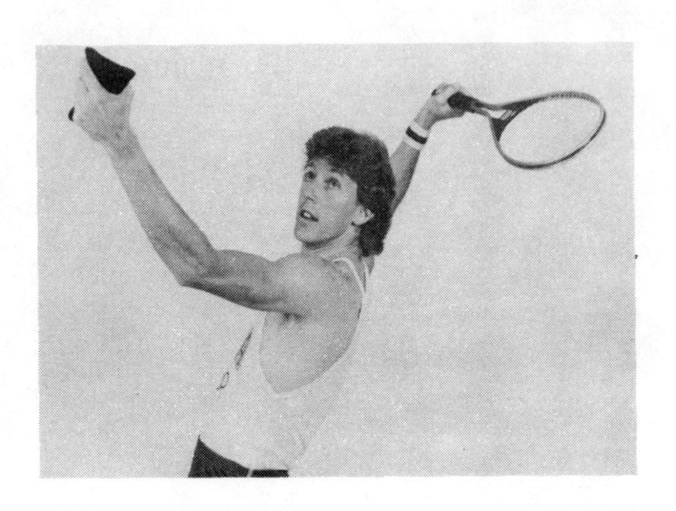

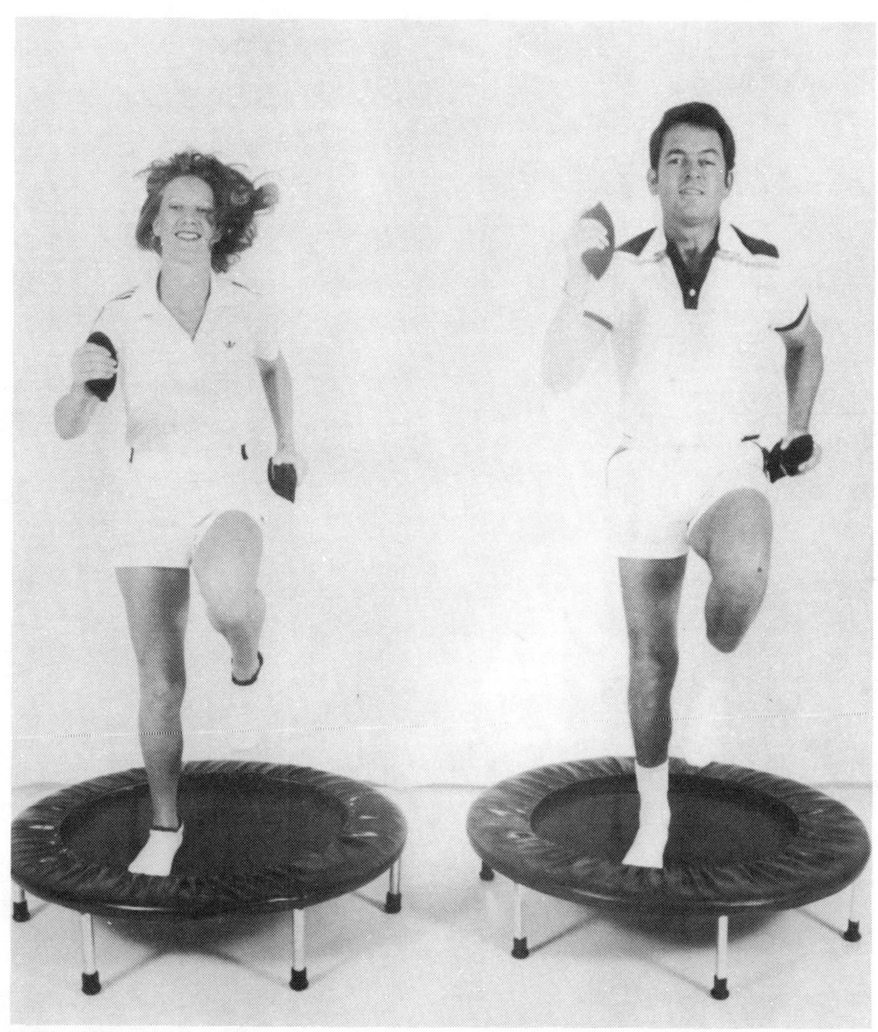

Beth and Roger Chaney

Satisfied Rebound Enthusiast

"Being an athlete and a coach for most of my life, I understand the importance and value of physical training. My wife, Beth, and I were introduced to the rebound unit over one year ago. We have made this apparatus an integral part of our daily lives.

"Disciplining oneself to exercise daily is a vital key for fitness improvement and well being. We enjoy the various training routines five to six days a week with or without the use of resistance weights. Our best results, however, have been achieved when we combine stretching, diet, weight training and other sports activities with our mini-trampoline workouts.

"Because of our noticeable improvement in over-all fitness and health, we are extremely excited to share our experiences with others."

Roger Chaney
Athletic Department
Ambassador College
Pasadena, CA 91123

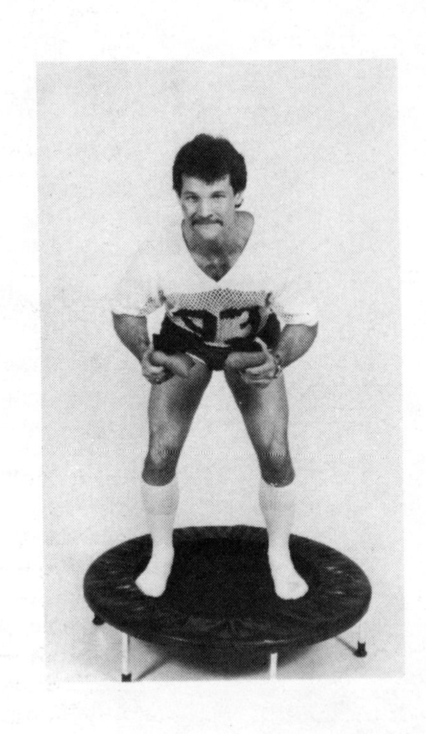

About the Models

Most of the models used in this book are members of our fitness and athletic training centers. They are part of the ever growing, enthusiastic group of people that believe in rebound exercise with Sanbagging. We hope you will try these programs as they have and achieve all-around fitness and health.

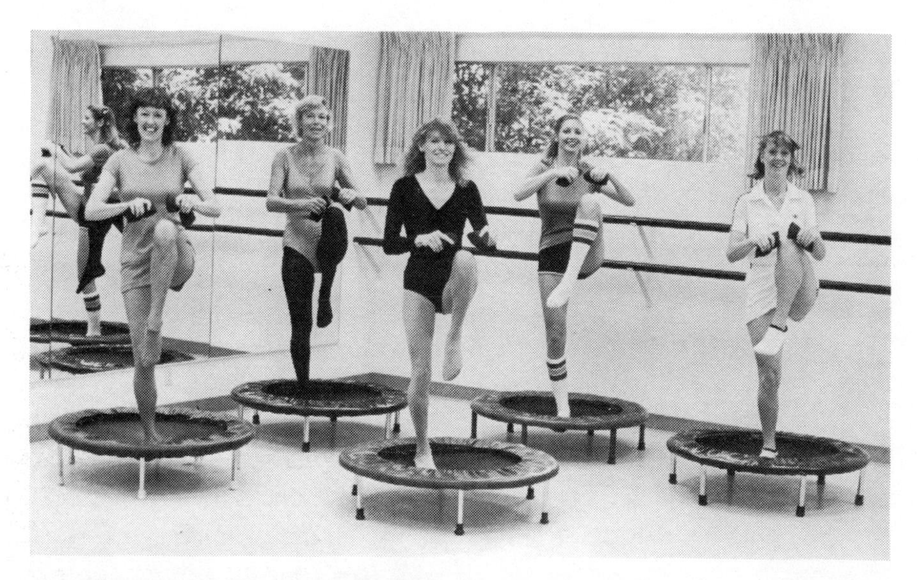

Donald L. Allen — Tennis pro, age group tennis champion
Hainsley L. Best, Jr. — Body builder, gymnast
James C. Butts — Silver medal, triple jump, 1976 Olympics (56′6¾″)
Beth Chaney — rebound exercise enthusiast
Roger Chaney — Athletic coach, rebound exercise trainer
Nancy J. Collins — Aerobic dance instructor
Eileen R. Dennis — Cheerleader, writer
Barb Egbert — Physical education instructor, author
Siew Eng Foo — Martial artist
Lynn Grimditch — Actress, all around athlete
Wayne Grimditch — 16 national titles, 3 world titles, water ski championships, Superstars winner, 1978.
Todd Grinolds — All around athlete
Denise A. Guthy — Fitness director
Richard A. Guthy — Fitness director
Greg Joy — Silver medal, high jump, 1976 Olympics, world record holder, 1978 (7′7″)
William J. Kessler — Doctor of Chiropractics, minister Worldwide Church of God
Jack LaLanne — "Mr. Fitness," author, TV personality, humanitarian
Joseph R. Mangan — Coach, founder of Southern California Striders
T. J. McCavitt — Actor, all around athlete
Mike Mentzer — Bodybuilder, Mr. Universe, 1979
Robin J. Morelli — Former cheerleader, mother-to-be
Keith S. Nelson — Actor, high jumper
Sandy Nelson — Rebound exercise enthusiast; daughters: Krisi, 10 yrs.; Amy, 8 yrs.; Becky, 5 yrs.; Julie, 2 yrs.
Bob Orosz — Ohio State football player, champion bench presser.
Brenda J. Hollingsworth-Pickett, Jr. — Dancer, martial artist; daughters: Akilah Nayo and Eshe Nayo, both 4 months old.
Eugene Pickett, Jr. — Captain, USA martial arts team
Lorraine Rapp — Fitness enthusiast
Dan Ripley — U.S.A. Olympic team member 1980, former world record holder pole vault (18′5¾″)
Debbie Smith — Rebound exercise enthusiast
Dwight E. Stones — High jumper, 10 world records, Olympic medalist, 1972 and 1976, Superstars runner-up, 1978
Kenneth L. Sutton — Speed roller skater, 2 gold medals, 1 silver in Pan American Games, 1978
George L. Throop, III — Professional baseball pitcher, Kansas City Royals, Houston Astros
Elaine A. Vernon — Rebound exercise enthusiast
Geary H. Whiting — Wrestler, weight lifter
Robert J. Wieland — Incredible athlete, "Strive for Success" lecturer and motivator
Marsha Whitley — Women's athletic director

Recommended reading list

For your total improvement

Miracles of Rebound Exercise, Albert E. Carter
Rebounding Aerobics, Morton Walker, DPM & Frank Angelo
Aerobics, Dr. Kenneth Cooper
As a Man Thinketh, James Allen
The Incredible Human Potential, Herbert W. Armstrong
Think and Grow Rich, Napoleon Hill
See You at the Top, Zig Ziglar
How to Win Friends and Influence People, Dale Carnegie
Aerobic Dancing, Jackie Sorenson
The Heart of a Champion, Bob Richards
Man's Search For Meaning, Victor Frankl
The Strangest Secret, Earl Nightingale
The Jack LaLanne Way to Vibrant Good Health, Jack LaLanne
The Education of a Bodybuilder, Arnold Schwarzenegger
Arnold's Bodybuilding for Women, Arnold Schwarzenegger
Acres of Diamonds, Russell Conwell
The Holy Bible

PROGRAM CARD

Men's and Women's Programs

PROGRAM

Sanbagging Your Way to Total Fitness

Exercise	Wt.	Reps/Time	Sets
Lymphatic Bounce	.45 kilo	30 sec.	1
Shuffle	.45 kilo	30 sec.	1
Jog Easy	.45 kilo	30 sec.	1
Bounce	.45 kilo	30 sec.	1
DAILY DOZEN			
Curl	.45 kilo	10	2
Press	.45 kilo	10	2
Upright Row	.45 kilo	10	2
Tricep Press	.45 kilo	10	2
Squeeze	.45 kilo	10	2
Curl & Press	.45 kilo	10	2
Side Raise	.45 kilo	10	2
Crossover	.45 kilo	10	2
Sprint High Knee	.45 kilo	15 sec.	2
Press Up & Out	.45 kilo	10	2
Pullover	.45 kilo	10	2
Jog Easy	.45 kilo	30 sec.	2

Goals

Set whatever goal you want, if you are overweight, do more reps. If you need to develop certain muscle groups, add more sets or add more "Sanbag Weight." With this handy program card, you can post your workout on a bulletin board, refrigerator door, mirror, etc. or, if you own a gym, then you can have them on file.

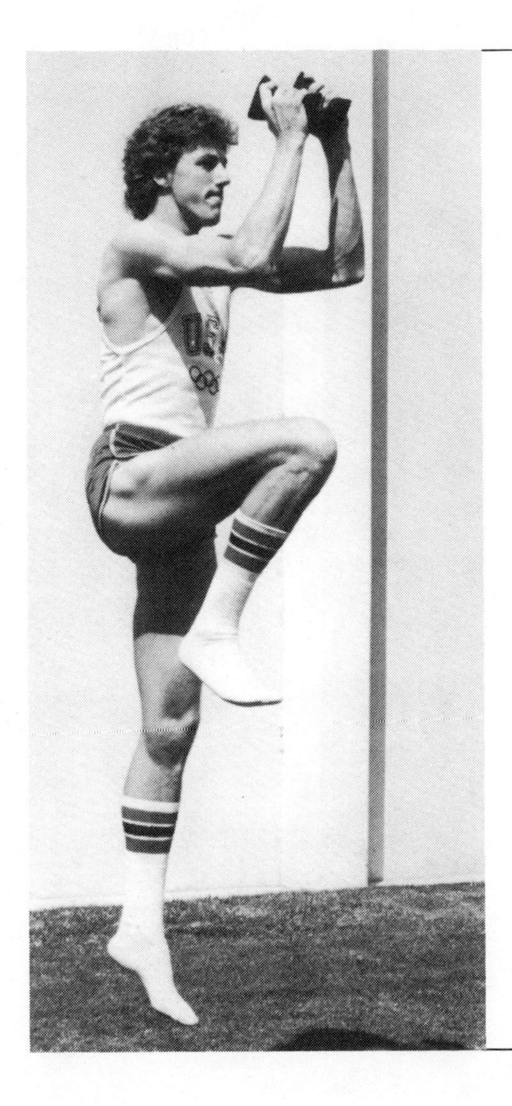

(Example Only)

GOALS CARD
FOR MEN AND WOMEN

Name ______________________________

Date Weighed and Measured ______________________________

PRESENT WEIGHT	**200**	**GOAL WEIGHT**	**190**
Measurements:			
Neck	16	Neck	15
Shoulders	52½	Shoulders	51½
Chest (Bust)	49	Chest (Bust)	49
Waist	35	Waist	33
Bicep	16½	Bicep	16
Hips	37	Hips	35
Thighs	27	Thighs	25
Calves	17	Calves	16

1. Write down your goals. It's been proven you are more likely to accomplish them if they are written down!

2. Write down weight and measurements **at least** once a week, or twice a week if you prefer.